B.S.A.V.A

MANUAL OF SMALL ANIMAL NEUROLOGY

Edited by

Simon J. Wheeler
B.V.Sc., Ph.D., M.R.C.V.S.

GW00634081

Published by the
British Small Animal
Veterinary Association
Kingsley House, Church Lane,
Shurdington, Cheltenham,
Gloucestershire GL51 5TQ

Printed by KCO, Worthing
West Sussex.

First Published 1989
Reprinted 1992

ISBN 0 905214 11 0

CONTENTS

PART 1   NEUROLOGICAL DIAGNOSIS

CONTENTS

ACKNOWLEDGEMENTS

The task of editing this manual has seemed, at times, to be endless. Without the help and support of a number of persons it is clear that this enterprise may have failed. From the outset, the advice of Colin Price, past chairman of the BSAVA Publications Committee, has been invaluable. His influence, particularly in liaising affairs in the UK, was significant. Latterly, he was succeeded by Simon Orr, who took on the role highly efficiently.

The help of Olivia Stagg has been vital in the coordination of the volume; her contribution was immeasurable.

I am grateful to the authors who gave of their time so generously. The pressures of practice and modern academic pursuit may differ, but both are considerable. Finding time to write book chapters is difficult and the effort is not always appreciated. I am particularly grateful to those authors who stepped in at a late stage.

The illustrations are the work of Barbara Davison, Linda LeFevre, Susan Rosenvigne and Catherine Parrish of The Biomedical Communications Unit of North Carolina State University. Michael Gorton Design are responsible for the layout of the Manual. The skill of all these people is gratefully acknowledged.

CONTRIBUTORS

JOHN BARKER, B.Vet. Med., M.R.C.V.S.
Eastfield Veterinary Clinic, Grimsby.

JEREMY V. DAVIES, B.Vet.Med., Ph.D., D.V.R., M.R.C.V.S.
Senior Lecturer Department of Surgery and Obstetrics,
The Royal Veterinary College,
University of London.

IAN D. DUNCAN, B.V.M.S., Ph.D., M.R.C.Path., M.R.C.V.S.
Professor of Neurology School of Veterinary Medicine,
University of Wisconsin.

RICHARD J. EVANS, M.A., Vet.M.B., Ph.D., M.R.C.V.S.
Lecturer Department of Clinical Veterinary Medicine,
University of Cambridge.

IAN R. GRIFFITHS, B.V.M.S., Ph.D., F.R.C.V.S.
Professor in Neurology Glasgow University Veterinary Hospital.

MICHAEL E. HERRTAGE, B.V.Sc., M.A., D.V.R., M.R.C.V.S.
Lecturer Department of Clinical Veterinary Medicine,
University of Cambridge.

PETER M. KEEN, B.V.Sc., Ph.D., M.R.C.V.S.
Reader Department of Pharmacology,
University of Bristol.

MARTIN P. C. LAWTON, B.Vet.Med., F.R.C.V.S.
Romford, Essex.

ROSE E. McKERRELL, B.A., Vet.M.B., M.R.C.V.S.
Research Fellow Department of Clinical Veterinary Medicine,
University of Cambridge.

PHILIPPE M. MOREAU, Dr. Vet., M.S.
Clinique Veterinaire Vanteaux, Limoges,
France.

SIMON M. PETERSEN JONES, B.Vet.Med., D.V.Ophthal., M.R.C.V.S.
Lecturer Royal (Dick) School of Veterinary Studies,
University of Edinburgh.

NICHOLAS J. H. SHARP, B.Vet.Med., M.V.M., Dip.A.C.V.S., M.R.C.V.S.
Research Assistant College of Veterinary Medicine,
North Carolina State University.

GEOFFREY C. SKERRITT, B.V.Sc., F.R.C.V.S.
Lecturer Department of Veterinary Anatomy,
University of Liverpool.

SIMON J. WHEELER, B.V.Sc., Ph.D., M.R.C.V.S.
Assistant Professor of Neurology College of Veterinary Medicine,
North Carolina State University.

FOREWORD

Reminiscence has been described as the pathos of distance but in truth it is both fascinating and salutary to look back over a period of time and to assess what has been achieved in a certain field of scientific endeavour. When the subject of small animal neurology is considered in this way it is pleasing to be able to record considerable satisfaction with the way it has advanced over the last four decades. Anyone delving into the history of small animal medicine and surgery would inevitably conclude that, up to the Second World War, documented information on spinal disorders in dogs was singularly lacking. And yet, in "A domestic treatise on the diseases of horses and dogs" published in 1810, Blaine records under the title of "Rheumatism" an account of a condition in dogs causing pain and paralysis which is instantly recognisable as intervertebral disc protrusion. There are a number of similar examples that could be quoted where a clinical syndrome has been recognised for many years but without there having been sufficient follow through to enable its cause to be elucidated. There are obviously many and various reasons for this, but suffice it to say that the essential elements involved in making progress are an unwavering curiosity, an unfailing energy and a willingness to collaborate with others to obtain a common goal.

The upsurge of interest in neurology which began in the 1950's was stimulated by an enthusiasm to understand and treat the condition whose clinical signs Blaine so accurately described more than a century before, namely, intervertebral disc protrusion. Few clinical sciences, however, develop in isolation and the contribution made by an improved knowledge of radiology was substantial so far as spinal disorders are concerned. Following these early excursions in the mysteries of the spine, such rapid advancement occurred that entire textbooks were devoted to the subject. Neurology is now a clinical speciality in its own right whereas previously it had tended to be a branch of orthopaedics. Being a relatively young subject the scope for discovering new entities and of introducing new treatments is boundless. Meanwhile, the evaluation of neurological cases has been revolutionised. In addition to a routine neurological examination, use is made of electrophysiological tests, radiography, myelography, and biopsy for histopathological study at both light microscope and electron microscope level.

The contents of this multi-author volume indicate the advanced level that small animal neurology has now reached. It wisely puts emphasis on neurological diagnosis, which is the essential prerequisite for the emerging neurologist, while the examples provided of neurological disorders reflect the variety of presentation likely to be encountered in clinical practice. Those now choosing neurology as their speciality will be rewarded with a satisfying life in clinical science and, by adding to the sum of clinical knowledge, will benefit the animals which they, as veterinarians, have pledged to serve.

L. C. VAUGHAN
Professor of Surgery, The Royal Veterinary College
University of London

CHAPTER 1

INTRODUCTION

Simon J. Wheeler, B.V.Sc., Ph.D., M.R.C.V.S.

The diagnosis and management of animals with neurological problems is a particularly challenging area of practice for most clinicians. The nervous system holds a special aura for many people, which may be due in part to the inaccessibility of its component parts for direct examination or because of the perceived complexities of the arrangements within the system. In essence, the nervous system is logically arranged and by adopting a systematic approach to a problem the clinician usually can reach a satisfactory conclusion, at least in terms of making a diagnosis.

APPROACH TO NEUROLOGICAL PROBLEMS

The steps in approaching a neurological problem may be summarised as follows:-

Determine the nature of the problem

Localise the lesion

Assess the severity and extent of the problem

Identify the aetiology

Evaluate treatment

Estimate the prognosis

These steps involve making a diagnosis both by locating the lesion and identifying the pathological changes involved. On the basis of these findings, the clinician can decide on the best form of medical or surgical treatment and also predict the prognosis. A rapid progression through these stages is desirable in most instances as, whilst many neurological conditions are amenable to treatment, prompt therapy is desirable to ensure the best possible outcome.

Determining the nature of the problem

This is the first step in the process. A full clinical examination should always precede any neurological evaluation as it is not uncommon for disorders of other body systems to mimic neurological presentations. This is particularly so in cases where there is apparent weakness of multiple limbs or where owners describe episodes of collapse or seizure-like activity. In the clinical examination, particular note should be made of abnormalities of the cardiovascular, respiratory and musculo-skeletal system.

The neurological examination

The neurological examination will provide information regarding the location and severity of the disorder. This information cannot be gained from the ancillary aids such as radiography but can only be obtained by a careful neurological evaluation. The performance of the neurological examination and the interpretation of the results is facilitated by the adoption of an ordered system of testing and of recording results. A typical proforma for recording the findings of a neurological examination is illustrated in Figure 1.1.

NORTH CAROLINA STATE UNIVERSITY
VETERINARY TEACHING HOSPITAL

NEUROLOGY EXAMINATION

Date ____________________

Time ____________________

I. Subjective:

II. Objective:

A. Observation (Circle or Describe):

Mental Status: ____________

Alert, depressed, stuporous, comatose

Posture: ____________

Normal, head tilt, tremor, falling, paraparesis, tetraparesis

Gait: ____________

Ataxia, dysmetria, circling

B. Palpation:

Muscular (tone, atrophy): ______

Skeletal: ____________

C. Postural Reactions:

L	Reaction	R
	Hopping	
	Front	
	Rear	
	Proprioception	
	Front	
	Rear	
	Placing, tactile	
	Front	
	Rear	
	Placing, visual	
	Front	
	Rear	
	Wheelbarrowing	
	Extensor Post. Thrust	
	Hemiwalking	

D. Cranial Nerve Reflexes:

L	Nerve, Function Test	R
	II + VII	
	Menace	
S M L	Equality of Pupil Size	S M L
	Stim. L. Eye	
	Stim. R. Eye	
	II — Fundus	
	III, IV, VI	
	Strabismus	
	VIII + III, IV, VI	
	Nystagmus	
	Oculovestibular	
	Responses	
	V Sensation	
	V Mastication	
	VII Facial Symmetry	
	V + VII Palpebral	
	IX, X	
	Swallowing	
	XII Tongue	

E. Spinal Reflexes:

L	Reflex, segments	R
	Triceps C7-12	
	Ext. Carpi Rad. C7-T2	
	Flexion, fore C6-T2	
	Patella L4-6	
	Cranial Tibialis L6-S1	
	Gastrocnemius L6-S1	
	Flexion, hind L6-S1	
	Perineal S1-2	

F. Urinary Function:

Evidence of voluntary urination? ______

Bladder distended? ______

Ease of bladder expression? ______

G. Sensation:

Hyperesthesia ______

Superficial Pain (Panniculus reflex ______

Deep pain ______

III. Assessment:

(Lesion localization, check one)

A. Peripheral nerve ______
(Name nerve)

B. Spinal Cord

Segment 1	______	C1-C5
Segment 2	______	C6-T2
Segment 3	______	T3-L3
Segment 4	______	L4-S3

C. Brain

Brain stem ______

Central vestibular ______

Peripheral vestibular ______

Diencephalon ______

(Thalamus, hypothalamus) ______

Cerebellum ______

Cerebrum ______

D. Generalized Neuromuscular

E. Normal ______

Reason(s) for Lesion Localization (localizing deficits):

IV. Plan:

Differential Diagnosis

Recommended Test

______________________ Student's Signature

______________________ Clinician's Signature

Key: 0 (absent), +1 (reduced), +2 (normal), +3 (increased), +4 (clonus)

Figure 1.1

In many instances, the complete picture in a particular case is not apparent on initial evaluation and subsequent examinations are required to crystalise the situation in the clinicians mind. There is nothing to be lost and much to be gained from making repeated neurological examinations. Also, it often is revealing to make a complete evaluation even where the problem seems to be restricted to a single location, as other deficits may be overlooked on first examination.

Identifying the aetiology

Identification of the aetiology usually can be accomplished by utilising ancillary aids such as radiography, CSF analysis and electrophysiological testing. Reaching a diagnosis is assisted by some consideration of the type, breed and age of the patient. However, the use of such information as the sole method of making a diagnosis will inevitably lead to mistakes and is a dangerous path to follow.

Evaluation of treatment methods

On the basis of the information gained, it is possible to decide on an appropriate course of treatment. The course adopted is dependent on a number of considerations. Whilst the aetiology of the problem is the most important, other factors may play a part, not least the wishes and expectations of the owner, the welfare of the animal and financial constraints. Various treatment regimes may be appropriate for a particular disorder and careful consideration of all the facets of a case is necessary to ensure that the most appropriate course is adopted.

Estimating the prognosis

Clearly, the nature of the disease has a significant influence on the prognosis, though other factors are important. The prognosis for cases with essentially similar neurological deficits is determined not only by the underlying pathological change, but also by the time course of the disorder and the duration of the deficits. For example, a dog with ataxia due to a disc protrusion carries a good prognosis for full recovery if the deficit has been present for only a few days, but if the ataxia has been present for a year, the chances of improvement are poor. Secondary problems which develop may significantly influence the outcome of an individual case, for instance, where a paraplegic dog develops a urinary tract infection. These factors must all be considered and it may be necessary to alter the prognosis as the disease progresses.

Arrangement of the 'Manual of Small Animal Neurology'

This manual is arranged in three sections, with the aim of assisting the clinician with the diagnostic process and providing some information on the treatment of neurological disorders.

> **PART 1** discusses general principles of the neurological examination and its interpretation, with further information given in **PART 2**, where identifiable neurological presentations are described and the examination, treatment and prognosis for particular conditions discussed.

> The commonly employed ancillary diagnostic tests and their interpretations are dealt with in **PART 1** along with a consideration of therapeutics of nervous system diseases. The reader is encouraged to read and understand the principles in **PART 1** prior to utilising the problem orientated approach in **PART 2**, where conditions are grouped and described on the basis of presenting signs.

> **PART 3** of the book is devoted to neurological disorders in cats and exotic species, which warrant special consideration as they may tend to become submerged in a general discussion of 'small animals'. These chapters are provided as additional information and should be read in conjunction with the general principles given in the preceding two sections and also used as reference.

This manual is intended to provide a ready reference to clinicians presented with animals with neurological disorders and to give a general grounding in the subject. It is not within the scope of the book to provide detail of such topics as neuroanatomy, pathology and surgical treatment, which are covered in detail elsewhere — see 'Further Reading' and references in each chapter.

It is hoped that the information provided in this manual will enable clinicians to approach neurological problems with confidence, thus ensuring the best possible outcome in individual cases.

FURTHER READING

DE LAHUNTA, A. (1983) *Veterinary Neuroanatomy and Clinical Neurology.*
W. B. Saunders Co., Philadelphia.
OLIVER, J. E., HOERLEIN, B. F. and MAYHEW, I. G., eds. (1987) *Veterinary Neurology.*
W. B. Saunders Co., Philadelphia.
SIMPSON, S. T. (1985) Nervous system. In *Textbook of Small Animal Surgery,* (ed. D. H. Slatter).
W. B. Saunders Co., Philadelphia.

CHAPTER 2

NEUROLOGICAL EXAMINATION OF THE CRANIAL NERVES

Philippe M. Moreau Dr.Vet., M.S.

The clinical evaluation of the cranial nerves is an important part of the neurological examination of the dog or cat, especially when brain disease is suspected. The objectives of this chapter are to describe the examination and the different signs of abnormal cranial nerve function.

Important information concerning the integrity of the brainstem and the precise localisation of lesions is obtained from the cranial nerve examination. Each of the twelve pairs of cranial nerves originate from the brainstem and innervate a specific region of the head (Figure 2.1.). The cranial nerves contain either sensory fibres (afferent fibres), motor fibres (efferent fibres) or both. Diseases affecting cranial nerves involve either the sensory pathways, the brainstem nuclei or the motor pathways.

Table 2.1. indicates the function and signs of dysfunction of the cranial nerves in the dog and cat. Table 2.2. lists the respective clinical tests as well as the normal or abnormal responses for each test.

As is usual practice, the cranial nerves (CN) will be referred to by number, expressed in Roman numerals. The reader is referred to Chapter 9 for more detailed assessment of the eyes and associated structures.

GENERAL CONSIDERATIONS

In practice, the evaluation of the cranial nerves (CN) is simple and quick. The animal is first assessed for normal posture of the head, head tilt often being associated with a vestibular problem (CN VIII). At the same time, symmetry of the face, ears, eyes and lips can be evaluated. The muscles responsible for facial expression are innervated by the trigeminal (CN V) and facial (CN VII) nerves. Anomalies that can be seen are:

Muscular atrophy often seen in the temporal or masseter muscles, (CN V, motor branch)

Abnormal drooping of the ears, lips or eyelids (CN VII) often accompanied by the inability of the animal to move these structures voluntarily.

Abnormal position or movement of the eyes (CN III, IV, VI and VIII)

Abnormal size of the pupils (CN III, parasympathetic branch)

After observing and palpating the head, the clinician tests the palpebral reflex and the menace response.

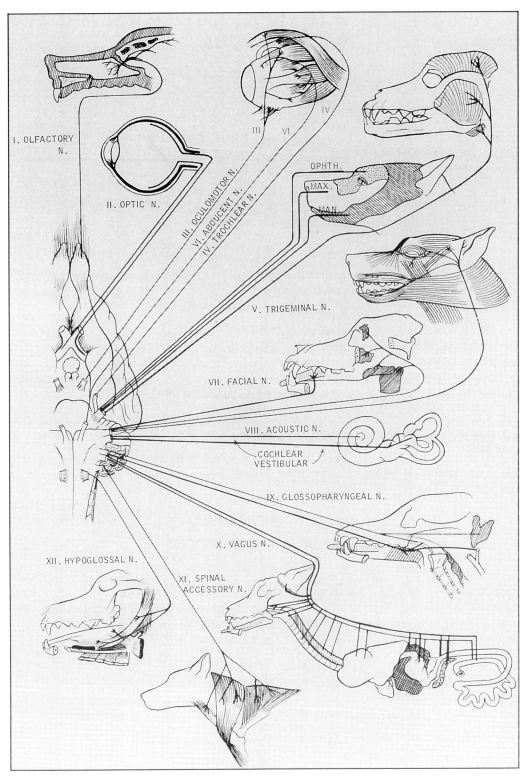

Figure 2.1
Origin and distribution of cranial nerves in the dog.

*(From GREENE, C. E. and OLIVER, J. E. (1983) Neurological examination
In Textbook of Veterinary Internal Medicine, Vol. 1. 2nd ed. (Ed. S. J. Ettinger)
W. B. Saunders Co., Philadelphia. (Reproduced by permission).*

The palpebral reflex is elicited by touching the medial canthus of the eye with the tip of a finger. If sensation is present (CN V) the animal reacts with a motor response (CN VII) by blinking (Figure 2.2.).

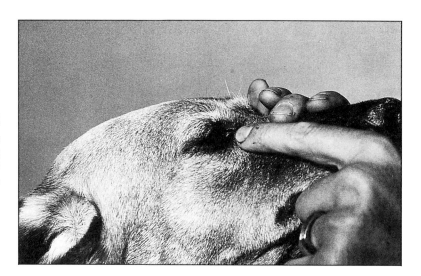

Figure 2.2

The palpebral reflex is generally elicited by touching the medial canthus of the eye with the tip of the finger.

The menace response is stimulated by abruptly approaching a hand or a finger towards the eye (simulating a blow to the eye) in order to test the patient's vision (Figure 2.3). One must be careful not to touch the ocular structures or to cause excessive air movement towards the eye which would elicit a different reflex, the palpebral reflex. In a normal animal this test evaluates the integrity of vision (CN II) as well as the motor pathway (CN VII) of the lids, normally causing a blinking of the eyelids.

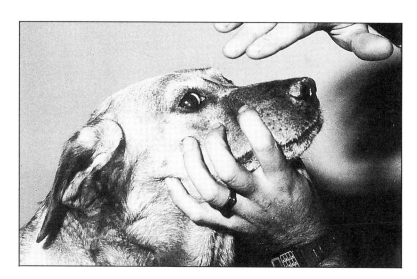

Figure 2.3

The menace reflex is performed by abruptly approaching a hand towards the eye to test the patient's vision.

Other tests to evaluate eyesight may be useful. Visual placing function may be tested in small dogs or cats where the animal is held and slowly brought up to a table. A normal animal raises and extends its thoracic limbs in response to the approach of the obstacle. One can test each eye separately by covering each eye alternately and repeating the test.

Vision can also be evaluated by the pupillary light reflex. This test is performed in dim light using a high intensity light source. By directing the beam towards the fundus of the eye, an immediate reflex is elicited with constriction of the pupil in the eye being examined (direct response) and also in the opposite eye (indirect or consensual response). In order for the reflex to be present, retinal vision and the parasympathetic fibres (CN III) that innervate the smooth muscle fibres of the iris must function adequately (Figure 2.4.).

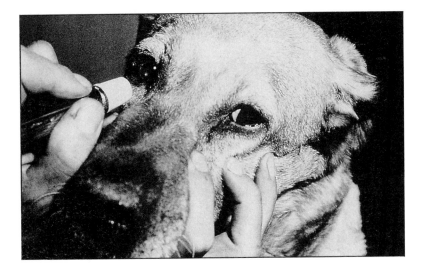

Figure 2.4

The pupillary light reflex tests both vision and the parasympathetic response.

The corneal reflex is performed by gently touching the corneal surface with a moistened cotton swab or with the finger. The animal reacts by blinking and retracting the globe. This test evaluates corneal sensitivity (ophthalmic branch of CN V) as well as the motor innervation of the eyelids (CN VII) and retractor muscles of the globe (CN VI) (Figure 2.5.).

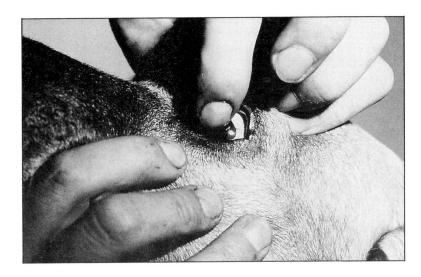

Figure 2.5

The corneal reflex is evaluated by gently touching the cornea. The animal normally reacts by blinking and retracting the globe.

Symmetry of the palpebral fissures should be present, indicating that the nerves controlling the extraocular muscles of the eye (CN III, IV and VI) function normally. The globes are then examined to determine whether or not a retracted globe is present (enophthalmia) which often is associated with an anomaly of sympathetic innervation (Horner's syndrome). At the same time, one looks for spontaneous movements of the eye (nystagmus) indicating abnormality of the vestibulocochlear tracts (CN VIII).

By moving the head from side to side and then up and down, one elicits rhythmic lateral and vertical movements of the globe (physiological nystagmus) respectively. These movements are normal and correspond to the oculocephalic reflex which tests the nerves controlling the position of the globe (CN III, IV, VI, VIII) (Figure 2.6). At the end of each movement, the head should be stabilised and cessation of nystagmus should be verified. If the eyes continue to move, a positional nystagmus exists, most often associated with a lesion of the vestibulocochlear nerve (CN VIII). Aberrant eye movements unrelated to head motion are called 'doll's eyes movement'. This condition is usually related to severe lesions involving cranial nerves III, IV, VI and VIII.

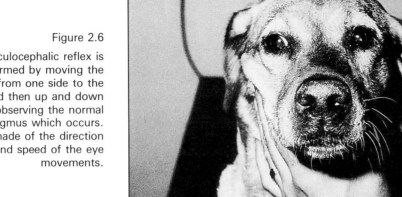

Figure 2.6

The oculocephalic reflex is performed by moving the head from one side to the other and then up and down and observing the normal nystagmus which occurs. Note is made of the direction and speed of the eye movements.

To evaluate facial sensitivity, one pinches the muzzle and the temporal regions of the head. Normally, the animal should blink in response to this stimulus, though some react more violently! In a stoical animal one may use haemostats to provide the stimuli and observe the motor innervation of this region (CN VII). By going over the face, one successively evaluates the ophthalmic branches (temporal region), the maxillary branches (nasal region), and the mandibular branches (buccal region) of the trigeminal nerve (sensory) as well as the facial nerve (motor) (Figure 2.7 a, b and c).

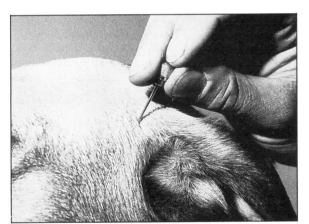

Figure 2.7 (a)

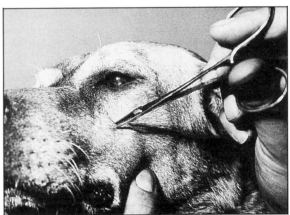

Figure 2.7 (b)

Figure 2.7 (a, b and c)

To test sensation of the face and the branches of the trigeminal nerve use a needle or haemostat.

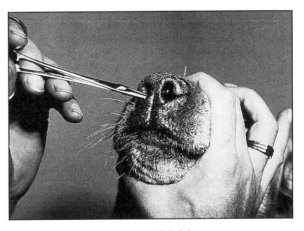

Figure 2.7 (c)

The oculocardiac reflex is performed by applying digital pressure to both globes simultaneously in order to provoke a reflex bradycardia. This test permits evaluation of the sensory response to pressure (CN V) and the parasympathetic reflex (CN X) (Figure 2.8.).

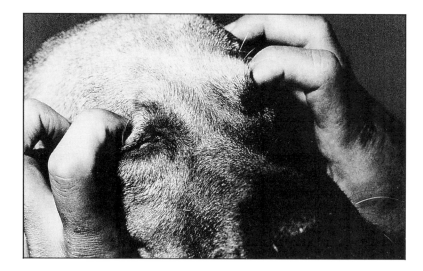

Figure 2.8

The oculocardiac reflex is performed by simultaneously applying digital pressure on both globes and measuring the ensuing reflex bradycardia.

By opening and closing the mouth one can evaluate jaw tone which is indicative of the integrity of the nerves to the muscle of mastication (CN V). To examine the tongue and the associated nerves (CN IX, X, XII) one first stimulates the tip of the nose (by moistening it, for example) in order to elicit a reflex licking (Figure 2.9). The symmetry of tongue movement is observed at the same time. Pulling gently on the tongue will test the muscle tone. The pharyngeal reflex is elicited by inserting a finger or tongue depressor towards the pharynx to stimulate a swallowing or gag response (Figure 2.10.).

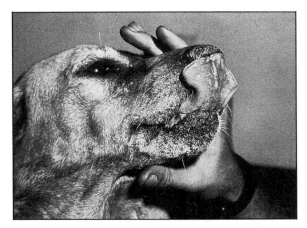

Figure 2.9
Stimulation of a licking reflex after sniffing a piece of cotton soaked in alcohol (to test the olfactory nerve and to observe the tongue movements).

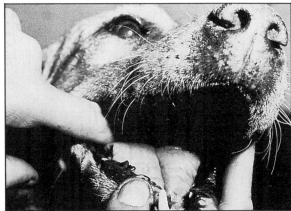

Figure 2.10
The pharyngeal reflex elicits a swallowing response by inserting a finger (or tongue depressor) into the pharynx.

To finish the cranial nerve examination, one palpates the trapezius and brachiocephalicus muscles to verify their symmetry and lack of atrophy (CN XI). Table 2.3 reviews tests commonly performed to evaluate cranial nerve function.

The cranial nerve examination should be performed frequently in order to become familiar with each test and the normal and abnormal responses. By performing these tests the examiner improves his clinical ability and his diagnostic skill. An *'aide-memoire'* provides an objective recording scheme for the examination (Figure 2.11). The cranial nerve examination does not require extensive knowledge of the anatomy of the brain and it takes much less time to perform the examination than to read its description. In order to precisely localise a neurolgical lesion it is advisable to understand the role, anatomy and pathology of the cranial nerves as well as the clinical signs associated with their dysfunction.

Figure 2.11
Example of a formulary for the neurologic examination of the head.

Legend	0	Absent		3.	**Cranial Nerves**	*Nerves tested*	*Response*
	+	Hypo			Palpebral reflex	V, VII	
	+ +	Normal			Menace reflex	II, VII	
	+ + +	Hyper			Pupillary light reflex	II, III,	
	+ + + +	Clonic			Consensual stimulation		
					Ipsilateral stimulation		
1. Observation					Pupillary symmetry	III	
Mental Status	*Abnormal*	*Normal*			Symmetry of eye position		
	Depressed				(strabismus)	III, IV, VI	
	Stupor				Corneal reflex	V, VI, VII	
	Coma				Facial motor response	V, VII	
Posture	*Abnormal*	*Normal*			nasal region		
	Head tilt	L R Tremors			temporal region		
	Paresis/paralysis				buccal region		
	tetra				Mastication	V	
	hemi	L R			Spontaneous nystagmus		
	hind legs	L R			Jerking nystagmus	VIII	
	fore legs	L R			Pendulus nystagmus	(cerebellum)	
Movement	*Abnormal*	*Normal*			Position nystagmus	VIII	
	Ataxia	cranial caudal			Oculocephalic reflex		
	Dysmetria				'Doll's Eyes'	III, IV, VI, VIII	
	Circling	L R			Pharyngeal reflex	IX, X	
2. Palpation	*Abnormal*	*Normal*			Tongue position	XII	
Muscle	Atrophy				Oculocardiac reflex	V, X	
Skeleton							

CN1   OLFACTORY NERVE

FUNCTION

The olfactory nerve is responsible for the conscious perception of smell.

ANATOMY AND CLINICAL EXAMINATION

The chemoreceptors in the nasal mucosa detect different odours and transmit the sensory information to the axons of the olfactory nerve. The nerve fibres that dispatch this information are numerous and form an important part of the rostral brain in carnivores, especially in the dog. The olfactory nucleus is situated in the olfactory bulb which is located rostral to the olfactory peduncles in the encephalon.

Absence (anosmia) or decreased (hyposmia) sense of smell often is difficult to evaluate in an animal whether it be part of the history (decreased appetite; little or no interest in food) or the neurological examination. A cotton ball soaked in alcohol or some highly scented food may be used to stimulate a licking reaction or aversion of the head, which is a sign of odour perception. It is important to note that an animal which sniffs does not necessarily perceive odours.

PATHOLOGY AND CLINICAL SIGNS

Lesions of the olfactory nerve are not easy to detect and are relatively rare. Chronic rhinitis with involvement of the olfactory mucosa is the most frequent cause of hyposmia. In the cat, upper respiratory infections frequently are associated with anorexia, which may disappear when the animal is offered odorous food (sardines etc.). Tumours of the nasal cavity also may be responsible for a lack of odour perception.

CN II   OPTIC NERVE

FUNCTION

The optic nerve is responsible for sensory visual perception and the sensory component of the pupillary light reflex.

ANATOMY AND CLINICAL SIGNS

Light and visual information are perceived by nervous cells in the retina which transmit this via the optic nerve to the optic tracts of the diencephalon. The axons reach the lateral geniculate nucleus where they have two options: some continue towards the reflex pathway and those responsible for conscious perception travel to the occipital cortex (Figure 2.12.).

The retina and the optic disc are the only structures that can be examined directly. Because the sensory and motor fibres responsible for vision and eye movement travel through the brain to the occipital cortex and brainstem, diseases involving the brain often have repercussions on vision. The tracts and nervous centres responsible for sight are represented in Figure 2.12.

Lesions of the lateral geniculate nucleus, the optic radiations or the occipital cortex result in a loss of vision without affecting the pupillary reflexes. If the lesion is unilateral (trauma, haemorrhage, etc.) the eye opposite the lesion is affected (contralateral). Bilateral lesions (encephalitis, hydrocephalus, etc.) cause complete blindness.

Lesions of the retina, optic nerve, optic chiasm or optic tracts cause both visual and pupillary light reflex deficits. Lesions of the retina and optic nerve are often bilateral (retinal atrophy, optic neuritis); lesions of the optic tracts are rare.

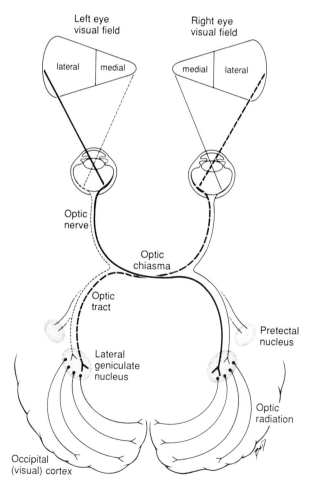

Figure 2.12
Tracts and nervous centres
responsible for sight

20

PATHOLOGY AND CLINICAL EXAMINATION

Injury to the optic nerve can be suspected from the history (animal bumps into furniture, etc.). The clinical tests used are the menace response and the pupillary light reflex.

The menace response examines both the optic nerve and the facial nerve which carries the motor fibres resulting in a blink response. The pupillary light reflex simultaneously tests the optic nerve and the oculomotor nerve, whose parasympathetic fibres constrict the iris. In small animals, visual placing is another valid clinical test for vision. One must be careful in interpreting reflexes and repeat the tests several times before the animal is declared blind. If the animal does not blink in response to the menace test but is still able to close his eyes in response to the palpebral reflex, for example, (indicating a functional facial nerve), one can suspect a deficit of the optic nerve or its associated structures.

The pupillary light reflex permits a more precise localisation of the lesion. A blind animal with non-responsive dilated pupils generally has a lesion of the retina, optic nerve, optic chiasm or optic tracts. Absence of vision in an animal with a normal pupillary light reflex indicates a lesion caudal to the pretectal nucleus or a lesion of the lateral geniculate nucleus, optic radiations or the occipital lobe of the cortex. Figure 2.13 shows the pathway of the pupillary light reflex. Localisation of lesions is discussed further in Chapter 9.

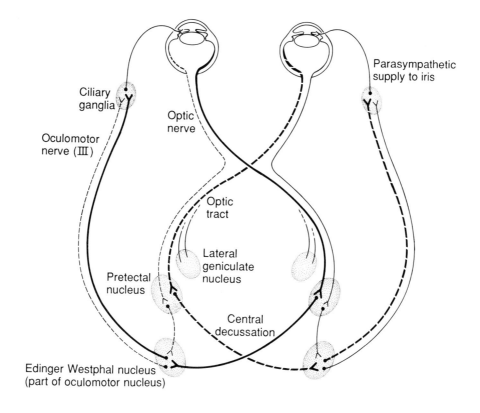

Figure 2.13
Pathways of pupillary light reflex

Numerous diseases may affect vision and can be classified as congenital, infectious, traumatic, neoplastic, metabolic, toxic or idiopathic. Congenital problems include optic nerve hypoplasia, hydrocephalus, lissencephaly and lysosomal storage diseases. Central nervous system (CNS) infections can result in a loss of vision with normal pupillary light reflexes. Other problems are often present such as ataxia, postural reflex deficits, seizures, etc. Cranial trauma can cause contusions, haemorrhage and cerebral oedema which in turn can trigger visual problems. Neoplasms affecting sight include primary and secondary tumours. Visual deficits may be associated with metabolic or toxic disorders such as cerebral anoxia, for example, following a cardiorespiratory arrest, hypoglycaemia, thiamine deficiency (in cats), heat stroke, certain intoxications (such as by products containing lead) and osmolarity disorders (diabetic ketoacidosis). See Chapters 8 and 9 for a full discussion.

CN III   OCULOMOTOR NERVE

FUNCTION

The oculomotor nerve controls pupillary constriction by the intermediary of its parasympathetic motor fibres. It is also responsible for the motor innervation of the extraocular muscles: dorsal, medial and ventral recti, the ventral oblique and the levator palpebrae.

ANATOMY AND CLINICAL SIGNS

The oculomotor nerve originates from a nucleus located in the rostral ventromedial portion of the mesencephalon. The fibres of CN III innervate most of the extraocular muscles, the upper eyelids and the constrictor muscle of the pupil via its parasympathetic branches.

Sympathetic responses are elicited by emotional reactions such as fear or attack. The sympathetic fibres innervate the smooth muscle of the periorbital fascia and the eyelids including the third eyelid. Lesions of this pathway provokes pupillary constriction (myosis), retraction of the globe (enophthalmus), a narrowing of the palpebral fissure (ptosis) and protrusion of the third eyelid. This group of signs is known as Horner's syndrome. In general, Horner's syndrome is not associated with a loss of vision. The most frequent causes are cranial trauma, lesions of the cervical spinal cord (down to T3) as well as tumours or surgical procedures in the neck area which may injure the sympathetic trunk (Figures 2.14, 2.15, and Chapter 9).

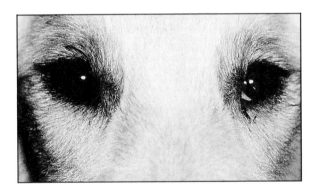

Figure 2.14
Left unilateral Horner's syndrome in a dog
after cervical and thoracic trauma showing
miosis, ptosis, enophthalmia and protrusion of the
third eyelid in the left eye

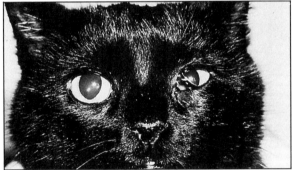

Figure 2.15
Cat with left side Horner's syndrome
following head trauma

Abnormal eye movement and position may be due to lesions of the oculomotor nerve (Figure 2.16 a and b). Eye movement is controlled by upper motor neurons (UMN) from the cortex and brainstem vestibular reflexes. It is co-ordinated by the synergistic and antagonistic action of the extraocular muscles innervated by CNs III, IV and VI. The centre responsible for this control is the medial longitudinal fasciculus that is located in the centre of the brainstem between the nuclei of CN III and CN VI. A lesion in this area can induce a lack of eye movement in response to head movements (absence of physiological nystagmus). The eyes remain fixed in the orbit as the head is moved. This is sometimes called 'Doll's Eye' phenomenon and often accompanies cranial trauma and cerebral haemorrhage. Such a loss of physiological vestibular nystagmus indicates the presence of extensive brainstem lesions at the level of the vestibular nuclei, the medial longitudinal fasciculus or both.

PATHOLOGY AND CLINICAL EXAMINATION

Lesions of the nucleus or tracts of the oculomotor nerve produce a ventrolateral strabismus due to a paralysis of the extraocular muscles and a ptosis of the upper eyelid caused by paralysis of the levator palpebrae. Moreover, loss of parasympathetic function causes dilation of the pupils which are also unresponsive to light stimulus.

Oculomotor nerve lesions at the level of the ciliary ganglion and short ciliary nerves or lesions of the constrictor muscle of the pupil are manifested by exaggerated constriction of the pupil in response to a light stimulus on the affected side. Sight is unchanged and both eyes are usually involved.

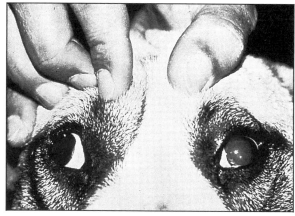 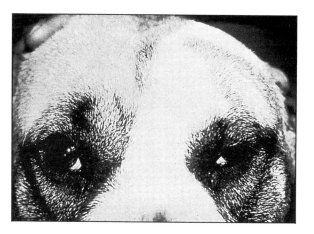

Figure 2.16 (a)
Dog with medial rectus paralysis in left eye.
The animal is looking towards the right but its left eye
does not follow the right one.

Figure 2.16 (b)
The dog is now looking straight and one can notice the
ptosis in the left eye. The diagnosis is unilateral
oculomotor paralysis on the left.
(Courtesy of Dr. Richard A. LeCouteur, Colarado State University)

Lesions of the retina, optic nerve or optic chiasma are detected by a lack of pupillary constriction on the affected side in response to a direct light stimulus; however, the iris constricts when a light is shone into the normal eye (normal indirect or consensual response). Sight is also affected in the injured eye. The most common causes of damage to the oculomotor nerve are trauma, infection or neoplasia. Usually other nerves are also involved.

The examination of the oculomotor nerve should be carefully conducted and repeated several times because excited and frightened animals often have dilated pupils which do not respond to light stimulus, due to excess sympathetic stimulation. See Chapter 9 for further discussion.

CN IV   TROCHLEAR NERVE

FUNCTION

The trochlear nerve innervates the dorsal oblique muscle.

ANATOMY AND CLINICAL SIGNS

The nucleus of the trochlear nerve is small and is located in the caudal portion of the mesencephalon, caudal to the nucleus of the oculomotor nerve. Isolated anomalies are rare, difficult to diagnose and not of major interest in veterinary medicine.

CN V   TRIGEMINAL NERVE

FUNCTION

The trigeminal nerve innervates the muscles of mastication and is the sensory pathway to the cutaneous elements of the face.

ANATOMY AND CLINICAL EXAMINATION

The nucleus of the trigeminal nerve is not well defined anatomically but is located in the pons in the lateral reticular formation at the level of the rostral cerebellar peduncles and dorsal to the trapezoid body. The motor axons pass through the trigeminal ganglion and the oval foramen to join the maxillary nerve tracts and innervate the maseter, temporal, rostral digastric, pterigoid and mylohyoid muscles. Bilateral involvement produces paralysis of jaw muscles with inability to close the mouth voluntarily(Figure 2.17). Unilateral lesions can result in decreased jaw tone. These lesions are often accompanied by an atrophy of the masseter and temporal muscles which appears approximately one week after nerve injury (Figure 2.18).

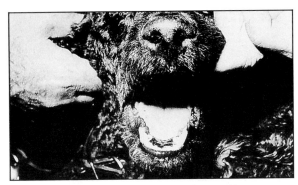

Figure 2.17   Dog showing dropped jaw
due to bilateral CN V paralysis

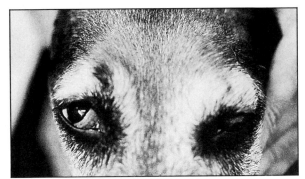

Figure 2.18   Unilateral CN V paralysis shows
atrophy of temporal muscles

The sensory pathways of the face are distributed in three branches. The maxillary branch innervates the nasal region; the ophthalmic branch provides sensation to the ocular region and cornea; and the mandibular branch innervates the buccal area. Each branch should be tested for sensory responses. To determine sensitivity of the skin of the face it should be thoroughly tested with a needle or haemostats (Figure 2.7, a and b). In certain animals it is necessary to pinch the skin to obtain a response but for the most part a slight stimulus is satisfactory. If no response is obtained, the nasal region is tested because it is particularly sensitive (Figure 2.7 c). The corneal and palpebral reflexes utilise the sensory pathways of the trigeminal nerve. They also permit evaluation of the motor responses of the facial and abducent nerves by the corneal reflex and the facial nerve by the palpebral reflex (see Tables 2.1 and 2.2). Touching the internal surface and hairs of the external ear stimulates the maxillary branch of the trigeminal nerve and normally elicits a twitching of the ear (especially in the cat) controlled by the motor pathway of the facial nerve.

PATHOLOGY

Included among the diseases involving the sensory and motor function of the trigeminal nerve are infection, trauma, neoplasia and vascular disorders. Generally, other cranial nerves are involved in addition. A deficit in motor function is manifested by decreased muscular tone with or without complete paralysis and inability voluntarily to close the mouth (dropped jaw) (Figure 2.17).

Certain polyneuropathies can involve the trigeminal nerve as well as other nerves and result in atrophy of the corresponding muscles (Figure 2.18). The diagnosis can be confirmed by electromyography. It should be noted that the most frequent causes of atrophy of the muscles of mastication are eosinophilic myositis and fibrosing myositis. In these cases one must distinguish between a primary muscular disorder and a neuropathy.

CN VI   ABDUCENT NERVE

FUNCTION

The abducent nerve innervates the lateral rectus and the retractor bulbi muscles.

ANATOMY AND CLINICAL SIGNS

The abducent nerve originates from the small abducent nucleus situated in the rostral part of the peduncular region, near the facial nerve nucleus and ventral to the floor of the fourth ventricle. Clinical examination of CN VI includes an examination of the position and movement of the eyes (oculocephalic reflex) and the corneal reflex described above. Lateral strabismus and the inability to retract the globe are rare and often associated with disorders of other cranial nerves.

CN VII   FACIAL NERVE

The facial nerve is composed of motor tracts which innervate the facial muscles and sensory fibres to the palate and cranial two thirds of the tongue (providing the sense of taste)

ANATOMY AND CLINICAL SIGNS

The facial nerve nucleus is situated ventrolaterally in the peduncular region caudal to the trapezoid body near the attachment of the cerebellar peduncles to the cerebellum. The axons cross the floor of the fourth ventricle before leaving the skull via the stylomastoid foramen and innervating the muscles of the ears,

Table 2.1 Cranial Nerve Function

	Nerve	Function	Signs of Dysfunction
I.	Olfactory	Sensory (olfaction)	Anosmia (Absence of smell) Hyposmia (decreased smell)
II.	Optic	Sensory (vision)	Blindness (total or partial)
III.	Oculomotor	Motor: external ocular muscles (dorsal, medial and ventral recti, ventral oblique and levator palpebrae)	Ptosis Strabismus (ventro lateral)
		Parasympathetic fibres for construction of the iris use the oculomotor pathway.	Mydriasis Fixed pupil
IV.	Trochlear	Motor: dorsal oblique muscle	Strabismus (dorso-medial)
V.	Trigeminal	Sensory: skin of face Motor: muscles of mastication	Facial anaesthesia Dropped jaw if bilateral; atrophy of muscles.
VI.	Abducens	Motor: lateral rectus and retractor bulbi muscles.	Medial strabismus Inability to retract the globe
VII.	Facial	Motor: muscles of facial expression (ears, eyelids and lips)	Falling, ears, drooping lips, inability to close the lids
		Sensory: rostral two thirds of the tongue	Hypoesthesia of rostral tongue
		Parasympathetic fibres to lacrimal and salivary glands (mandibular and sublingual)	Decreased tears secretions (Keratitis Sicca)
VIII.	Vestibulocochlear	Sensory: hearing balance	Deafness or decreased hearing Head tilt, circling, nystagmus, i.e. vestibular syndrome.
IX.	Glossopharyngeal	Sensory: pharynx Motor: pharyngeal muscles	Dysphagia Regurgitation
X.	Vagus	Sensory: larynx, pharynx, abdominal and thoracic organs Motor: larnyx, pharnyx Parasympathetic fibres to thoracic and abdominal organs	Dysphagia Salivation disorders Change or lack of barking Regurgitation Cardiac or gastrointestinal signs
XI.	Accessory	Motor: trapezius muscles	Atrophy of neck muscles
XII.	Hypoglossal	Motor: muscles of the tongue	Paralysis and atrophy of tongue.

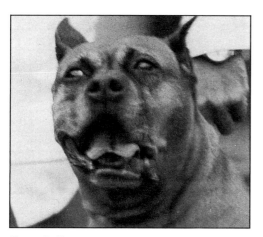

eyelids, nose, cheeks, lips and caudal portion of the digastricus muscle.

Clinical tests which serve to evaluate the trigeminal nerve are used for the facial nerve which controls the motor response of these reflexes (menace response, corneal and palpebral reflexes, pinching the lips, stroking the hair of the external ear). Normally, if the facial nerve is affected, pinching the lips produces a painful reaction (transmitted by CN V) but the lips remain immobile due to impairment of the motor response (transmitted by CN VII). In general, one also observes a lateral deviation of the muzzle towards the normal side, while the ear and lower eyelid droop on the affected side (Figure 2.19). Taste can be evaluated using

Figure 2.19
Seven year old female Boxer with idiopathic unilateral paralysis of the facial nerve on the left.
One notes drooping lips on the affected side and a facial muscle retraction on the right.

Table 2.2: Clinical Tests of Cranial Nerves

Nerve	Clinical Test	Response
I. Olfactory	Smelling a non-irritating substance (e.g. alcohol)	Animal sniffs or licks his nose (normal response)
II. Optic	1. Throw a piece of cotton wool in front of animal 2. Simulate a blow to eye (menace response) by abruptly moving hand towards eye without touching it. 3. Observe animal's movements in a room with reduced light. 4. Evaluate pupillary light reflex by directing a light beam towards the fundus.	1. Animal's attention is (normal) or is not (abnormal) attracted. 2. Eyelids will (normal) or will not (abnormal) close. 3. Animal bumps into obstacles or stays against the wall 4. a) Light in affected eye: absence of direct and consensual pupillary light reflexes. b) Light in normal eye; normal pupillary reflexes, both pupils constricting.
III. Oculomotor	1. Evaluation of pupillary light reflexes. 2. Observe eye movements while head is moved laterally (oculocephalic reflex)	1. A. Unilateral lesion a) light in affected eye — direct pupillary reflex absent. b) light in normal eye — direct pupillary reflex present —consensual reflex absent. B. Bilateral lesion — absence of direct and consenual pupillary. 2. Eye movements should be symmetric and a horizontal nystagmus should appear (normal).
V. Trigeminal	1. Pinching skin of ears, lips and muzzle to evaluate mandibular and maxillary branches and around eye for ophthalmic branch 2. Corneal reflex (gently touch cornea) tests ophthalmic branch. 3. Palpebral reflex (touch medial canthus) 4. Test jaw tone	1. Movement of skin or a painful response (normal) 2. Blinking and retraction of globe (normal). 3. Blinking (normal) 4. Animal resists opening jaw and closes immediately (normal)
VI. Abducens	Corneal reflex (gently touch cornea)	Globe retracts in orbit (normal)
VII. Facial	1. Prick face with a needle or pinch with haemostats. 2. Corneal reflex (see trigeminal n.) 3. Palpebral reflex (see trigeminal n.) 4. Schirmer tear test (evaluation of lacrimal secretions)	1-2-3. With intact sensory perception (trigeminal n.) but absent motor function (facial n.) the animal may have a pain response without moving the skin.
VIII. Vestibulocochlear	1. Auditory reflex (clapping hands behind ear) 2. Oculocephalic reflex (see oculomotor n.)	1. Jumping of animal, movement of external ear or blinking 2. If unilateral lesion exists, one may observe a spontaneous or positional nystagmus.
IX. Glossopharyngeal	Pharyngeal or swallowing reflex (stimulate pharynx with finger = 'gag reflex')	Animal reacts by swallowing
X. Vagus	1. Pharyngeal or swallowing reflex (see glossopharyngeal n.) 2. Oculocardiac reflex (digital pressure on both globes and observation of cardiac rhythm.	Cardiac rhythm slows (reflex bradycardia) (normal)
XI. Accessory	Palpation of neck muscles	Muscular atrophy
XII. Hypoglossal	Retraction reflex (pulling on tongue)	Animal resists pulling and retracts tongue Tongue atrophy (uni-or bilateral)

a cotton swab, by applying atropine to the surface of the tongue. The animal does not react on the affected side while he immediately responds to the bitter taste by salivating and retracting the tongue on the intact side.

The Schirmer tear test can be performed to verify the normal function of the parasympathetic facial nerve fibres which innervate the lacrimal gland (See Chapter 9).

PATHOLOGY AND CLINICAL EXAMINATION

Unidentified causes are, in the author's experience, most often responsible for isolated paralysis of the facial nerve, followed by traumatic or infectious causes and tumours. Other problems such as polyneuropathies of toxic, metabolic or immunologic origin also are described. Usually, the facial nerve is affected along with other nerves. For example, an otitis media or interna can affect the facial nerve as it traverses the middle ear. Additionally, one may observe a unilateral Horner's syndrome with simultaneous involvement of the vestibulocochlear nerve. To confirm involvement of the middle or inner ear, a thorough examination of the auditory canal (under general anaesthesia) to verify the integrity of the tympanic membrane, as well as radiography of the tympanic bulla, should be performed. Samples should be taken for culture and long term systemic antibiotic therapy should be administered. Antibiotics known to be toxic to the auditory apparatus include gentamycin, streptomycin and other aminoglycosides and are to be avoided both topically and systemically. If otitis externa is diagnosed, the auditory canal should be thoroughly cleaned and treated with an antibiotic solution. Oil based solutions should not be used if the tympanic membrane is punctured.

Brainstem lesions (due to trauma, infection, neoplasm, etc) often involve the facial nerve. In such cases, signs of brain stem involvement (ataxia, decreased postural reactions, etc) accompany the facial paralysis.

Unfortunately, the cause of isolated facial paralysis or paralysis associated with other cranial nerve problems is not always clear. Unilateral or bilateral facial paralysis of 'idiopathic origin' is often encountered. After ruling out an infectious cause (no fever, normal blood count, etc) corticosteroids sometimes are helpful.

CN VIII   VESTIBULOCOCHLEAR NERVE

FUNCTION

The vestibulocochlear nerve is composed of two branches: the cochlear branch which mediates hearing, and the vestibular nerve which is responsible for orientation of the head and body with respect to gravity.

ANATOMY AND CLINICAL EXAMINATION

The dorsal and ventral cochlear nuclei, located on either side of the peduncular region, receive the axons that transmit acoustic information originating from the ear. Numerous nervous pathways involving many synapses conduct signals towards the auditory centre for reflex activity as well as to the cortex for conscious perception of sound. The auditory zone of the cerebral cortex is situated in the temporal lobe.

The cochlear branch is tested by stimulating hearing with a loud, sharp sound behind the ear and observing the animal's reaction. The history often provides valuable information regarding the animal's ability to hear. Unilateral involvement is always difficult to establish clinically through the use of simple tests. Sophisticated methods, including brainstem auditory evoked response (BAER), exist to measure the electrical activity of the brainstem in response to auditory stimuli.

There are four vestibular nuclei situated on each side of the caudal part of the peduncular region, adjacent to the lateral wall of the fourth ventricle. Numerous projections leave the vestibular nuclei and travel towards the spinal cord (via the vestibulospinal tract), the brainstem (via the reticular formation) and the cerebellum (via the caudal cerebral peduncles). Through these pathways, the vestibular system coordinates eye, trunk, limb and head movement.

Anomalies affecting the vestibular branch produce characteristic signs. Usually, vestibular problems are unilateral and are manifested by ataxia, nystagmus and a head tilt to the affected side. Vestibular abnormalities are also responsible for circling and difficulty in maintaining equilibrium with falling to the side of the lesion, and possibly hemiparesis.

Table 2.3:
Tests commonly employed to evaluate Cranial Nerves

Reflex	Technique	Nerves Tested
Menace response	Simulate a blow to the eye by abruptly approaching a hand towards the eye without actually touching it.	Optic n., Facial n., (CN II, VII)
Pupillary light reflex	Shine light source in the back of the eye	Optic n., Oculomotor n., (CN II, III)
Corneal reflex	Gently touch the cornea with the finger or a cotton swab soaked in sterile saline solution	Trigeminal n., Facial n., Abducent n. (CN V, VI, VII)
Palpebral reflex	Touch medial canthus of eye with finger	Trigeminal n., Facial n., (CN V, VII)
Auditory reflex	Clap hands or snap fingers behind ears	Vestibulocochlear n. (CN VIII)
Oculocephalic reflex	Move head laterally from left to right and observe eye movements during and after displacement.	Vestibulocochlear n. Oculomotor n.(CN III, VIII)
Pharyngeal	Insert finger toward the pharynx and observe swallowing	Glossopharyngeal n. Vagus n. (CN IX, X)
Oculocardiac reflex	Apply digital pressure on globes by pushing simultaneously on upper eyelids and measuring variation in cardiac rhythm.	Trigeminal n. Vagus n. (parasympathetic) (CN V, X)

Table 2.4
Clinical Signs of Vestibular Syndrome

	Central	Peripheral
Head tilt	yes	yes
Asymmetric ataxia	yes	yes
Nystagmus	yes	yes
Positional nystagmus	yes	no
Absence or decreased proprioceptive reflexes	yes	no
Paresis	yes	no

Two forms of nystagmus must be differentiated. One is called 'jerk nystagmus' and consists of an involuntary rhythmic eye movement composed of a rapid phase (eye movement in one direction) followed by a slow recuperatory phase (movement of the eyes in the other direction). The rapid phase is usually directed away from the side of the lesion and indicates the description of the nystagmus (right nystagmus, for example). A jerk nystagmus is observed in lesions of the cranial nerves or the brainstem region where their nuclei are located. Another form of nystagmus is called 'pendular nystagmus'. This form is less frequent and is manifested by weak ocular oscillations that have no rapid or slow components. Pendular nystagmus is seen in certain cerebellar diseases and sometimes in animals with visual problems. In this chapter, only jerk nystagmus will be considered.

By performing the oculocephalic reflex (successive movements of the head from left to right), eye mobility and a physiological nystagmus are observed. In the case of an anomaly, the eyes remain immobile or the nystagmus may be exaggerated (persistent ocular movement while the head is prevented from moving). If an abnormal horizontal nystagmus exists, the direction of the rapid phase indicates the side of the lesion, with the rapid phase occurring away from the affected side.

Another test is frequently performed in people, where nystagmus is observed after rotation of the body, and can be used in certain small sized animals. The animal is placed on a chair or stool which is rapidly turned. A physiological nystagmus (or vestibular nystagmus) is induced. Once rotation is stopped, a short post rotatory nystagmus in the opposite direction of turning occurs. Both directions are tested; different intensities and durations of post rotatory nystagmus can appear with unilateral lesions. Furthermore, if a peripheral lesion of the vestibular branch exists, a decrease or absence of post rotatory nystagmus is noticed after having turned the animal towards the side opposite the lesion.

PATHOLOGY AND CLINICAL SIGNS

Cochlear Branch

Partial or even complete unilateral deafness is difficult to detect clinically in domestic animals. Complete bilateral deafness generally is associated with problems of the ear itself. Given the multiple nervous pathways which transmit information to the cortex, a large margin of security exists and central lesions necessary to cause such signs must be extensive.

Congenital deafness occurs most often in white animals, notably white cats with blue eyes and Old English Sheepdogs with depigmented irises. Congenital deafness also has been described in Cocker Spaniels, Dalmatians and Bull Terriers.

The most common causes of lesions of the cochlear branch are chronic otitis interna, cranial trauma, ototoxic medications (aminoglycoside antibiotics, for example) and degenerative disorders. Elderly patients who progressively lose their hearing have a degeneration of the organ of Corti (spiral organ) or the chain of ossicles of the middle ear.

Vestibular Branch

Equilibrium disturbances or a vestibular syndrome may be due to either lesions of the brainstem nerve centres and the central vestibular tracts (central vestibular syndrome) or lesions of the peripheral nerves (peripheral vestibular syndrome). It is of clinical importance to determine the origin of the syndrome (central vs. peripheral). The clinical signs of a vestibular syndrome are well recognised, (head tilt, circling, ataxia, etc). Table 2.4 lists the principle clinical signs which differentiate between central and peripheral vestibular syndrome (Figure 2.20).

Diseases resulting in a vestibular syndrome most often are associated with degenerative or multifocal inflammatory lesions. The most frequent causes are infection (bacterial, viral or protozoal), haemorrhage (post traumatic, intoxication or platelet problems), tumours (reticulosis, metastases from mammary gland, prostatic or other tumours), cerebral emboli and idiopathic causes. Clinical signs seen include serious neurologic problems with abnormal postural reactions and cranial nerve function, behavioural changes, seizures and ataxia.

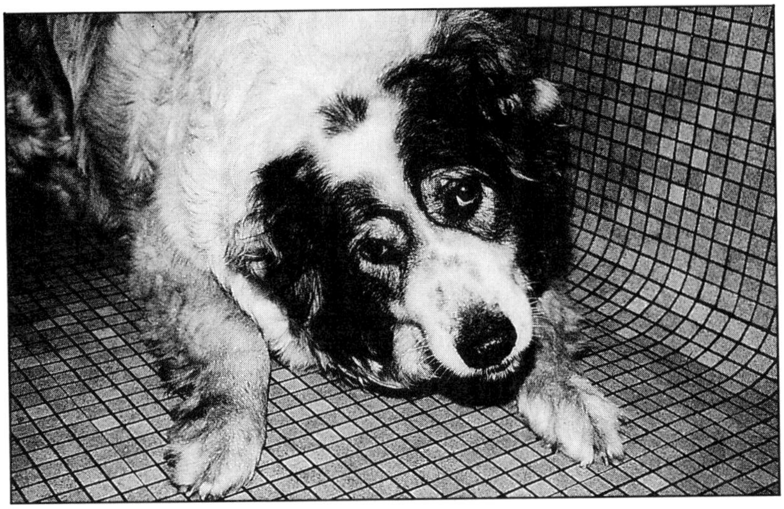

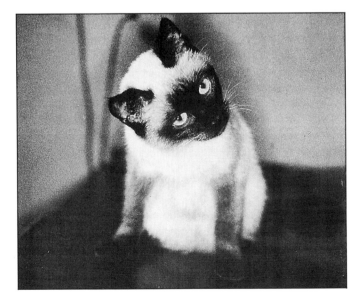

Figure 2.20

Dog with a right head tilt, ataxia, circling to the right and right positional nystagmus. These signs illustrate a vestibular syndrome.

Cerebral emboli often are suspected clinically; nevertheless, most neurologists consider their frequency over estimated. Acute idiopathic vestibular syndrome in the cat and dog is encountered commonly in clinical practice. In the cat, this problem appears abruptly with no apparent cause (Figure 2.21). It does not seem to be associated with an infectious process and no histopathological lesions underlie the disorder. Most often the signs are unilateral, the animal has no symptoms of otitis and, apart from the neurological problem, is in good health. The diagnosis is made by excluding other causes, especially otitis interna and central infections. No specific treatment exists but affected cats generally improve spontaneously in two or three days. Supportive therapy is sometimes useful (vitamin complexes, fluids). Also, in the elderly dog, an acute idiopathic vestibular syndrome is encountered. The signs are similar to those seen in the cat. The disease is not associated with an infectious agent and the cause is still unknown. This syndrome is often, erroneously, interpreted as cerebral embolus ('stroke'); no specific lesions are found at necropsy. Like the cat, the dog often recovers spontaneously in 48—72 hours. However in some cases, residual deficits remain. There is no treatment except for supportive therapy. Corticosteroids (dexamethasone for 4—6 days at 0.1 mg/kg bid, halving the dose every two days) may help reduce secondary inflammation.

Problems resulting in a peripheral vestibular syndrome are more common. The principal cause is ear infection (otitis interna or media). Animals with severe chronic ear infection, may demonstrate central signs. After excluding auricular disorders, the differential diagnosis can include tumours originating from the nerves (neuronoma, neurofibroma) or of surrounding cranial tissue, trauma, intoxication and congenital vestibular syndrome (described in the German Shepherd, Dobermann, Siamese and Burmese cats). It is not uncommon to speak of an idiopathic origin if no cause can be determined.

Figure 2.21

Idiopathic vestibular syndrome in a young Siamese cat.

Complementary examinations which help establish an aetiologic diagnosis of vestibular syndrome include an otoscopic examination, skull radiographs (of the tympanic bullae in particular), cerebrospinal fluid analysis as well as blood tests. Other analyses include FeLV and FIP tests, toxoplasmosis titre, and finally, for those who have access to them, electroencephalograms and computed tomography examinations (Figure 2.22, 2.23).

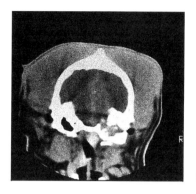 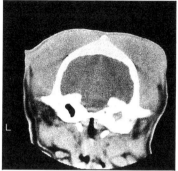

Figure 2.22

CT scan of a dog with a right central vestibular syndrome. An intracranial tumour was suspected clinically. The CT examination showed a severe inner ear infection with complete bone erosion and involvement of the brain.

(Courtesy of Dr. J. Lang, University of Berne, Switzerland).

Left   Right

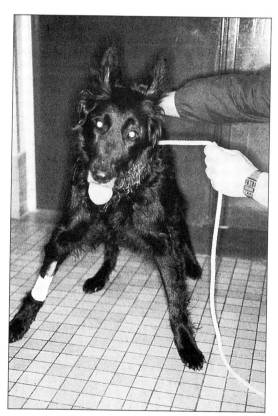 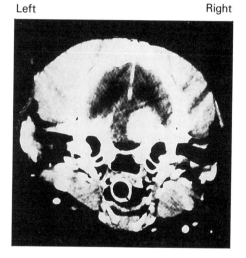

Figure 2.23 (a and b)

Nine year old female Groenendael with progressive trunkal ataxia, pacing towards the right, left head tilt, and postural deficits on the right. A right central vestibular syndrome was diagnosed. A computed tomographic examination shows an intracranial tumour in the right posterior fossa. This was a meningioma. The left head tilt may be explained by a cerebellar displacement by the tumour and presence of a so-called paradoxical vestibular syndrome of cerebellar origin.

CN IX GLOSSOPHARYNGEAL NERVE

FUNCTION

The glossopharyngeal nerve is the motor pathway to muscles of the pharynx, in conjunction with certain fibres of the vagus nerve. For this reason, it is useful to consider the examination of these nerves simultaneously. Moreover, the glossopharyngeal nerve supplies sensory innervation to the caudal third of the tongue, the pharyngeal mucosa and is responsible for taste. Also, this nerve carries parasympathetic fibres to their zygomatic and paratoid salivary glands.

ANATOMY AND CLINICAL EXAMINATION

The glossopharyngeal, vagus and accessory nerves originate from a common nucleus, the nucleus ambiguus. This is formed by a group of neurons situated in the ventrolateral zone of the medulla. The glossopharyngeal nerve emerges from the jugular foramen.

The integrity of the glossopharyngeal nerve is evaluated by testing the pharyngeal reflex. A finger or tongue depressor is inserted into the back of the mouth to induce deglutition (Figure 2.10).

PATHOLOGY AND CLINICAL SIGNS

Lesions affecting the glossopharyngeal nerve generally are associated with infectious diseases, trauma or tumours affecting the brainstem. Clinical signs seen in CN IX disorders include dysphagia and regurgitation of undigested food. Often other cranial nerves are involved and central signs can be present (Figure 2.24).

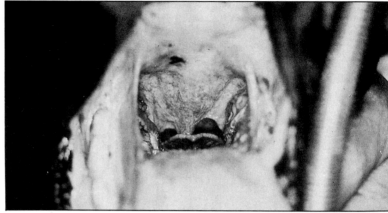

Figure 2.24
Nine year old Male Boxer with chronic swallowing difficulties associated with a right sided pharyngeal paralysis due to a unilateral glossopharyngeal lesion. Other cranial nerves involved in this case included V, VII and VIII. The aetiology was an oligodendroglioma.

Symptoms of rabies and pseudorabies (Aujesky's disease) often include problems of deglutition, salivation and voice changes. These aetiologies should, therefore, always be included in the differential diagnosis. Certain neuromuscular diseases are characterised by dysphagia as well as by other signs of peripheral nerve involvement, which could be due to polyneuropathies, botulism or myasthenia.

CN X   VAGUS NERVE

FUNCTION

Like CN IX, the vagus nerve innervates the pharynx and the larynx. The main function is to provide parasympathetic innervation to all the thoracic and abdominal viscera, except those of the pelvic region, which are supplied by nerves arising from the sacral parasympathetic nuclei.

ANATOMY AND CLINICAL EXAMINATION

Sensory and motor activity of the vagus nerve is tested at the same time as that of the glossopharyngeal nerve, by the pharyngeal reflex. Parasympathetic activity is evaluated by testing the oculocardiac reflex. This is performed by simultaneously applying digital pressure on the two globes and pushing the eyelids into the orbit. Normally, a reflex bradycardia will be elicited due to sensory stimulation by the trigeminal nerve and motor response by the vagus nerve (Figure 2.8).

PATHOLOGY AND CLINICAL SIGNS

Infectious, vascular, traumatic and neoplastic processes involving the brainstem can affect the vagus nerve. Other central signs usually are present such as motor difficulties or proprioceptive losses as well as anomalies of other cranial nerves. Signs described by the owner can include difficulties in swallowing, voice change, an abnormal snoring noise during respiration or symptoms of dyspnoea. These signs are most often associated with a certain degree of laryngeal paralysis. Other diseases can cause paralysis of the larynx and should be included in the differential diagnosis.

CN XI   ACCESSORY NERVE

FUNCTION

The accessory nerve is the motor nerve of the trapezius muscle and part of the sternocephalicus and brachiocephalicus muscles.

ANATOMY AND CLINICAL SIGNS

The motor fibres of the accessory nerve originate in the ventral roots of the cervical segments (C_1 to C_5) and the medulla. The fibres course towards the back of the neck and innervate the trapezius muscle and a portion of the sternocephalicus and brachiocephalicus muscles. These muscles participate in shoulder and upper limb movement and support the neck laterally.

Paralysis of this nerve is rarely seen clinically. Nevertheless, in a case of a lesion, one sees atrophy of the above mentioned muscles, with an eventual deviation of the neck towards the affected side (Figure 2.25).

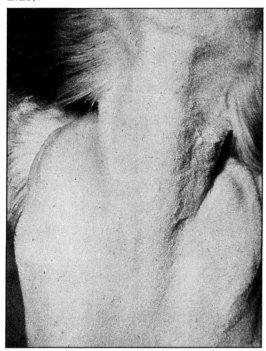

Figure 2.25
Dog with unilateral paralysis of right accessory nerve resulting in atrophy of the trapezius, sternocephalicus and brachiocephalicus muscles.
(Courtesy of Dr. Richard A. LeCouteur, Colorado State University, U.S.A.).

CN XII   HYPOGLOSSAL NERVE

FUNCTION

The hypoglossal nerve is the motor nerve to the intrinsic and extrinsic muscles of the tongue.

ANATOMY AND CLINICAL SIGNS

The neurons forming the hypoglossal nerve originate in the hypoglossal nucleus in the medulla at the level of the fourth ventricle. Lesions affecting part of these neurons can cause a dysfunction of the tongue in swallowing, prehension and mastication.

To evaluate the integrity of CN XII, the tongue and its motor activity are observed. All deviations and dysfunction should be noted. A licking reflex can be elicited by wetting the nose and the motor ability of the tongue can be studied. A deviation of the tongue must always be carefully interpreted. Acute unilateral paralysis induces a deviation of the tongue towards the unaffected side. When the lesions are several days or weeks old, a progressive fibrosis occurs and atrophy of the tongue is seen with retraction or deviation towards the affected side.

Anomalies of CN XII are most often the result of trauma or neoplastic disorders of the face.

ADDITIONAL READING

CHRISMAN, C. L. (1982). *Problems in Small Animal Neurology.* Lea & Febiger Co. Philadelphia.

DELAHUNTA, A. (1977) *Veterinary Neuroanatomy and Clinical Neurology.* W. B. Saunders Co. Philadelphia.

GREENE, C. E. and OLIVER, J. E. (1983). Neurological Examination. In *Textbook of Veterinary Internal Medicine (2nd ed.)* Ettinger, S.J. (ed.). W. B. Saunders Co., Philadelphia.

HOERLEIN, B. F., (1978). Peripheral nervous system. In *Canine Neurology (3rd ed.)* Hoerlein B.F. (ed.) W. B. Saunders Co. Philadelphia.

MOREAU, P. M. (1985). Examen neurologique du chien et du chat: les nerfs crâniens. *Pract. Med. Chir. An. Comp.* **20** (1), 5-22.

MOREAU, P. M. (1985). Examen des nerfs craniens chez le chien et le chat. *Rec. Mid. Vét.* **161** (11), 883-901.

OLIVER, J. E. and LORENZ, M. D. (1983). *Handbook of Veterinary Neurologic Diagnosis.* W. B. Saunders Co. Philadelphia.

REDDING, R. N. and BRAUND, K. G. (1978). Neurological Examination, in *Canine Neurology (3rd ed.)* W. B. Saunders Co. Philadelphia.

SHELL, L. (1982). Cranial nerve disorders in dogs and cats. *Compendium on Continuing Education for the Practicing Veterinarian.* Vol. **4** (6), 458-467.

VENKER-VAN HAAGEN, A. J. *et al.* (1978). Spontaneous laryngeal paralysis in young Bouviers. *J.A.A.H.A.* **14**, 714-720.

CHAPTER 3

NEUROLOGICAL EXAMINATION OF THE LIMBS AND BODY

Ian R. Griffiths B.V.M.S., Ph.D., F.R.C.V.S.

PRINCIPLES UNDERLYING THE NEUROLOGICAL EXAMINATION

Before describing the practical details of the examinations and their interpretation it is essential to understand what the clinician is attempting to achieve. The obvious questions which ideally should be answered are: − a) where is the problem, b) what is causing it, c) how severe is the damage, d) what is the prognosis. (a) and (c) usually can be determined from the clinical examination while (b) often requires further information such as history and ancillary tests.

Upper and lower motor neurones and sensory fibres in relation to limbs

The lower motor neurone (LMN) has its cell body located in the ventral horn of the grey matter with the axon running in the ventral nerve root and peripheral nerve to supply the appropriate muscle. The motor unit is the basic functional unit comprising the LMN and muscle fibres which it supplies. Limb muscles are invariably innervated by fibres originating in more than one spinal segment. The upper motor neurone (UMN) can, oversimplistically, be regarded as a neurone originating in some motor centre in the brain and travelling down the spinal cord to synapse, via interneurones, with the LMN (Figure 3.1.).

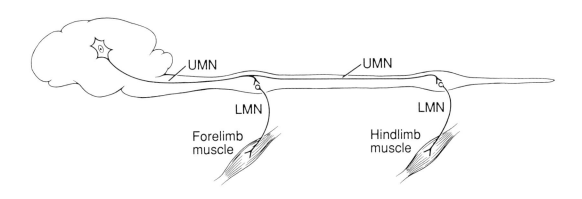

Figure 3.1
Diagramatic representation of upper (UMN) and lower (LMN) motorneurones supplying the limbs.
The UMN is shown as a single neuronal pathway and no interneurones are included.

The LMN is the final common pathway for motor activity, whether voluntary or reflex. Most of our clinical tests examine local limb reflexes that require afferent fibres and perhaps interneurones to complete the reflex arc. The type of peripheral receptor and afferent fibre will vary according to the nature of the reflex and the stimulus used to initiate it (eg noxious stimuli or muscle stretch) (Figures 3.1 & 3.2).

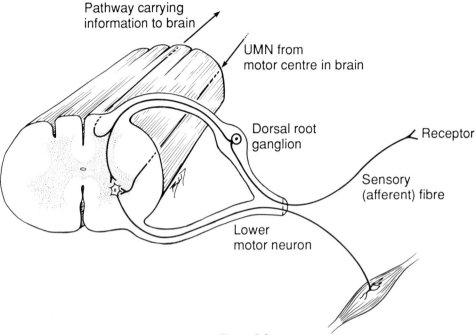

Figure 3.2

Representation of a simple reflex arc which serves a clinically-testable reflex. Damage to either the LMN or the sensory fibre or both will interrupt the reflex. This feature is used in separating lesions in these neurones from those in the UMN or in sensory pathways in the spinal cord.

The effect of lesions on these pathways

These are best appreciated by reference to Figure 3.2 and Table 3.1.

Motor problems (eg weakness or paralysis in limb(s)) should be classified as either UMN or LMN in type. The major clinical differentiation is their effect on muscle tone, local reflexes and muscle bulk. Variation in the severity of damage can cause gradation of signs. In acute LMN lesions, the depression or loss of tone and reflexes occurs early, while atrophy takes up to three weeks to become evident. In more chronic LMN lesions atrophy can be obvious by the time the animal is first presented.

Table 3.2 compares the effects of LMN and afferent fibre lesions. Some effects such as reflex loss may be common to both. In many peripheral nerve diseases or injuries, both sensory and motor fibres are damaged, causing a combination of the signs.

Table 3.1. Differentiation of upper and lower motor neurone lesions

| | LMN | | UMN | |
	Complete	Partial	Complete	Partial
Motor Function	Paralysis	Paresis	Paralysis	Paresis
Muscle tone	Absent	Decreased	Present but may be altered in character	
Local reflexes	Absent	Depressed	Present but may be altered in character	
Muscle atrophy	Severe*	Less severe	Minimal	Minimal
*The atrophy will take some time, 2—3 weeks +, to become clinically obvious.				

*Reproduced by permission from In Practice (1982) **4**, 44*

INITIAL NON-NEUROLOGICAL EXAMINATION

It is assumed that general systemic examinations will be performed. In many instances these are best done before the neural examination as systemic disease can affect these tests even if the nervous system does not appear directly involved. For example, a dog with severe cachexia or hypovolaemic shock will not react to neurological testing in a similar way to one in which these features are absent.

There are also certain non-neurological conditions which, on superficial examination, may be confused with nervous disease. Following acute trauma, pelvic fractures or bilateral limb fractures can produce a state somewhat resembling paraplegia due to a spinal injury. Acute bilateral anterior cruciate rupture can also lead to confusion and in all instances the femoral pulses should be checked. The moral, therefore, is to make sure there are no orthopaedic or vascular problems which could be misdiagnosed.

NEUROLOGICAL EXAMINATION

Disturbances in gait are one of the most common reasons for neurological investigation, usually presenting as a motor problem (paresis or paralysis), inco-ordination (ataxia) or a combination of these. The first stage of the physical examination usually involves ascertaining the animal's ability to make co-ordinated movements. Often, this can be achieved by watching the animal walk or attempt to walk. If this is not possible it can be supported as necessary so that any movement, however weak, can be noted. At the end of this stage it should be possible to determine which limbs are involved, if there is lateralisation of signs and if weakness and/or ataxia is present. It can sometimes be difficult to distinguish the effects of weakness and ataxia on the gait. Ataxia due to spinal or peripheral lesions commonly produces a swaying, swaggering gait, with occasional hypermetria and catching of limbs. It gives the impression of misapplied power and is best observed at a slow steady pace rather than a faster walk. Pure motor signs can be seen in diseases like myasthenia gravis and motor polyneuropathies. In such instances, the animal has a stiff, stilted gait taking shorter strides, often has a degree of postural tremor and usually collapses or rests after a short distance. The movements, however, remain co-ordinated. In many conditions both ataxia and weakness are present.

Table 3.2
Comparison and differentiation of lower motor neurone
and sensory neurone lesions

	LMN	SENSORY
Motor Function	Paralysis/paresis	Present but may be ataxic
Sensory Function	Normal	Deficit*
Local reflexes	Absent/depressed	Absent/depressed*
Muscle tone	Absent/reduced	Probably reduced*
Muscle atrophy	Severe	Mild

*The exact sensory deficit and the involvement of reflexes and tone will depend on type(s) of sensory fibre affected. e.g. if large diameter primary afferents from spindles are involved, the patellar reflex and muscle tone would be affected.

Following acute trauma where a spinal injury is suspected the animal should not be encouraged to move until the nature of the damage is known. Some indication of motor function may be gained by watching spontaneous attempts to move, but efforts to support the animal and encourage it to move could lead to further spinal damage.

Motor function can also be assessed in the tail but it is important to ensure that tail wagging is spontaneous. Reflex wagging can occur after spinal cord injuries if the dog is handled around the hind end. Axial weakness may be indicated by the inability to hold up the head and support the trunk, resulting in a 'floppy dog'.

More specific examination of motor function can then be made. By lifting a contralateral limb the strength of the ipsilateral extensor muscles can be assessed. For example, weakness in the triceps would lead to dropping of the elbow. Some of the flexor groups can be tested for their ability to move the limb against gravity, for example, in attempting an ocular placing reflex the elbow joint is flexed to lift the lower limb onto the table surface. The wheelbarrow test (where the weight is taken on both forelegs during walking while the rear end is supported) and the hopping test (where the weight is taken on a single forelimb during walking) are very useful to unmask latent paresis in the forelegs. Weakness is usually demonstrated by the dog knuckling on that limb, the head and neck dropping, and the animal tending to somersault. The weakness can be the result of UMN, LMN, muscle and sometimes orthopaedic problems.

Co-ordination can be examined further by turning the animal in circles, especially on a slippery surface, and by walking up or particularly down steps. Tests such as hemistepping are also useful. Co-ordination of gait and movements requires intact unconscious proprioceptive information from the limbs as well as other inputs from eyes, vestibular system etc. These inputs and the resultant adjustment of motor function are mediated via the cerebellum. Other tests are designed to look at conscious proprioception, that is, the conscious awareness of limb position and movement which depends on connections to the somatosensory cortex. These tests are paw position sense, reflex stepping and sway response. Paw position is tested by turning the foot so that the dorsum of the paw is in contact with the ground. A normal animal will return the foot to a normal position immediately whereas one with a proprioceptive deficit may leave the foot in the inverted position. The reflex step is tested by placing a sheet of paper beneath the foot and pulling it sideways; the normal animal rapidly returning the foot to a standing position. The weight of the animal's body should be supported during these tests and each limb assessed individually. The sway response is tested by pushing the trunk sideways and observing the animal regain a normal upright position. Animals with neurological deficits may find this difficult or even fall over. In spinal cord and peripheral nerve disease it is common for any defects in conscious proprioception to be accompanied by abnormalities in unconscious proprioception though this is not always so. The conscious proprioceptive tests do require a motor response and it is therefore pointless to perform them if the animal has insufficient motor function to return the limb to the correct position.

EXAMINATION OF INDIVIDUAL LIMBS

A general visual examination may reveal worn nails or scuffed paws suggesting dragging or knuckling of the limb. Atrophy is detected by vision and palpation. Determine if the atrophy is generalised or selective, taking into account the duration of the disease and the animal's general physical state. If a unilateral condition is present, compare side to side.

Muscle tone and local limb reflexes are assessed with the animal lying relaxed on its side. In most instances sufficient relaxation can be achieved but, in tense animals, muscle tone and the patellar reflex can be markedly affected.

Muscle tone.

This is the resistance to passive stretch and depends chiefly on the stretch reflex. It is assessed by flexing or extending a joint to stretch an appropriate muscle, for example, flexing the stifle joint will stretch the quadriceps muscle. The resistance to stretch is graded subjectively by the clinician as being within normal range, increased or decreased. Increased tone can be subdivided into: a) spasticity where the tone increases after an initial period of stretch (the free interval) during which resistance is normal; b) rigidity where there is no initial free interval. This differentiation of spasticity and rigidity is perhaps not so important in veterinary neurology as in human medicine. In these states of hypertonia, the resistance will usually decrease after initially increasing. This can be a gradual lessening of resistance or involve a sudden collapse of the limb — the clasp knife phenomenon.

Spasticity is usually associated with UMN lesions either in the spinal cord or brain stem. Rigidity may be seen in certain muscle diseases such as Cushing's disease myopathy or the polyneuromyositis of Toxoplasma gondii and in the interneuronal destruction caused by ischaemia of the intermediate grey matter.

Hypotonia is seen in LMN lesions or in sensory neuropathies affecting the larger diameter afferent fibres. It should be remembered that in many neurological disorders, muscle tone is within normal limits.

Patellar reflex.

This is an example of a phasic stretch reflex initiated by tapping the patellar ligament, thus causing a synchronised activation of the muscle spindles. The response is a twitch-like muscle contraction of the quadriceps muscle causing the lower leg to move forward before relaxing. At the end of this contraction/relaxation there are almost imperceptible oscillations as the movement is damped down. The afferent and efferent pathways are in the femoral nerve and the central connections lie in segments L_4, L_5 and L_6. In most relaxed dogs the reflex is obtained easily but is more difficult in pups, cats and tense dogs. The test should be performed in the uppermost leg with the stifle slightly flexed to provide some stretch to the muscle. If there is some doubt as to whether a response is present or not, perhaps because the dog is tense, then the lower limb should be tested as this often is more relaxed. As this limb is against the surface of the table it is difficult to observe the character of the response but its presence or absence can be verified. In young pups, the reflex may also be tested by suspending the pup under the forelimbs and allowing the hind limbs to dangle.

In UMN lesions the reflex usually is present but may be altered in character. In severe, acute spinal injuries, the response may be decreased for several days following the damage. Typically, in UMN lesions, the response may be exaggerated with a tendency to oscillate at the end of the relaxation phase, that is, clonus. Less commonly, clonus may be observed when muscle tone is increased. Under these circumstances there is a rhythmic series of contractions, mainly during the relaxation phase of the response.

The reflex is depressed or absent in LMN lesions or those involving the larger diameter sensory fibres. As femoral nerve lesions are relatively uncommon, this situation is usually seen in polyneuropathies or in diseases or injuries affecting the lumbar enlargement and appropriate nerve roots, for example fractures of L_4 or L_5, or nerve root tumours. The reflex may also be depressed or absent in some cases of degenerative myelopathy where there is involvement of larger diameter afferent fibres in the dorsal nerve roots.

In some sciatic nerve lesions, the patellar reflex, while present, may oscillate excessively due to the paralysis of the antagonistic hamstring muscles.

Pedal reflex.

This is also known as the flexor or withdrawal reflex and involves the withdrawal of the limb from a painful stimulus. The receptors are the free nerve endings in the skin, sensitive to noxious stimuli and the afferent pathways are in small myelinated fibres. The motor output is to all the flexor muscle groups in the limb and therefore involves several peripheral nerves and spinal cord segments. The stifle and hock flexors are innervated chiefly from segments L_6, L_7 and S_1, via branches of the sciatic nerve. The hip flexors have more widespread innervation mainly from lumbar segments and the femoral nerves.

To test the reflex, the inter-digital skin is squeezed between the index finger and thumb (in some cases it may be necessary to place forceps across the animal's nail), at the same time putting slight longitudinal tension on the limb so that it must be withdrawn against such tension. This allows some assessment of the strength of the flexor groups. It is important to observe that all the flexor groups are functional as it is not unusual to uncover selective weakness in muscles, most commonly in the hock flexors.

In UMN lesions, the reflex should be present but it is common to find a prolonged contraction continuing after the cessation of the noxious stimulus. In addition to the withdrawal reflex, other reflex activities may be noted: a) the crossed extensor reflex in which there is extension of the contralateral limb as the ipsilateral limb is flexed, b) reflex tail wagging which also occurs while the toes are being pinched.

In LMN lesions, all or parts of the reflex may be lost depending on the location of the damage in the cord or peripheral nerves.

Anal reflex.

Although not a limb reflex, this function should be assessed as it gives information regarding the integrity of the sacral segments and nerve roots and is obviously important for faecal continence. It should be observed if the anus is closed or gaping and the perianal skin should be flicked. This will result in a wink-like contraction of the sphincter, usually accompanied by a downward movement of the tail head and an upward movement of the vulva. Finally, and if necessary, anal tone can be assessed during a rectal examination. In LMN lesions involving the sacral segments or cauda equina, the reflex may be lost and the anus may be flaccid.

Local reflexes in the forelegs.

Tendon reflexes − biceps and triceps tendon jerks − can be elicited but are inconsistent in normal dogs. It is probably not worthwhile performing these tests. The pedal reflex is obtained in the same manner as for the hind-legs, noting if there is flexion of shoulder, elbow and carpal joints.

OTHER FUNCTIONS TO BE ASSESSED

Panniculus Reflex.

This is the well known twitch of the skin over an animal's back in response to a stimulus over that area. The effector organ is the panniculus carnosus muscle innervated by the lateral thoracic nerve, which originates from the caudal brachial plexus and receives its fibres from segments C_8 and T_1. The receptive field is a saddle-shaped area over the chest wall and flank extending to, or just caudal to, the iliac crest. Although there is an output for the reflex at C_8 / T_1, the afferent side is organised on a dermatomal basis with inputs at many segmental levels from about T_3 to L_1 representing the area of skin over the trunk. Interneurones, probably located in the ventrolateral white matter, connect the afferent and efferent pathways (Figure 3.3).

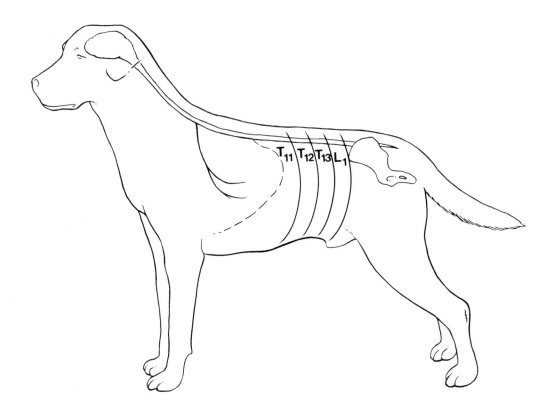

Figure 3.3
Outline of the panniculus reflex to show the single outflow at $C_8 - T_1$ the caudal borders of dermatomes $T_{11} - L_1$. These have been identified by matching the level of 'cut off' of the reflex to underlying cord damage as determined at post-mortem. If, for example, a lesion was present at T_{12} then T_{11} would be the intact segment immediately rostral to this and the panniculus 'cut-off' would be just behind the last rib as indicated.

Using a light pin prick, the skin is stimulated about $2-3$ cm lateral to the mid-line starting at the level of the iliac crest. The response should be a twitch of the skin which usually is stronger ipsilaterally but can be bilateral. This twitch should be distinguished from the lordotic movement of the back that sometimes occurs in response to the prick and represents a withdrawal reflex from a painful stimulus. If the panniculus reflex is not present at the level of the iliac crest the stimulation should proceed rostrally until a line is found above which the twitch occurs. This level represents the caudal border of the last intact dermatome. Sometimes, reflex tail wagging is noted as the skin is stimulated behind this level.

Damage to the outflow can also occur either with cord lesions at C_8/T_1 or, more commonly, avulsion of these nerve roots (brachial plexus root avulsion). In such circumstances, the skin twitch is absent over the whole of the receptive area, ipsilaterally in the case of root avulsions and perhaps bilaterally with cord damage. With nerve root avulsions a strong consensual response usually is evident.

The panniculus reflex can, therefore, often be used to locate the site of damage either to the spinal cord or nerve roots/brachial plexus. In thoracolumbar cord lesions the cut-off represents the caudal border of the last intact dermatome cranial to the lesion indicating that the rostral extent of the damage is the next caudal segment. The caudal levels of dermatomes can be determined by various experimental or clinical methods and show some variation according to the technique used and the sensory modality tested. Figure 3.3 illustrates the caudal borders of dermatomes around the thoraco-lumbar area as determined by the site of 'cut off' of the panniculus reflex correlated with the location of the underlying cord lesion. (This map does not necessarily correspond to one obtained using other methods, for example, electrophysiological recordings from nerve roots.)

If an animal has lost pain sensation behind a cord lesion it is usual to find the panniculus 'cut off' and level of pain sensory loss correspond, but the two functions are not inter-related and it is common to find animals with intact pain sensation and interruption of the panniculus reflex. The panniculus reflex will only show abnormalities if the lesion is within the appropriate anatomical area, i.e. $C_8 - L_1$. Therefore, cervical cord, lower lumbar and sacral problems should have an intact reflex. In certain circumstances lesions can also occur between C_8 and L_1 and leave the panniculus reflex intact. Very mild damage is often not associated with panniculus loss and some diseases may spare the interneurones concerned with the reflex. For example, in degenerative myelopathy, degeneration occurs in the thoracic and lumbar white matter, but the panniculus reflex invariably is intact. In traumatic or compressive myelopathies between C_8 and L_1, it would be highly unusual for the panniculus not to be affected with a lesion sufficient to cause more than moderate paraparesis.

Assessment of pain sensation.

The appreciation of pain is obviously subjective and whether an animal is feeling pain must be inferred by its response to noxious stimuli. The quality and intensity of pain can be modified at a number of levels in the CNS. As can be commonly observed, individuals respond differently to apparently identical stimuli. In a single animal some comparisons can be made between fore and hind limbs or left and right sides.

Assessment of pain sensation requires a noxious stimulus and an evaluation of the animal's response. In regard to limbs, the interdigital skin is usually pinched between finger and thumb. A greater stimulus can be provided by gripping the nail with forceps. It is advisable to stimulate both medial and lateral sides of the foot. Forcep pressure can also be used on the tail. The use of pin prick needs careful evaluation. If it can be shown that a response is absent from stimulation in one area and present from another similar area, this may have value. However, failure to respond to pin prick should not be taken as evidence of absent or diminished pain sensation.

In general terms, one is looking for a response from the 'front end' of the animal. This may involve yelping, snarling, attempting to bite, turning to look at the stimulated site, licking the lips, or even a 'hurt expression' of the eyes. The response will vary from dog to dog. A movement (e.g. a withdrawal) of the stimulated area from the noxious stimulus will probably be the result of a local reflex and should not be taken as evidence of pain sensation.

Over the limbs, loss of pain sensation may occur as the result of a cord/nerve root problem or peripheral nerve lesions. Cord or root damage will cause loss in a dermatomal pattern corresponding to the caudal border of the last intact dermatome.

Bladder function

Bladder control and continence are obviously most important and may be impaired in spinal cord or cauda equina lesions. The local parasympathetic innervation of the bladder is from the sacral segments via the pelvic nerves while the urethral sphincter is also innervated from these segments via the pudendal (pudic) nerve. Besides local segmental innervation of the bladder, long supra-spinal reflexes to centres in the reticular formation are necessary for micturition. Spinal cord injury rostral to the sacral segments (the equivalent of an UMN lesion) may damage these connections resulting in inability to urinate. The damage, which must be bilateral, usually results in urinary retention and overflow — a large volume distended bladder with dribbling of urine. Injuries to the sacral segments, sacral nerve roots or pelvic nerves (LMN) can either cause a similar situation or a small volume bladder also with incontinence (see Chapter 12).

Following damage rostral to the sacral cord, recovery may occur or an automatic bladder, emptying reflexly to raised intracystic pressure, may develop. Full recovery following LMN lesions can occur but is less likely.

The involvement of the bladder following cord injury and disease depends markedly on the type and severity of the lesion and in many instances function is unaffected. In many types of polyneuropathy, bladder control is spared.

Bladder function can be assessed by

a. Asking the owner or watching if the animal can pass urine in a stream (many dogs with loss of control will void urine if picked up in such a way as to increase intra-abdominal pressure).

b. Looking for evidence of urine wetting around the prepuce or vulva (inability to move could also cause this).

c. Manual pressure on the abdomen causing expression of urine which ceases once the pressure is withdrawn.

d. Dribbling of urine.

For a fuller discussion of bladder function see Chapter 12.

Sympathetic function.

The cell bodies of the preganglionic fibres lie in the thoracic and rostral lumbar segments. After synapsing in sympathetic ganglia, many post- ganglionic fibres supply peripheral blood vessels. Structures in the head receive their sympathetic innervation from the first few thoracic segments via the vagosympathetic trunk. Central sympathetic fibres descend from various brain stem nuclei to synapse with the preganglionic fibres and it is these descending fibres which may be damaged in cord disease.

Two major effects may be noted.

a. Skin hyperthermia due to loss of vascular tone and increased skin blood flow. In cervical lesions this can affect the head, body and limbs whereas in thoracic lesions the body and limbs caudal to the lesion are involved.

b. Horner's syndrome following cervical cord, T_1 nerve root, vagosympathetic trunk or post-ganglionic (usually middle ear) lesions. A complete Horner's syndrome consists of myosis (the pupil will respond to changes in light intensity), ptosis of the upper lid, protrusion of the membrana nictitans and slight enophthalmos. In T_1 nerve root lesions, usually caused by brachial plexus avulsion, a partial Horner's syndrome with myosis is the usual evidence of sympathetic damage (See Chapters 2 and 9).

In other peripheral nerve injuries the affected limb may also appear warmer due to sympathetic damage. In most instances, skin hyperthermia, due to either central or peripheral lesions, is seen only in the acute stages and later resolves. Also, in many cases of cord disease or injury, the sympathetic system remains intact.

Schiff-Sherrington phenomenon

Following damage (usually severe) to the upper thoracic cord the forelimbs may become rigidly extended, with marked increase in extensor tone. Even when the toes are pinched the withdrawal may be sluggish because of the extension. Voluntary movement is still present although it is markedly reduced by hypertonia. This extension of the limbs is known as the Schiff-Sherrington phenomenon and is associated with either direct damage to the rostral thoracic cord or extension of damage from a more caudal level into the upper thoracic segments, for example, in the ascending syndrome following thoracolumbar disc protrusions. The Schiff-Sherrington phenomenon is almost invariably an indication of poor prognosis.

Paradoxical respiration

During normal inspiration, the rib cage is tensed and rotated outward and forward by the action of intercostal and other muscle groups, while the diaphragm flattens. These procedures decrease endothoracic pressure and cause the inward movement of air. If all or the majority of the chest wall is paralysed, respiration is achieved by diaphragmatic movement while the thoracic wall moves passively with changes in thoracic pressure. The chest wall therefore moves inward during inspiration. Paradoxical respiration is seen with high thoracic cord lesions which sever the descending pathways to intercostal motorneurones or extensively damage the motorneurones themselves. It may well be concurrent with the Schiff-Sherrington phenomenon.

PROCEDURE FOR NEUROLOGICAL EXAMINATION OF SPINAL CORD AND PERIPHERAL NERVES

(Following history and systemic examinations)

Procedure

1. Watch the animal walk and stand (support if necessary).

2. More specific tests of weakness (hopping, wheelbarrow, etc.).

3. Conscious proprioceptive tests (paw position, sway, reflex stepping)

> Great care
> in acute
> spinal injuries

4. Lie animal on side for local hind-limb examination

    a. Muscle tone

    b. Patellar reflex

    c. Pedal reflex — at the same time check conscious pain sensation

    d. Muscle atrophy

5. Forelimb examination

    a. Muscle tone

    b. Pedal reflex — check conscious pain sensation

    c. Atrophy

6. Panniculus reflex

7. Skin temperatures (compare left to right — front to hind)

8. Horner's syndrome (and cranial nerve examination)

9. Other signs e.g. Schiff – Sherrington, neck pain, paradoxical respiration.

10. Bladder function

LOCALISATION OF CORD AND NERVE LESIONS CAUSING LIMB SIGNS

After obtaining the history and watching the animal walk (if appropriate) some judgement on localisation can be formed on the basis of probability.

a. **'Motor signs (weakness/paralysis) and/or ataxia in fore and hind limbs'**

    — spinal cord lesions in cervical cord or brain, or a diffuse peripheral nerve problem (polyneuropathy)

b. **'Motor signs more pronounced in forelimbs than in hind-limbs'**

    — probably cervical cord problem or, less likely, a bilateral peripheral problem in forelegs.

c. **'Motor signs and/or ataxia in hind-limbs with normal foreleg function'**

    — Spinal cord lesions below brachial outflow or bilateral peripheral problem in hind limbs.

d. **'Monoparesis/plegia'**

    — most probably peripheral nerve problem in that limb.

Brain lesions will not be described further here as they are discussed in Chapters 2 and 8.

Assuming that a motor problem is present, the next stage is to ascertain whether it is UMN or LMN or a combined UMN/LMN deficit. This is based on the presence or absence of local limb reflexes, muscle tone and atrophy as discussed above and in Table 3.1. This categorisation of the motor problem allows further definition of the lesion as indicated in Table 3.3 and Fig.3.4. Other tests or signs may then be used for more precise localisation as indicated in Table 3.4.

LMN signs in a limb can be caused by lesions within the vertebral canal damaging the cell bodies, proximal motor axons and ventral nerve roots or by more peripheral, extraspinal problems. Bilaterality of signs does not always indicate a central lesion as many polyneuropathies are bilaterally symmetrical. Extraspinal problems are less likely to be associated with urinary or faecal signs.

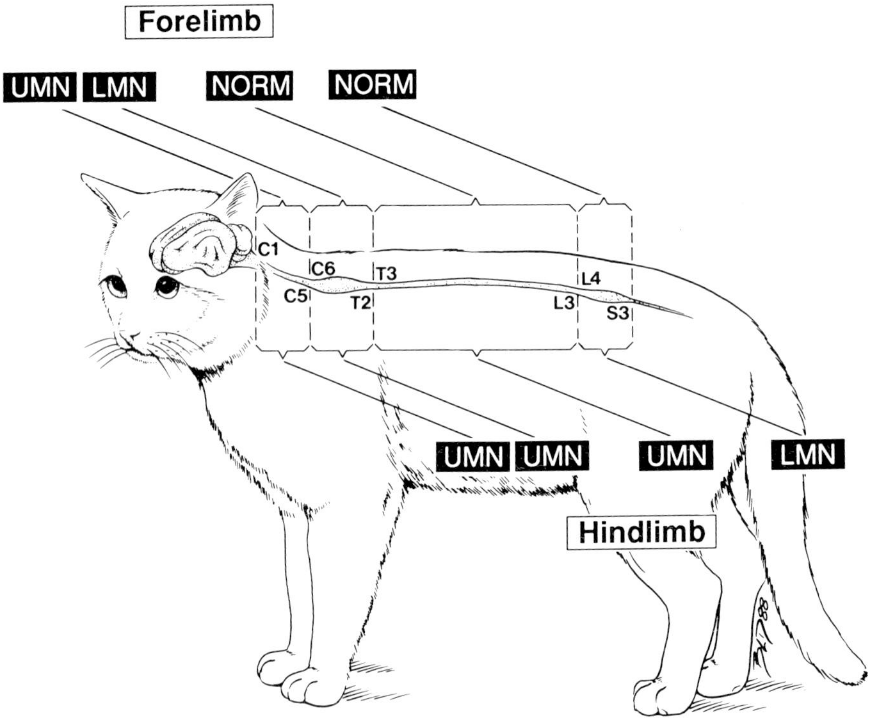

Figure 3.4
To be used in conjunction with Table 3.3. The diagram of the spinal cord segments indicates how damage at a particular area can affect motor function in fore or hind-limbs in terms of causing an upper or a lower motor neurone type of dysfunction. (From Wheeler S.J. (1989) Spinal Tumours in Cats. In *Veterinary Annual* **29**, 270-277, reproduced by permission).

Table 3.3

Type of Motor Problem	Probable location(s) of lesion
1. UMN signs FL and HL	Cervical cord or brain
2. LMN signs FL UMN signs HL	Lower cervical cord
3. LMN signs FL Normal HL	Cervical nerve roots or peripheral nerves in FL
4. Normal FL UMN signs HL	Thoracic or upper lumbar cord
5. Normal FL LMN signs in HL	Lower lumbar/sacral cord or cauda equina or peripheral nerves in HL.
6. LMN signs FL and HL	Peripheral polyneuropathy
FL = Forelimb HL = Hindlimb	UMN = Upper motor neurone type deficit LMN = Lower motor neurone type deficit

LOCALISATION OF SENSORY SIGNS

In some spinal and peripheral disorders ataxia is the predominant sign. This results from defects in proprioceptive transmission to or within the CNS or within the central co-ordinating unit — the cerebellum. In this chapter we will be concerned with localisation of spinal and peripheral forms.

Where a peripheral nerve problem is causing ataxia it is likely that there will also be conscious proprioceptive deficits, loss of muscle tone and depression or absence of the patellar reflex (Figure 3.2 and Table 3.2). The pedal reflex and pain sensation are usually spared as they are mediated by small diameter fibres on the afferent side. Using presence/absence of tone and tendon reflexes it should be possible to distinguish spinal and peripherally located ataxia. With an ataxia of spinal origin there may be additional signs such

Table 3.4
Signs used for localisation of lesions

The signs listed are those useful for localisation and not the entire range of signs. e.g. loss of bladder control could occur depending on the severity of the lesion but would not be a particularly useful localising sign. It is also possible that some or all of the signs might not be present in certain conditions.

Motor Sympathetic Others	**Upper cervical cord** UMN type in FL and HL (sometimes FL more severe than HL). Horner's syndrome. Skin hyperthermia over head and body. Neck pain/stiffness.
Motor Sympathetic Panniculus	**Lower cervical cord and T$_1$** UMN type HL LMN type in some muscles of FL Horner's syndrome. Skin hyperthermia over head and body Absent if C$_8$/T$_1$ involved. Loss of pain sensation is unlikely in cervical lesions as damage of such severity is likely to cause respiratory failure.
Motor Sympathetic Respiration Panniculus Sensation	**Upper thoracic cord** UMN type HL FL possibly normal. Could be Schiff-Sherrington phenomenon present Skin hyperthermia behind lesion Paradoxical Restricted to area immediately caudal to shoulder May also be restricted.
Motor Sympathetic Panniculus Sensation	**Middle, lower thoracic cord and L$_1$** UMN type HL FL normal Skin hyperthermia behind lesion Cut off at level of last intact dermatome May also be restricted.
Motor Panniculus Sensation	**L$_2$ and L$_3$** UMN type HL FL normal Intact May also be restricted.
Motor Anal reflex Sensation	**L$_4$ — Sacral segments** LMN type in some muscle groups of hind limbs Lost if sacral segments involved May be restricted in dermatomal distribution over limbs
	Cauda equina syndrome* Mild distal hind-limb weakness and proprioceptive defects Urinary and faecal incontinence Loss of anal reflex Paralysis and anaesthesia of tail Loss of perineal sensation Lumbo-sacral pain *The combination of signs will vary with the cause of the problem.

as those involving the panniculus reflex, sympathetic function etc., as listed in Table 3.4. Whether such localising signs are present or not depends largely on the pathological changes. Gross tissue destruction due to injury, compression or inflammation will often show localisation while more subtle degenerative disorders do not.

Estimating the severity of the lesion

There is no all-embracing strategy for estimating the severity of damage which is applicable to every type of condition. The severity at any particular stage is judged by the degree of functional deficit which may not be a static parameter but can increase or decrease as the lesion progresses or resolves. In essence, the cord consists of white and grey matter and, while a gross oversimplification, the white matter can be regarded as transmitting impulses rostrally or caudally and the grey matter as relaying these impulses to and from the periphery.

Using this scheme the clinically-important segments of grey matter are those innervating the limbs, respiratory muscles, bladder and sphincters — essentially the cervical and lumbar enlargements. Damage to these segments will denervate clinically-important muscles. The severity can be judged by the degree of LMN damage — paresis or paralysis, depressed or absent reflexes and the amount of atrophy. As neurones are not replaced, any marked or progressive loss will have serious consequences.

Table 3.5

A system for evaluating the severity of white matter damage to spinal cord segments following injury or compression. It is based on assessment of motor and bladder function and deep pain sensation behind the level of the lesion.

1.	Weakness. Varying from mild to severe paresis.
2.	Paralysis. Paraplegia or quadriplegia of an UMN type.
3.	Paralysis (as in 2) and loss of bladder control (usually urinary retention and overflow).
4.	Paralysis and loss of bladder control (as in 3) and loss of deep pain sensation. (This level of severity is not usually compatible with survival in cervical cord injuries.)

In evaluating white matter damage we need to choose assessable functions which are normally transmitted across the damaged segment. Usually, motor and bladder function and deep pain sensation are used. With increasing severity of damage these functions tend to be impaired and lost in that order. This scheme is particularly useful for cord injuries and compression and such cases could be graded as in Table 3.5.

Cervical cord injury or compression often causes less severe signs than lesions in the thoracolumbar area. One obvious reason is the different vertebral canal/spinal cord diameter ratios. It is highly unlikely that a cervical cord lesion with loss of pain sensation caudally would not also be associated with respiratory failure. Cervical cord damage often results in motor deficit (quadriparesis or plegia) and occasionally in loss of bladder control. Damage to the cervical enlargement will also cause grey matter destruction and LMN signs in the forelegs. As mentioned above, this often has more serious consequences than damage confined solely to white matter.

In thoracolumbar lesions (e.g. disc protrusions) we are concerned essentially with white matter damage, the severity of which is judged as described above in Table 3.5.

In injuries and compressions the prognosis usually correlates with the severity and the scheme indicated in Table 3.5 will provide a good guide of this damage. However, this system cannot be transferred directly to other disease categories such as inflammatory and degenerative myelopathies. For example, a dog with a disc protrusion could be paraplegic and recover completely whereas dogs with viral myelitis or degenerative myelopathy might only be paretic and yet have a very poor or hopeless prognosis.

ANCILLARY DIAGNOSTIC AIDS

INTRODUCTION

This chapter covers some of the ancillary diagnostic aids available to the clinician which are useful in the identification of nervous system diseases. The indications for the tests, their performance and the interpretation of results are discussed. The chapter covers the following topics:

Part 1.

Haematology, Biochemistry, Cerebrospinal fluid analysis and other clinicopathological investigations.

Richard J. Evans

Part 2.

Electromyography and nerve conduction studies

Ian D. Duncan

Part 3.

Electroencephalography

John Barker

Part 4.

Urodynamic studies

Nicholas J. H. Sharp

Part 5.

Muscle and nerve biopsy

Simon J. Wheeler

HAEMATOLOGY, BIOCHEMISTRY, CEREBROSPINAL FLUID ANALYSIS AND OTHER CLINICOPATHOLOGICAL INVESTIGATIONS

Richard J. Evans M.A., Ph.D., Vet. M.B., M.R.C.V.S.

THE ROLE OF CLINICAL PATHOLOGY IN NEUROLOGICAL INVESTIGATIONS

Clinical pathological determinations have two roles in the investigation of patients with signs of nervous dysfunction. In some cases, apparent nervous signs will be due to disturbance of neural or muscular function secondary to a systemic disease or to a generalised metabolic disturbance. In such cases, clinical pathology is essential in the identification of the underlying cause and this is the major role for such tests. Clinical pathology is limited in value in diseases which directly involve nervous tissue. Diagnostically helpful changes in the peripheral blood are only seen rarely in primary neurological conditions. Faecal examination rarely is helpful, as parasitic infections which affect the CNS generally are not patent at the time when CNS signs become apparent. The occurrence of seizures or tetany, episodic or persistent weakness, collapse, coma, multifocal or variable signs are all circumstances where the clinician should investigate the possibility of an underlying generalised or systemic disease being present (Table 4.1). Clinical pathological investigation also may be required to monitor the consequences of nervous or muscular diseases.

CLINICAL PATHOLOGY IN GENERALISED DISORDERS INDUCING NEUROLOGICAL SIGNS

The generalised disorders which may induce or mimic neurological dysfunction may be divided into eight overlapping categories:

Disturbance of oxygen transport

Inflammatory disease

Acquired disturbance of intermediary metabolism

Acquired electrolyte or acid-base disturbances

Inherited metabolic disorders

Intoxications

Haematopoietic neoplasia involving the CNS

Diseases of muscle

Acquired systemic disturbances, and the signs to which they give rise are detailed in Table 4.1. The underlying causes of these changes are give in Table 4.2.

Table 4.1

Clinical signs which may be seen in association with
some important metabolic derangements

Hypoxia
Cyanosis
Neuromuscular weakness
Ataxia
Collapse
Seizures
Coma

Hypoglycaemia
Dullness/depression
Neuromuscular weakness
Collapse
Seizures
Coma

**Hyperglycaemia/hyperosmolarity/
ketoacidosis**
Polydipsia/polyuria
Depression
Coma
Neuromuscular weakness
Arrythmias
Shock

Blood hyperviscosity
Polydipsia
Episodic variable neurological signs
Transient disorientation
Transient weakness
Transient collapse
Convulsions

Hypernatraemia
Peripheral and pulmonary oedema
Polydipsia/polyuria
Coma
Neuromuscular weakness
Paresis
Seizures

Hyponatraemia
Anorexia
Disorientation
Neuromuscular weakness
Incoordination
Collapse
Seizures
Cyanosis
Shock

**With normal extracellular
fluid volume**
Often asymptomatic

**With diminished extracellular
fluid volume**
Low pulse volume
Decreased skin turgor
Diminished intraocular pressure

**With expanded extracellular
fluid volume**
Generalised or pulmonary oedema

Hyperkalaemia
Cardiac arrest
Vomiting
Diarrhoea
Anorexia
Bradycardia
Weak pulse
Depression
Neuromuscular weakness
Paralysis
Disorientation
Ileus

Hypokalaemia
Dullness/depression
Disorientation
Severe neuromuscular weakness
Tetany
Failure of urine concentration
Polyuria/polydipsia
Cardiac arrythmias
Coma

Hypercalcaemia
Polyuria/polydipsia
Depression
Neuromuscular weakness
Cardiac arrythmias
Lameness/Bone pain/Pathological
   fractures

Hypocalcaemia
Tetany
Weakness
Seizures

Uraemia
Polyuria/polydipsia
Anorexia
Depression
Muscle weakness
Tremors
Seizures
Tetany
Vomiting
Diarrhoea
Uraemic odour
Failure of urine concentration

Hyperammonaemia
Signs may be prominent after
   high-protein meal
Anorexia
Depression
Aimless walking
Head pressing
Seizures
Hysteria
Aimless/unpredictable aggression
Coma
Polydipsia/polyuria
Vomiting
Diarrhoea
Cortical blindness
   (may be transient)

Table 4.2

Some conditions resulting in systemic derangements

Local or generalised hypoxia

Cardiac insufficiency
Haemorrhage
Vagal syncope
Airway obstruction
Severe anaemia
Toxic conversion of haemoglobin to
    derivatives not supporting oxygen
    transport
Hyperviscosity
Vascular spasm
Thrombosis
Embolism

Hyperviscosity

Polycythaemia
Plasma cell myeloma (IgM secreting)
Haemagglutinin disease

**Hyperglycaemia/hyperosmolarity/
    ketoacidosis**

Uncontrolled diabetes mellitus

Hyperosmolarity

Hypernatraemia
Hyperglycaemia
Uraemia

Hypoglycaemia

Functional islet cell tumours
    (insulinomas)
Insulin overdose
Hypoadrenocorticism
Hepatic failure
Glycogenosis
Starvation
Neonatal glycogen depletion
Exercise

Hypernatraemia

Excess dietary sodium intake coupled
    with water restriction
Diabetes insipidus or mellitus
    plus water restriction

Hyponatraemia

Vomiting
Diarrhoea
Hypoadrenocorticism

Hyperkalaemia

Hypoadrenocorticism
Renal failure
Urinary tract obstruction
Acidosis
Iatrogenic
    (potassium-containing infusions)
Muscle necrosis

Hypokalaemia

Vomiting
Diarrhoea
Insulin administration
Potassium-losing diuretics
High-dose corticosteroid therapy
Hyperaldosteronism
Acute renal failure

Hypercalcaemia

Primary hyperparathyroidism
Lymphosarcoma
Multiple myeloma
Other osteolytic neoplasms
Dietary excess plus vitamin D
    supplementation

Hypocalcaemia

Lactation tetany
Acute pancreatitis
Ethylene glycol poisoning

Uraemia

Decompensated renal failure
Acute renal failure

Hyperammonaemia

Hepatic failure (acute or chronic)
Congenital portosystemic shunts
Acquired portosystemic shunts

GENERAL CLINICAL PATHOLOGY

HAEMATOLOGICAL EXAMINATION

Haematological examination may reveal a leukocytosis in cases of encephalitis, abscessation and, particularly, in meningitis. Fungal and protozoal infections may be associated with leukocytosis or with normal white cell values in peripheral blood. Leukopaenia progressing to leukocytosis may be encountered in toxoplasmosis. In feline infectious peritonitis (FIP), generally there is a mild neutrophilia with a left shift, a moderate, non-regenerative anaemia and hypergammaglobulinaemia. Leukopaenia may be due to underlying bone marrow disorders, may be associated with distemper or with overwhelming bacterial infections.

Care must be exercised in interpretation of findings, as haematological changes may result from treatment. Corticosteroid therapy will induce a stress leukogram. More unusual changes may also be encountered, for example, haemolysis and diffuse intravascular coagulation (DIC) can result from muscle damage occurring during surgery.

When distemper encephalitis is suspected, examination of buffy coat or conjunctival smears for inclusion bodies may be of value, though these often have disappeared by the time the animal shows neurological signs.

Routine haematological examination may reveal the presence of polycythaemia, or the greatly increased plasma protein concentrations seen in myeloma.

SEROLOGY

When toxoplasmosis is suspected, determinations of antibody titres to *Toxoplasma gondii* may be valuable. Titres of antibody against FIP may be of some value in cats where this disease is suspected.

BIOCHEMICAL INVESTIGATIONS

A variety of systemic disorders may result in functional neurological signs, and often are detectable by biochemical examination of blood.

Hepatic failure with hyperammonaemia may result in encephalopathy. Where this is suspected, liver state and function should be investigated. Liver enzymes, (ALT, AST, GGT & ALP) are of limited value since they may not be elevated in chronic conditions which are slowly progressive. Indices of the functional capacity of the liver are much more helpful. The serum albumin concentration may be lowered, cholesterol may be increased and the one-stage prothrombin time may be increased. If any of these abnormalities is noted, or if suspicion remains, determination of the clearance of the dye sulphobromophthalein (BSP) is particularly valuable in establishing if there is any impairment of hepatic function. Ammonia estimation has been used to detect hyperammonaemia but there are considerable difficulties in making accurate determinations. Plasma bile acid (bile salt) determinations may prove of value in these circumstances since they are very sensitive indicators of impaired hepatic function (Evans and Heath, 1988). In such cases, ammonium biurate crystals may be present in the urine. Liver biopsy is required to establish the nature of any hepatic pathological change.

Seizures may occur in severe uraemia. Determination of plasma urea, creatinine and phosphate will confirm this suspicion.

Both hyperglycaemia and hypoglycaemia may result in coma, thus, the determination of blood glucose is essential in the comatose animal. Urinalysis will reveal the presence of glucosuria in hyperglycaemic coma and of ketonuria in ketotic coma. In severe hyperglycaemia, hyperosmolarity may contribute to the coma and measurement of plasma osmolality may be helpful. Transient hypoglycaemia in cases of insulinoma and in glycogen storage diseases may give rise to collapse. In cases of insulinoma, the fasting blood glucose is low and the amended insulin to glucose ratio (AIGR) is raised. Assay of plasma glucose at the time when signs are manifest is important in animals with episodic weakness or collapse.

Hyponatraemia may give rise to muscle weakness and may result from hypoadrenocorticism and from diuretic therapy.

Hyperkalaemia may give rise to listlessness, disorientation, neuromuscular weakness and severe abnormalities of cardiac conduction which may be fatal. It may be associated with acidosis, renal failure, diabetes mellitus, severe dehydration and abrupt withdrawal of steroid therapy.

Hypocalcaemia may give rise to tetany, which can be confused with seizures or tetany of neurological origin.

Blood lead concentration determinations are of value in suspected lead poisoning.

URINE ANALYSIS

The situations in which analysis of urine is of value are limited. The finding of urine with specific gravity below 1.012 is a significant finding, raising the suspicion of diabetes insipidus, possibly central in origin. This may be investigated further by performing a water deprivation test. The finding of glucose in the urine suggests that significant hyperglycaemia is present and ketones indicate the presence of ketoacidosis. Ammonium biurate crystals may be present in the urine of animals with hepatic dysfunction.

CEREBROSPINAL FLUID EXAMINATION

Changes in the composition of the cerebrospinal fluid (CSF) may reflect the involvement of the central nervous system (CNS) parenchyma, the meninges, the choroid plexus or the axial skeleton in a disease process. However, the conditions where CSF examination will provide useful diagnostic information are limited. In a significant proportion of cases of inflammatory disease and of neoplasia, it may provide useful data. In trauma, haemorrhage, degenerative disorders, cord compression and hydrocephalus, CSF examination may provide helpful information but other investigations, notably radiology, will be required. In many cases, it still will not be possible to establish the diagnosis unequivocally. Patients will need to be selected with care if maximum benefit is to be gained from its use. It is important to consider the history, the clinical signs and the results of physical and neurological examinations to identify the type of disease likely to be present before performing a CSF collection.

INDICATIONS AND CONTRAINDICATIONS

The main indications for analysis of CSF are suspicion of inflammatory disease or neoplasia, though failure to find tumour cells does not rule out the possibility of neoplastic involvement. It should be remembered that collection of CSF is not without risk, particularly in small breeds of dogs and cats. There are several contraindications to the collection of CSF:

Raised intracranial pressure

This may be evident on examination by evidence of papilloedema or by progressive disorientation leading to profound depression, pupillary dilation and coma. The performance of a CSF tap in the face of raised intracranial pressure may lead to brain herniation, either of the occipital lobes under the tentorium cerebelli or of the brain stem through the foramen magnum. In the presence of haemorrhage, further bleeding may be induced which may itself lead to herniation or to meningeal irritation.

Mechanical instability in the cervical or cranial region

Fractures of the upper cervical region or skull, or subluxations of the cervical vertebrae render the neuraxis liable to trauma during the manipulations necessary for CSF collection from the cisterna magna.

Foramen magnum herniation or lesions which distort the brain stem

These may predispose the brain stem to trauma by the spinal needle in performing cisterna magna puncture. Such lesions should be suspected where there is paralysis of cranial nerves nine to twelve, where there are progressive changes of pupillary diameter or the degree of consciousness, or where there is anisocoria of central origin.

Anaesthetic risk

Any situation where general anaesthesia is considered unnecessarily risky is a contraindication to CSF collection.

EQUIPMENT

For the collection of CSF, a spinal needle with a stilette usually is utilised. A 20 gauge, 1.5 inch needle, is used for most cases. Smaller needles may be needed in very small dogs and cats, and larger needles may be used in giant breeds. A syringe and sample collection pots (see below) also should be to hand.

If CSF pressure is to be measured, a three-way tap and CSF manometer are required. However, the value of this determination is very doubtful and the author rarely performs it. The normal values quoted are very variable, even in a single individual, being affected by gaseous anaesthesia, occlusion of the jugular vein and variations in CO_2 tension. Normal pressures of 170 mm of water for the dog and 100 mm of water in the cat have been cited (Mayhew and Beal, 1980).

COLLECTION TECHNIQUE

In small animals, the cisterna magna is the site of choice for collection of CSF samples, though lumbar collection sites may also be used. General anaesthesia is required for the great majority of CSF collections and strict asepsis is essential.

Collection from the cisterna magna

Anaesthesia is induced and the patient intubated, preferably with a kink-proof endotracheal tube. The caudal aspect of the vault of the skull and the dorsal aspect of the neck should be clipped to a level well behind the dorsal spine of the axis. The patient is positioned in lateral recumbency with the occiput and dorsum of the neck parallel and close to the edge of the table. For a right-handed operator, the animal should be placed in right lateral recumbency. The skin is prepared and the operator should scrub hands and don sterile gloves. An assistant holds the head so that the neck is flexed at a right angle with the sagittal axis of the skull parallel to the table surface (Figure 4.1). Adoption of this position may kink the endotracheal tube, so it may be wise to deflate the cuff at this stage.

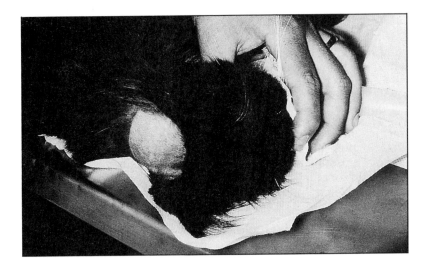

Figure 4.1

Position for CSF collection from the cisterna magna

There are two separate methods available for identifying the site for puncture, both requiring the correct identification of certain landmarks (Figure 4.2). The bony prominence of the occipital protuberance is palpated. The longitudinal midline runs from this point to the dorsal spine of the axis and is identified as a groove in the soft tissues of the dorsal aspect of the neck. The wings of the atlas also are identified. Here the methods of cisternal puncture vary importantly and are described separately.

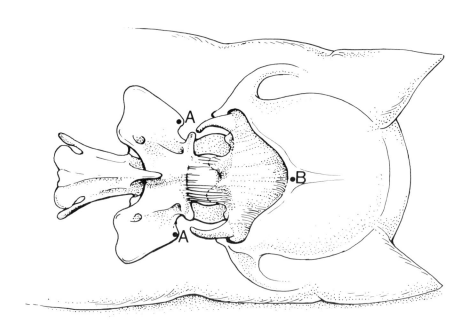

Figure 4.2

A — prominent wings of atlas   B — occipital protuberance

METHOD 1 An imaginary line is drawn between the wings of the atlas and the point where it transects the midline is noted. The site for puncture is in the midline, midway between this point and the occipital protuberance and slightly caudal to a depression in the soft tissues which lies just behind the protuberance. It is a temptation to make the puncture in this depression, but doing so invariably leads to the needle hitting bone. The needle is inserted perpendicular to the skin and advanced in this manner.

METHOD 2 The point of insertion of the needle is the intersection of the line joining the wings of the atlas and the dorsal longitudinal midline. The needle is inserted at an angle such that the point is directed rostrally, toward the angle of the jaw, and advanced in this direction.

The two methods are designed to achieve the same result, though there are significant differences in the performance of the puncture and one should be selected and adhered to. The needle is advanced through the layers of soft tissue until the dura is penetrated and the subarachnoid space entered. It is important to know where the point of the needle is relative to the dura and this can be achieved in one of several ways. A popping sensation is felt when the needle penetrates the atlanto-occipital membrane and the dura in many cases, though this is not universal. Thus, using this as the only estimate of depth may lead to the needle being advanced too far, penetrating neural tissue with potentially catastrophic results. It is suggested that each time the needle is advanced the stilette is removed to ascertain whether CSF flows. Alternatively, once the skin and superficial soft tissues are penetrated, the stilette may be removed and the needle advanced, the hub of the needle continually being observed for the appearance of CSF. Whilst this method carries the theoretical risk of a soft tissue plug obstructing the needle and preventing CSF flow, this is considered the safest by many. Should the needle hit bone, either it may be 'walked' off the bone or it may be withdrawn completely and a fresh attempt made. If dark, venous blood appears in the needle, the needle usually is lateral to the midline and should be repositioned.

Collection from the lumbar cistern

Cerebrospinal fluid collection may be performed by puncture of the subarachnoid space in the lumbar region (Kornegay, 1981). The procedure may be performed with the animal either in lateral or in ventral recumbency, though the former is usual. The skin is clipped and prepared and the animal is positioned with the spine flexed. In the dog, the needle is introduced in the $L_6 - L_7$ intervertebral space and in the cat at the $L_7 - S_1$ space, in each case just cranial to the appropriate spinous process. The needle is advanced perpendicularly, redirecting it should it hit bone, until CSF flows. In this way, a sample is collected from the dorsal subarachnoid space. Alternatively, the needle may be passed through the nervous structures to the floor of the spinal canal and CSF collected from the ventral subarachnoid space. The former method is preferable. The technique is more difficult than cisterna magna puncture.

Collection of samples

Whichever site is used, once CSF flows freely, samples may be collected. It is preferable to allow the CSF to drip from the needle into collection pots. Occasionally, it may be necessary to apply gentle syringe suction to collect a sample, particularly in small patients and at the lumbar cistern. In such cases, the collection should be by very slow withdrawal, as the application of significant suction increases the likelihood of haemorrhage occurring. If there is initial blood contamination, particularly with passive flow, allowing the flow to continue and discarding the early portion of fluid usually will allow the collection of an uncontaminated specimen. Should this fail, the needle should be removed and the tap repeated, possibly on a different occasion. Blood contamination makes meaningful laboratory examination extremely difficult.

Failure of CSF flow generally is due to incorrect needle placement, although lowered pressure resulting from anaesthesia may be responsible. In some cases, although flow begins, it ceases before an adequate sample is collected.

Normal CSF is low in protein and cell content, does not clot and can be collected in sterile plain tubes. In disease, the cell count may be higher and bacteria may be present, protein concentrations may be high and the presence of fibrinogen may lead to clotting. Therefore, it is wise to be prepared to collect CSF into EDTA pots for cytology and into oxalate/fluoride pots if glucose concentration is to be determined. Sterile plain pots are required for microbiological investigation. Paediatric 1 ml pots should be used due to the small volumes of fluid available. If the specimen is to be sent to a laboratory for cytological examination, it must be preserved by the addition of an equal volume of 4% formalin solution or of 50% or 95% ethanol. Alternatively, smears may be made by one of the techniques described below. They either may be air-dried or fixed for 10—20 minutes in absolute ethanol and the laboratory informed of which method is used.

LABORATORY EXAMINATION OF CSF

This consists of evaluation of the following:

Colour
Turbidity
Specific gravity
Protein concentration
Presence of globulins (Pandy, Nonne-Apelt or quantitative examination)
Red cell count
Nucleated cell count and differential count
Coagulation

The colour and turbidity of the fresh specimen are most easily assessed and recorded by the clinician at the time of collection. Where infection, particularly meningitis, is suspected the following additional investigations may be performed:

Gram stain
Ziehl-Neelsen stain
Indian ink or other negative staining
Glucose concentration determination.

Measurement of CSF glucose is most valuable when accompanied by determination of plasma glucose.

TECHNIQUES OF EXAMINATION

Colour

This is assessed by inspection against a uniformly illuminated, plain white background and compared with distilled water.

Turbidity

This is assessed by visual examination. If discolouration makes the judgement difficult, placing a pencil or ruler behind the specimen is helpful. In clear but discoloured samples, the outline of the object and the printing on it will be clearly perceptible. If there is turbidity, these features will be obscured.

Cell counts

Cell counts are performed using an improved Neubauer haemocytometer unless the cell counts are extremely high, in which case a Coulter or other automatic cell counter may be used. When using the haemocytometer method, the fluid may be counted without dilution or after dilution by 1 in 10 or greater with white cell counting fluid, depending on the cellularity. Both sides of the chamber are filled. It is important not to introduce air bubbles or to allow fluid to spill over into the troughs. Red cells and nucleated cells usually are distinguishable by their appearance. In cases of doubt, a little crystal violet or methylene blue may be added to the counting fluid. It then will be possible to identify white cells by their stained nuclei. The cells in all nine of the large squares making up the ruled area of the chamber are counted on each side and the mean calculated. If the count was made using undiluted CSF, the result is multiplied by 1.1×10^6 to calculate the cells per litre. If there was dilution, the result must be multiplied by ($1.1 \times$ dilution factor) to obtain the count.

Cytological examination

The nucleated cells may be differentiated by examination of stained smears. The stains commonly used are the Romanowsky stains used for blood films (Giemsa, May-Grunwald-Giemsa, Leishman's, Wright's). Cells are very labile in low protein fluids such as CSF and specimens for cytological examination must be prepared within 30 minutes of collection, or the material must be fixed. Smears may be prepared by one of a number of techniques.

1. **Centrifugation** of the specimen in a conical centrifuge tube (80-100g for 5 minutes) followed by resuspension of the sediment in 100 μl of autologous serum. The resuspended sediment is smeared using a spreader to pull the fluid along the slide, as in the preparation of a blood film.

2. **Sedimentation** of the cells directly on to the slide from the CSF sample may be achieved in two ways:

    ### Passive gravitational sedimentation.

    A flanged cylinder about 1—2 cm in diameter and 1—2 cm high is applied to a slide and anchored to it with a ring of silicone grease. (A suitable cylinder may be prepared from the barrel of a 5 ml syringe). An intervening filter paper in which a hole has been made to match the internal diameter of the cylinder may be used to absorb the fluid with the cylinder attached to the slide with bulldog clips. Cerebrospinal fluid (1—3 ml, depending on cellularity and the capacity of the cylinder) is put into the cylinder and the assembly placed in a refrigerator for two hours. During this time, any cells will sediment out and adhere to the slide. The cylinder and filter paper (if used) are removed and the slide dried, fixed and stained in the usual manner.

    ### Cytological centrifuge.

    This method only will be available in large laboratories with a considerable throughput of samples. Good cell adhesion and spreading is obtained, but there are suggestions that some cells may be lost selectively onto the filter paper.

    Direct smearing, as for blood films, is applicable only to samples of extremely high cellularity.

Approaches not involving the use of fixed, stained smears.

Wet preparations under a coverslip may be examined by dark field or phase contrast microscopy, or by transmitted light after the addition of methylene blue. This is an insensitive technique and is suitable only for highly cellular samples. The cells are clustered rather than spread out, making differentiation difficult.

Membrane filtration may be employed to deposit the cells on Millipore or similar filters. The cells from a large volume of CSF are concentrated and trapped in the filter, but again they are clustered together. Romanowsky stains cannot be used and these preparations commonly are stained by Papanicolaou's method or with haematoxylin and eosin. Differentiation of the cells requires more experience than with Romanowsky-stained smears and can be particularly difficult for tumour cells. This technique is suited best to referral laboratories, particularly for samples sent as fixed suspensions in formalin or methanol.

Having prepared the smear, a differential count should be performed. In smears from normal animals, and in many cases of CNS or meningeal disease, few cells will be present, even after concentration. In such cases, all available cells on the smear must be examined and included in the differential count. A few pathological samples will have sufficient cells present for a differential count to be made on one or two hundred cells. Differentiation is made using the same morphological criteria and nomenclature as for cells in the blood. Macrophages or tumour cells may be encountered in some specimens.

Specific gravity.

In view of the limited sample volumes available, specific gravity is best determined using a refractometer. The sample should be centrifuged to remove any suspended cells and the supernatant used.

Protein concentration.

The concentration of protein in the CSF is low compared with plasma and an approximate determination may be made using dipsticks of the type used for assessing urine protein. Increased total CSF protein may be detected qualitatively by shaking the sample. In normal circumstances, a very slight amount of foam, if any, is formed and any that does develop breaks down within five minutes. Increased protein levels result in moderate to marked foam formation and the foam is stable for over five minutes.

Accurate determinations of CSF protein concentration may be made by the Coomassie blue dye-binding method or by turbidimetry with sulphonylsalicylic acid (SSA) or trichloroacetic acid (TCA). These methods require careful calibration and quality control and are limited to referral laboratories.

Globulins

Normally, the majority of CSF protein is albumin and in pathological states, increases generally are due to globulins. The detection of globulins is performed using a qualitative test.

The Pandy test.

A solution of 10 mg of carbolic acid crystals is made in 100 ml of distilled water and one drop of this phenol solution is placed in a small test tube. A single drop of CSF is added and the mixture examined visually. With normal CSF, the mixture remains clear, though a faint inhomogeneity may be detectable, this being a negative result which is given a score of 0. Where globulins are increased, definite white or grey turbidity develops which is qualitatively scored on a scale of $1+$ to $4+$.

The Nonne-Apelt or Ross-Jones test.

One ml of saturated ammonium sulphate solution is put into a small test tube and 1 ml of CSF is layered carefully over this. The tube is allowed to stand for three minutes, after which it is examined visually. With normal CSF, there is no ring detectable at the interface, while in the presence of increased globulins, a grey ring of precipitate is formed.

Quantitative determination of globulins.

This is made by electrophoresis after concentration of the sample by dialysis against glycerol. The results are unreliable quantatively but qualitative examination of the trace from scanning the electrophoresis strip will give some indication of the extent of globulin increase and of the fractions present.

Coagulation.

This occurs in the presence of fibrinogen and is detected visually. Fibrin strands or a solid coagulum may be seen.

Glucose.

Glucose concentration may be measured by any technique applicable to blood, glucose oxidase methods being the most specific. Approximate values can be obtained using dipsticks intended for the measurement of plasma glucose. CSF glucose determinations are of most value if combined with simultaneous determination of plasma glucose.

Microbiology.

In bacterial, fungal or protozoal meningitis, encephalitis or myelitis, organisms may be present in the CSF. Microscopic examination of sedimented smears stained by the Gram and the Zeihl-Neelsen methods may be of value. In the case of yeast infections, Indian ink or nigrosin may reveal organsims by negative staining. Micro-organisms also may be encountered when making cytological examination of Romanowsky stained smears.

Bacterial or fungal culture is indicated when the CSF is turbid, clots are present, the nucleated count is high or when organisms are seen on stained smears.

CSF enzymology.

There are reports of the determination of CSF aspartate amino-transferase (AST), alanine amino-transferase (ALT), creatinine kinase (CK), lactate dehydrogenase (LDH) and ß-glucuronidase (see Coles, 1980 for review). Any leakage of these enzymes from damaged brain tissue is confined to CSF and there is no effect on levels measured in plasma or serum. However, the changes encountered are small and correlate poorly with the pathological process and are of limited value.

NORMAL FINDINGS FOR CEREBROSPINAL FLUID

If normal, the CSF is colourless and free from turbidity, resembling water. The nucleated cell count of cisterna magna CSF in the normal dog is less than 5×10^6 cells per litre, with lumbar CSF cell counts reported to be lower (Bailey and Higgins, 1985). The cells encountered are predominantly lymphocytes, though occasional macrophages or monocytes will be seen. Normal CSF is free of micro-organisms and sterile on culture. The specific gravity of normal canine and feline CSF is in the range of 1.004—1.006. The total protein concentration of cisterna magna CSF is in the range of 8—30 mg/dl in the dog and 8—20 mg/dl in the cat, but lumbar samples have a higher level of protein (Bailey and Higgins, 1985). Albumin comprises 80—95% of the total protein, the residue being globulins. There is no fibrinogen in normal CSF and it does not clot. The glucose concentration is in the range of 2.7—4.2 mmol/l in dogs and 3.2—4.3 mmol/l in cats and is approximately 80% of the plasma glucose concentration.

ABNORMAL CSF FINDINGS AND THEIR INTERPRETATION

Appearance.

Discolouration — the most commonly encountered is the bright red of fresh blood and usually indicates contamination at the time of puncture. Such specimens are rarely diagnostic due to the difficulty in interpretation.

Dull red or brown discolouration is a rare finding and indicates recent or chronic haemorrhage preceding collection. The finding of evidence of erythrophagocytosis (see below) and of crenated red cells on cytological examination is helpful confirmatory evidence. The specimen may be turbid or clear. After centrifugation, the supernatant will be clear but discoloured.

Yellow discolouration (xanthochromia) is an uncommon finding. The colouration is due to bilirubin and indicates haemorrhage more than 48 hours previously. Possible causes are given below (see Cytological abnormalities). Xanthochromia can also be a consequence of severe jaundice or can be associated with hydrocephalus and with very high CSF protein concentrations.

Grey or grey-green discolouration is associated with suppuration, particularly in acute pyogenic meningitis. The presence of suppuration will be confirmed by the finding of pus cells on cytological examination.

Clots or fibrin flecks indicate blood contamination, severe, often suppurative inflammation or haemorrhage. Turbidity is common, often with reddening due to the presence of blood. When white, grey or grey-green in colour it indicates the presence of cells, organisms or fibrin. The nucleated cell count must be greater than 500×10^6 cells per litre to render CSF turbid. Usually, this is due to suppuration but rarely it may be due to exfoliation of tumour cells, particularly in lymphoid neoplasia. The finding of turbidity or clots is an indication for microbiological examination.

Cytological abnormalities.

When large numbers of red cells are present, it is necessary to attempt to establish whether these represent pathological haemorrhage or contamination at the time of sampling. Evidence of erythrophagocytosis in the form of macrophages laden with red cells, haemosiderin or bilirubin suggests that the red cells result from pathological haemorrhage. The finding of residual xanthochromia after centrifugation of the sample also supports this conclusion. However, in many cases it can be difficult to ascertain the significance of the presence of blood. Where there is reasonable certainty of pathological haemorrhage, this may be associated with:

> Trauma
> Intracerebral haemorrhage
> Subarachnoid haemorrhage
> Severe, acute inflammation
> Acute disc extrusion with haematomyelia
> Necrotic or erosive neoplasia

Other rare causes include:

> Leptospirosis
> Cryptococcosis
> Toxoplasmosis
> Ischaemic myelopathy
> Haemostatic disorders, particularly coagulopathies.

When there is contamination with blood, it can be very difficult to evaluate and interpret the WBC and protein findings. A formula relating the ratio of white to red cells in the CSF to that in a simultaneous sample of blood can be applied to correct the CSF white cell count.

$$WBC_{csf} = WBC_{observed} - \frac{WBC_{blood} \times RBC_{observed}}{RBC_{blood}}$$

However, doubt has been cast on the general validity of this formula and it is, at best, a crude approximation (Wilson and Stevens, 1977). It is preferable to wait a few days after collecting a contaminated sample to repeat the tap in the hope of collecting diagnostic CSF.

An increase in the nucleated cells of the CSF is known as **pleocytosis**. Such an increase may be due to elevated numbers of mononuclear cells which are present in CSF. Also, there may be neutrophils, erythrophagocytes or other abnormal cells present. When neoplastic cells are found, often it is not possible to determine the lineage to which they belong, though on occasion large numbers of neoplastic lymphocytes are present, associated with lymphoma of the CNS.

An increase solely in mononuclear cells is a relatively uncommon finding and is suggestive of:

Viral infections	Uraemia
Toxoplasmosis	Intoxications
Distemper encephalitis	Post-vaccinal reactions
Feline infectious peritonitis	Reticulosis
Cryptococcosis	Granulomatous meningoencephalitis
Other chronic infections	Discospondylitis

Fungal infections may show an increase in CSF mononuclear cells alone, but the pleocytosis they induce is rather variable.

In globoid cell leukodystrophy, the characteristic enlarged, foamy macrophages known as globoid cells may be found (Roszel, Steinberg and McGrath, 1982).

An increase in neutrophil numbers is always indicative of pathological change and may be seen in:

Bacterial meningitis ⎫
Bacterial encephalitis ⎬ neutrophilic pleocytosis
Bacterial myelitis ⎭
Abscessation
Early viral infections
Acute distemper
Feline infectious peritonitis
Other CNS inflammatory conditions
Discospondylitis
Acquired hydrocephalus
Necrotic tumours
Granulomatous meningoencephalitis (GME).

Meningeal diseases have the greatest effect on neutrophil counts, which are highest in purulent meningitis. The presence of neutrophils, particularly in large or increasing numbers, is an unfavourable prognostic sign. In GME, a mononuclear pleocytosis may be seen, but in many cases up to 30% of the cells are neutrophils (Vandevelde and Spano, 1977; Bailey and Higgins, 1986b). FIP can result in lymphocyte or neutrophil dominated pleocytosis.

The presence of bacteria on microscopic examination or culture, in the absence of neutrophils, suggests that the bacteria are due to contamination of the specimen.

Eosinophils are a relatively frequent finding, but their significance often is uncertain. They can be associated with fungal and parasitic conditions, notably cryptococcosis and toxoplasmosis. However, their presence correlates poorly with the underlying pathological process (Vandevelde and Spano, 1977).

Abnormal specific gravity

A specific gravity above 1.007 raises suspicions of the presence of significant pathological change, for example, cervical stenosis with chronic cord compression often is associated with values in the range of 1.009 — 1.010. Disc extrusions may show values of 1.008 — 1.012 and parenchymal disease values of 1.007 — 1.012.

Protein abnormalities

Increased CSF protein usually is due to increased globulin levels. The protein concentration may be increased in:

Inflammation: Meningitis, Encephalitis, Abscessation, Toxoplasmosis, Distemper*

Haemorrhage
Neoplasia*
Seizures*
Fever*
Uraemia*
Ischaemic myelopathy*
Disc extrusion*
Degenerative myelopathy*
Myelomalacia*
GME*

In the conditions marked with an asterisk (*), the protein may be increased in the absence of pleocytosis, a situation termed albuminocytological dissociation.

Haemorrhage contributes approximately 1 mg/dl of protein to the CSF per 10^9/l of red blood cells. The largest increases in CSF protein (up to 5 g/l), usually accompanied by severe pleocytosis, are seen in infective meningitis. In FIP, there may be marked elevations in globulin in the CSF.

Abnormal glucose concentrations

CSF glucose concentration usually parallels that in plasma, consistently being about 80 — 85% of that level. Lowered values relative to plasma glucose, usually with a decrease to less than 50%, generally are indicative of pyogenic infection. Rarely, other severe inflammatory changes or advanced neoplasia may result in such a finding. Reduced CSF glucose with maintenance of the normal ratio to plasma glucose is seen in hypoglycaemia. Increased CSF glucose, with the normal relationship to plasma glucose, is seen in hyperglycaemia or diabetes mellitus. Slight increases are seen in some cases of encephalitis, in brain abscessation, with spinal cord compression and in neoplasia of the CNS.

Normal CSF findings in the face of disease

The CSF shows no detectable abnormality in many cases of disease of the CNS, despite the fact that the CSF may be affected in other animals with the same condition.

The CSF is normal in the majority of cases of:

Idiopathic epilepsy
Congenital hydrocephalus
Functional disorders
Metabolic disorders
Intoxications
Vertebral diseases
Myelomalacia

This is also true of a significant proportion of cases of:

FIP
Distemper encephalitis
Neoplasia
GME

CONCLUSION

Evaluation of CSF is of assistance in confirming the presence of CNS disease in a significant number of cases. However, its value is limited in many cases, as it infrequently provides conclusive information when attempting to distinguish between different causes of neurological disfunction. It is positively diagnostic in certain circumstances: finding pus cells or organisms in severe infective processes; finding pleocytosis or increased globulins in inflammatory disorders and the rare findings of neoplastic cells or of globoid cells. In many functional, metabolic and degenerative disorders, there will be no changes in the CSF. CSF changes may be poorly correlated with the type and severity of the lesion, though meningeal lesions have particularly marked effects on CSF composition. Some thoracolumbar and lumbar spinal cord lesions may result in changes in the lumbar CSF, but cisterna magna samples remain normal (Kornegay, 1981).

History, clinical examination and detailed neurological examination are the essential elements in reaching a diagnosis of nervous system disease. CSF examination is a useful adjunct to the interpretation of these evaluations, but rarely is diagnostic *per se.*

REFERENCES AND FURTHER READING

BAILEY, C.S. and HIGGINS, R.J. (1985) Comparison of total white blood cell count and total protein content of lumbar and cisternal cerebrospinal fluid of healthy dogs. *American Journal of Veterinary Research,* **46,** 1162.

BAILEY, C.S and HIGGINS, R.J. (1986a) Characteristics of cisternal cerebrospinal fluid associated with primary brain tumours of the dog: a retrospective study. *Journal of the American Veterinary Medical Association,* **188,** 415.

BAILEY, C.S. and HIGGINS, R.J. (1986b) Characteristics of cerebrospinal fluid associated with canine granulomatous meningoencephalitis: a retrospective study. *Journal of the American Veterinary Medical Association,* **188,** 418.

BICHSEL, P., VANDEVELDE, M., VANDEVELDE, E., AFFOLTER, U. and PFISTER, H. (1984) Immunoelectrophoretic determination of albumin and IgG in serum and CSF in dogs with neurological disease. *Research in Veterinary Science,* **37,** 101.

COLES, E.H. (1980) *Veterinary Clinical Pathology, 3rd Edition,* W.B. Saunders Co., Philadelphia.

EVANS, R.J. and HEATH, M.F. (1988) The laboratory assessment of hepatobiliary damage and dysfunction. In *Advances in Small Animal Practice,* **1,** 30. (Editor E.A. Chandler).

KORNEGAY, J.N. (1981) Cerebrospinal fluid collection, examination and interpretation in dogs and cats. *Compendium of Continuing Education,* **3,** 85.

MAYHEW, I.G. and BEAL, C.R. (1980) Techniques of analysis of cerebrospinal fluid. *Veterinary Clinics of North America, Small Animal Practice,* **10,** (1), 155.

ROSZEL, J.F., STEINBERG, S.A. and MCGRATH, J.T. (1982) Periodic acid Schiff-positive cells in the cerebrospinal fluid of dogs with globoid cell leukodystrophy. *Neurology,* **22,** 738.

SORJONEN, D.C., WARREN J.N. and SCHULTZ, R.D. (1981) Qualitative and quantitative determination of albumin, IgG, IgM and IgA in normal cerebrospinal fluid in dogs. *Journal of the American Animal Hospital Association,* **17,** 833.

VANDEVELDE, M. and SPANO, J.S. (1977) Cerebrospinal fluid cytology in canine neurologic disease. *American Journal of Veterinary Research,* **28,** 1827.

WILSON, J.W. and STEVENS, J.B. (1977) Effects of blood contamination on cerebrospinal fluid analysis. *Journal of the American Veterinary Medical Association,* **171,** 256.

Part 2

ELECTROMYOGRAPHY AND NERVE CONDUCTION STUDIES

Ian D. Duncan B.V.M.S., Ph.D., M.R.C.V.S., M.R.C.Path.

INTRODUCTION

The application of electrophysiological diagnostic techniques has become a cornerstone in the investigation of neuromuscular disease in small animals (Griffiths and Duncan, 1974; 1978; van Nes, 1986). Two principle electrodiagnostic techniques which utilise the same equipment, the electromyograph (EMG), are employed. These are: **electromyography,** the investigaton of the electrical activity of muscle, and measurement of **nerve conduction**. These techniques examine the integrity of the motor unit, the basic anatomical and physiological component of the neuromuscular system and the peripheral portion of sensory nerve fibres. The motor unit consists of the lower motor neurone (the motor fibre and its cell of origin which is found in the ventral horn of the spinal cord and in certain cranial nerve nuclei) and the muscle fibres that it innervates.

EQUIPMENT

The expense of EMG equipment has limited its use in the past to veterinary schools and large institutions. More recently, however, less expensive and second hand EMG's have become available and this has led to the acquisition of EMG's by certain specialist practices. The EMG essentially consists of an amplifier, oscilloscope screen and loudspeaker, with a stimulating unit to allow the performance of nerve conduction studies (Bowen, 1978). If more refined sensory nerve testing is to be performed, a signal averaging unit is required to filter out the background noise that is present at the high amplifications required to record sensory action potentials. Concentric needle electrodes are used to record EMG activity and a ground electrode must be used. For motor nerve conduction studies, two needle electrodes are used to stimulate the nerve and two similar electrodes to record the compound evoked muscle action potential (CEMAP).

ELECTROMYOGRAPHY

There are two parts to this examination, the evaluation of voluntary muscle activity and the testing for spontaneous activity in the resting muscle.

Voluntary activity

Voluntary activity is the electrical activity recorded in a muscle as it contracts, which is brought about by the firing of individual motor units. The individual **motor unit potentials** (MUP's) can be identified on the oscilloscope screen during minimal muscle contraction. The amplitude and duration of these MUP's are important parameters that are measured and compared with control values. As contraction increases, so the number of motor units and their frequency of firing increases, a phenomenon known as **recruitment**. Eventually, individual motor units become indistinguishable on the oscilloscope screen and this combined electrical activity constitutes the **interference pattern**. Voluntary activity is difficult to evaluate in small animals. It is possible to examine individual motor unit potentials and the interference pattern by inserting concentric needle electrodes into extensor or flexor muscles, with the animal standing or while inducing a withdrawal reflex respectively. In neuropathies, a loss of nerve fibres leads to a drop out of motor units and an incomplete interference pattern (Griffiths and Duncan, 1974). In a totally denervated muscle, no MUP's are detectable. Conversely, in a muscle which has been re-innervated, the motor units are often enlarged and so the MUP's are of a higher amplitude and longer duration.

Spontaneous activity

Spontaneous activity only can be accurately assessed in the anaesthetised animal. It consists of a variety of abnormal potentials which signify denervation of the muscle or a primary muscle disease. In the normal resting or anaesthetised state, no electrical activity is found, with two exceptions. **Insertion activity** is a short burst of activity which corresponds to the mechanical depolarisation of muscle fibres caused by the EMG electrode as it passes through the muscle. **End plate noise** is recorded within the area of the neuromuscular junction.

In denervated muscle, the insertion activity may be prolonged and is followed by abnormal potentials, most often fibrillations and positive sharp waves.

Fibrillations are brief, spontaneous potentials which have a low amplitude ($20-200\,\mu V$) and short duration ($1-5$ msec). On the loudspeaker, they are described as sounding like cellophane paper being wrinkled or like eggs frying. They arise from single muscle fibres and are triggered by needle movement, which frequently induces a rapid discharge of fibrillations.

Positive sharp waves have a saw toothed shape, a similar amplitude to fibrillations but are of a slightly longer duration. They also are triggered by needle movement and can occur in bursts at high frequency. Both fibrillations and positive sharp waves can be found in certain myopathies, for example, polymyositis, but they are most often signs of denervation.

High frequency discharges, often of positive sharp waves, can be seen in neuropathies.

Fasciculations represent the contraction of a single motor unit. They result from irritant lesions of ventral horn cells (for example, in canine spinal muscular atrophy) or in nerve root lesions (for example, in some cervical intervertebral disc protrusions). They fire randomly and appear similar to MUP's. Fasciculation may be visible in the animal as small rippling movements on the muscle surface.

Myotonic discharges are high frequency bursts of activity which wax and wane in frequency and amplitude, giving them the characteristic sound of a motor bike 'revving up'. They are induced by needle insertion and movement and by percussion of the muscle, though they can occur spontaneously. They are classically seen in myotonic disorders such as myotonia congenita in the dog (Duncan and Griffiths, 1986).

High frequency discharges which have a sudden onset and termination and that do not wax and wane are called **high frequency repetitive discharges.** They often are found in dogs with myopathy associated with Cushing's disease (Duncan and Griffiths, 1986).

NERVE CONDUCTION STUDIES

Techniques are available to measure conduction in both motor and sensory nerves.

Motor nerve conduction.

To record from motor nerve fibres, a mixed nerve (containing both motor and sensory fibres) is stimulated at proximal and distal sites. The compound evoked muscle action potential which results from this stimulation is recorded from a muscle innervated by the nerve. For example, in the hind limb, the sciatic nerve is stimulated at the greater trochanter and the tibial branch stimulated at the hock. The CEMAP is recorded from the interosseous muscles of the foot. By measuring the latencies from the two sites of stimulation and the distance between the stimulating electrodes, the nerve conduction velocity is calculated. The velocity is a representation of speed of conduction only along the fastest firing fibres. The amplitude, duration and shape of the CEMAP are recorded and reflect the number of fibres firing. A similar technique is employed in the fore limb using the ulnar nerve.

Sensory nerve conduction.

To measure sensory nerve conduction, a suitable sensory nerve is stimulated distally and a recording of the action potential made directly from the nerve proximally. In the fore limb, the lateral cutaneous radial nerve is used. The stimulation site is the digital branch on the dorsum of the foot and the recording made from the nerve in the mid-antebrachium where it runs close to the cephalic vein. The nerve conduction velocity is calculated from the distance between the sites and the latency. The amplitude, shape and duration of the action potential are also recorded.

Effect of neuropathy.

The nerve conduction velocity and evoked muscle action potentials are affected both by demyelination and axonal degeneration. In demyelination, NCV is slowed due to lack of the insulating sheath around the axon and loss of saltatory conduction. The CEMAP is no longer bi- or triphasic, but has many phases; the phenomenon of temporal dispersion. As demyelination progresses, nerve conduction will be blocked in certain fibres and the CEMAP will be reduced in amplitude.

In axonal degeneration, affected nerve fibres cannot conduct, so the CEMAP is reduced in size as there are fewer intact motor units. However, the NCV will remain approximately normal as long as some large diameter fibres are intact.

If the nerve is sectioned completely, it will continue to conduct at a normal velocity distal to the lesion for up to eight days, though the CEMAP gradually declines until the nerve no longer conducts. In sensory nerves, demyelination and degeneration have the same general effect.

These techniques only measure conduction in the mid and distal limb. To measure more proximal conduction, late waves are measured, in particular the **F-wave** and **H-reflex** (van Nes, 1986). These measure conduction through the ventral nerve root and the dorsal and ventral root respectively. They are of considerable use in evaluating lesions involving the nerve roots, for example, polyradiculo-neuritis.

To test the integrity of the neuromuscular junction, **repetitive nerve stimulation** of the motor nerves mentioned above can be used. The response to low frequency stimulation (3—5 Hz) is measured. In a healthy animal, this technique leads to a uniform amplitude of the CEMAP. In patients with myasthenia gravis, the CEMAP decreases to a lower amplitude after two or three stimuli. This decrement can be quantified.

REFERENCES

BOWEN, J.M. (1987) Electromyography. In *Veterinary Neurology* (Editors J.E. Oliver, B.F. Hoerlein and I.G. Mayhew), W.B. Saunders Co., Philadelphia.

DUNCAN, I.D. and GRIFFITHS, I.R. (1986) Neuromuscular Disease. In *Neurologic Disorders* (Editor J.N. Kornegay), Churchill Livingstone, New York.

GRIFFITHS, I.R. and DUNCAN, I.D. (1974) Some studies of the clinical neurophysiology of denervation in the dog. *Research in Veterinary Science,* **17,** 377.

GRIFFITHS, I.R. and DUNCAN, I.D. (1978) The use of electromyography and nerve conduction studies in the evaluation of lower motor neurone disease or injury. *Journal of Small Animal Practice,* **19,** 239.

VAN NES, J.J. (1986) An introduction to clinical neuromuscular electrophysiology. *Veterinary Quarterly,* **8,** 233.

CHAPTER 4
Part 3

ELECTROENCEPHALOGRAPHY

John Barker B.Vet. Med., M.R.C.V.S.

INTRODUCTION

Veterinary electroencephalography (EEG) is the use of a high-amplification recording system to display the summation of the electrical activity of the neurones of the accessible areas of the animal's cortex. This signal is attenuated by the skull table and the temporal muscles and recording is complicated by artifacts arising from the skull musculature, patient movements and from the general lack of co-operation of subjects. Recording techniques are directed towards achieving control of these variables whilst obtaining signals of diagnostic value. EEG is solely an ancillary aid to assessing cortical activity; it is no substitute for accurate and intelligent history taking or clinical 'hands on' neurological examination, and it requires considerable experience in its evaluation and interpretation. Unfortunately (and uniquely) in the U.K., this is not always appreciated by both clinicians and owners and the technique has been, and continues to be, used to 'screen' healthy animals for seizure disorders. There is no value in this and the practice is to be deplored.

METHOD

The following is a simple and standard technique derived from experimental and clinical experience to enable the recording of EEG quickly and successfully in the dog and cat. It is arranged sequentially as it would be carried out on a clinical case.

ELECTRODE ARRAY

Electrodes are placed on the animal's cranium in a predetermined pattern or an 'array'. This pattern must take into account the necessity of adequately covering the limited area of the cortex available in small animals, but must accept the limitations imposed by the small size of the calvarium, the attenuation of the signal arising from the relatively massive skull bones and overlying musculature and the need, in bipolar recording techniques, to achieve adequate electrode separation to allow some potential difference between the sites (Figure 4.3). These severe limitations mean that, in practice, seven electrodes will suffice to obtain reasonable recordings in the dog and cat. (Figure 4.4).

THE PATIENT

Very few patients are relaxed enough to record from directly, contrary to opinions expressed in the literature. In practice, the majority of dogs and cats will display head movements, eye blinks, ear movements or EMG artifacts and will resent electrode placement and restraint whether handled quietly or restrained in slings, restraint bags or the like. Practically, recording as a routine from conscious, physically restrained animals, is unprofitable. The exceptions to this are the small breeds, such as the Miniature Yorkshire Terrier or the Chihuahua, or very young animals with relatively under-developed skull musculature, in which the calvarium is exposed. Sedation with *acepromazine* alone or with *buprenorphine* has two potential benefits; a more tractable patient and enhancement of certain EEG abnormalities, particularly epileptic activity. Over more than a decade of using this technique, the author has not precipitated any adverse reactions in patients, even those suffering from severe

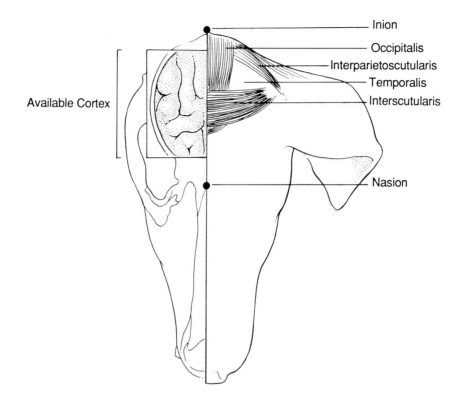

Figure 4.3

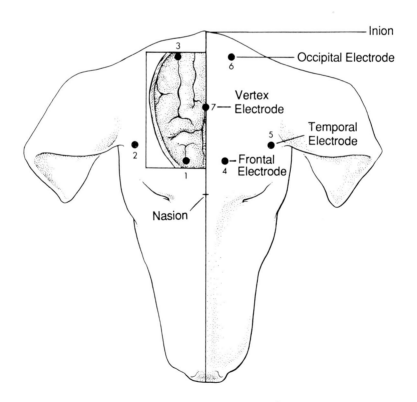

Figure 4.4

neurological problems. Various evocative techniques involving further drug adminstration or photic stimulation may be utilised during the recording session though their possible adverse effects should be carefully considered.

Prior to electrode placement, up to 0.5 ml of local anaesthetic is infiltrated under each electrode position using a 25g hypodermic needle. Once this has taken effect (the time can be used taking blood samples, carrying out examinations etc.) platinum needle electrodes are introduced subdermally. The electrode leads are held by the handler with a hand on the animal's neck, with sufficient slack to allow for sudden head movements without electrode displacement. Other electrode types need not be considered here — hypodermic needles, clips etc. have high impedance and poor recording characteristics, whereas silver/silver chloride disks do not justify the difficulty in securing them to the animal's scalp by any great degree of signal enhancement. A simple alligator clip screened earth lead is then attached to the point of a 0.9 inch, 25g needle thrust through a fold of flank skin. Once recording is underway, assessment can be made of the efficacy of the attempts to control artifacts, and further steps can be taken if required.

MONTAGE

The recording of EEG in animals is generally carried out using bipolar derivations, i.e., the two electrodes producing the signal for a given channel are both positioned over active cortical areas and the EEG machine amplifier (a 'push-pull' differential amplifier) 'sees' the potential difference between them. Unipolar derivations have one inactive electrode over an EEG quiet area, such as the nasal bones and the other over a cortical site. It follows that some selection of the electrode pairs can be made to produce the channels of EEG signal, and the pattern of these connections is known as a montage (Figure 4.5). Selection of different montages allows the comparison of different areas of cortex (e.g. frontal with occipital, left hemisphere with right, right temporal to left temporal, etc.). These montages can be prewired into the machine via a selector switch, or, less rigidly, can be selected during recording to best display the significant findings for that patient. It follows that a two-channel machine is thus somewhat limited in its capacity to allow simultaneous comparison of different areas of cortex and that at least four channels are required for clinical use. Two useful montages are shown (Figure 4.5).

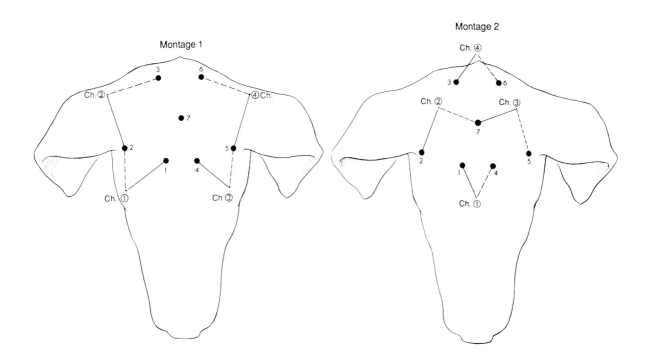

Figure 4.5

To allow some standardisation and reproduction of recordings made between different animals, or, more importantly, serial EEG of the same animal at different times, initial recording must use default values of the machine settings familiar to the operator and written on the record and any subsequent changes during the recording session must be clearly marked and a calibration signal included. Any drugs administered and possible extraneous sources of artifact such as movement or reactions of the animals should be noted to aid interpretation later. The whole process of obtaining an EEG recording must be an interactive one if useful results are to be obtained. EEG machine controls must be constantly adjusted to eliminate artifact (high frequency filters, time constants), to localise abnormalities to particular areas of the cortex (channel selectors) or to enhance desired signals (gain) (Figure 4.6).

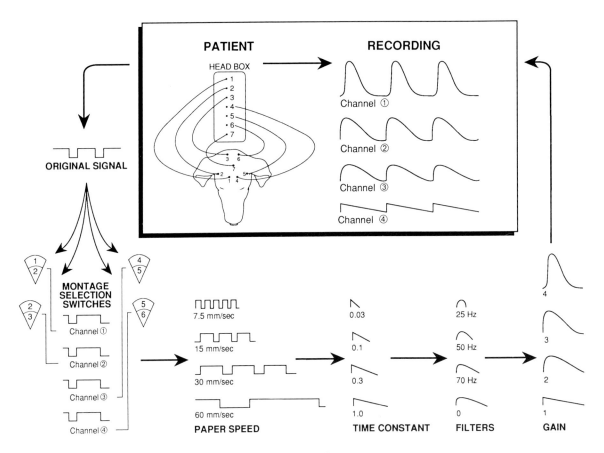

Figure 4.6

INTERPRETATION

Following a successful EEG recording session, the record should be read 'blind' if possible, rather in the manner of radiologist reading an X-ray film and a brief written description of the salient features of the dominant frequencies, focal abnormalities, response to drugs, etc. should be made. Interpretation of the recording with preconception of the expected findings and diagnosis is to be abhorred, since this has given rise to the inflated claims made for the technique in the past. Diagnosis of such conditions as cerebrovascular accidents from EEG findings, when the syndrome rarely, if ever, exists in the dog, underlies the importance of pathological investigation and illustrates the dangers inherent in preconception. In interpreting an EEG one is not looking for a definitive diagnosis (although in some cases this may be possible) but rather for an indication of the state of the animal's cortical activity at the time of recording. This state can vary from entirely normal and appropriate for its age, to a complete absence of apparent cortical activity. The presence of focal abnormalities or lateralising signals may allow more detailed assessment of the nature of the pathology (for example, acquired epileptic foci and neoplasia may be discrete, whereas viral encephalitic lesions are usually diffuse). The technique of serial EEG recordings over a period of time is of prognostic value in assessing response to therapy or recovery. The presence of a normal EEG may also be of value in the negative diagnosis of idiopathic epilepsy in certain breeds of dog, since such animals usually have entirely normal interictal EEG, whereas acquired epileptics frequently have focal changes.

Figure 4.7a is a recording from a conscious Labrador and illustrates the problems in recording from such an animal. There is marked muscle artifact in all channels, with periodic blink artifacts (electroculograph). Standard calibration data are shown beneath the trace. Compare this with Figure 4.7b which is the same animal under a sleep dose of methohexitone. The artifacts have disappeared and only slight slowing is superimposed. Figure 4.7c is a recording of a young Labrador in a state of profound depression.

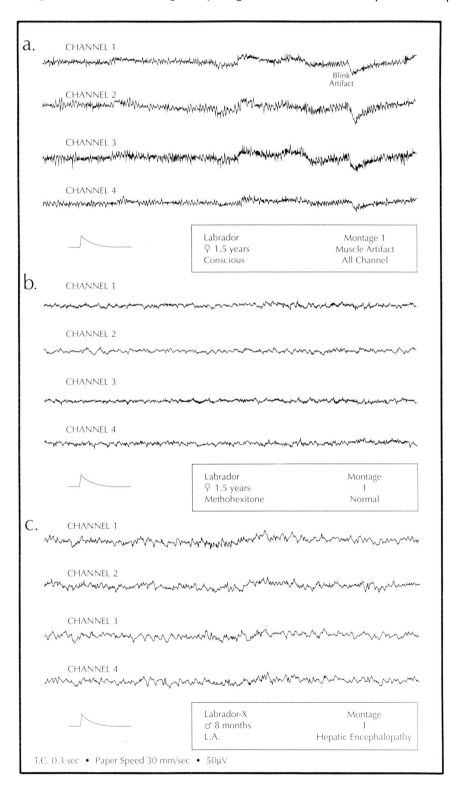

Figure 4.7

There is no artifact (local anaesthetic having been placed under the electrodes) and normal low voltage fast activity is replaced by excess slow activity, with runs of almost sinusoidal waves in all channels, reflecting the poor state of cortical function.

Figure 4.8a is a recording of a mature Labrador suffering clinical partial complex seizures. The low voltage fast activity is typical of an alert, mature animal and offers no indication of abnormality. Figure 4.8b is the same animal under methohexitone sleep and, compared with Figure 4.8a, shows increased slow activity, occurring in brief epochs. This is often seen in animals post-seizure, but is not diagnostic of 'idiopathic epilepsy'.

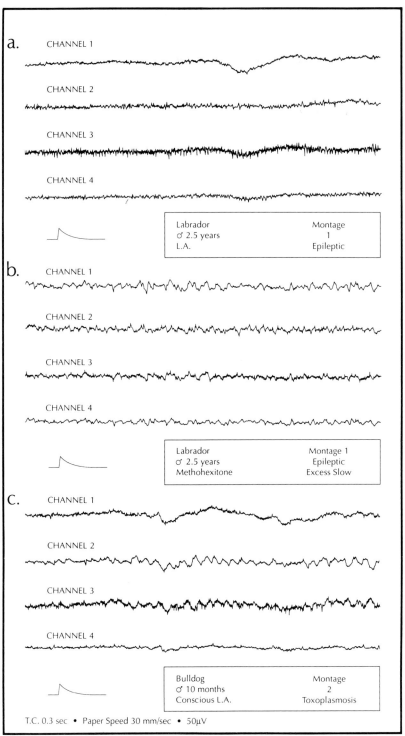

Figure 4.8

Figure 4.8c shows sinusoidal slow activity with little low voltage fast activity, often seen in chronic or recovering encephalitis cases. Methohexitone in this case (Figure 4.9a) enhances the basic waveform beautifully, but without altering the pattern shown in Figure 4.8c.

Figure 4.9b is case of acute distemper encephalitis and illustrates the lack of cortical detailed activity and shows well the irritative spike complexes, which may give rise to larval seizures in the EEG, occasionally associated with clinical signs during the recording session.

Figure 4.9c illustrates well the non-diagnostic nature of many EEG recordings. The trace shows marked, diffuse slow activity, but it would be impossible to arrive at a diagnosis of hypomyelinogenesis, the underlying pathological change in this case, from the EEG findings. This is the basic paradox of the technique, which must be acknowledged by its practitioners.

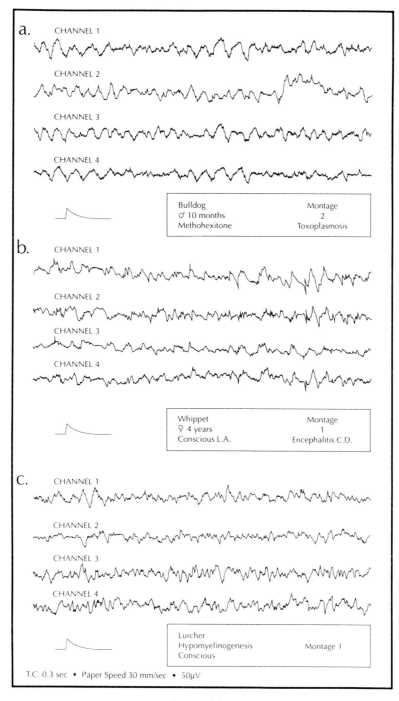

Figure 4.9

Part 4

URODYNAMIC STUDIES

Nicholas J. H. Sharp B.Vet. Med., M.V.M., Dip. A.C.V.S., M.R.C.V.S.

INTRODUCTION

Urodynamic studies comprise two basic techniques, the cystometrogram (CMG) and the urethral pressure profile (UPP). Each may be combined with electromyography (EMG) to simultaneously record function of the urethralis skeletal muscle, the so-called external urethral sphincter.

Although these are very valuable as objective means of assessing micturition, it should be stressed that less objective, but clinically very useful, information can be obtained from the neurological examination (see Chapter 12). Conscious control of micturition, the anal reflex and perineal sensation assess the sacral spinal cord segments and their integration with higher centres. In particular, the ability to pass a good stream of urine with low residual volume indicates normal detrusor function, which may obviate the need for a CMG. Likewise, the ability to retain urine normally without leakage implies correct function of the urethral sphincter mechanisms and should correlate to a normal UPP.

In addition to CMG and UPP, there are three more specialised techniques that will be briefly discussed: namely, electromyelography, evoked potentials and uroflowmetry. Of these, uroflowmetry is of most potential value because it is designed to assess the micturition process during the voiding process rather than in the static state.

CYSTOMETROGRAM

This is an objective measure of intravesicular pressure during the initiation of an induced detrusor reflex, although a normal sustained reflex is difficult to document. The CMG also provides information on the threshold volume and pressure, and the capacity and compliance of the bladder wall. Compliance can be affected either by fibrosis limiting the ability of the bladder wall to stretch, or due to inference with neural mechanisms (ß sympathetic control) of smooth muscle relaxation. The threshold volume necessary to initiate a detrusor reflex is approximately 20 ml/kg body weight. The absolute maximum volume that should not be exceeded is 35 ml/kg.

Sedation is required to perform a CMG and *xylazine* is the agent of choice because it does not interfere with the detrusor reflex. The drug both overcomes voluntary inhibition of micturition and any movement caused by the sensation of bladder distension, but its effect usually lasts no more than 45 minutes. The recommended dose of 1.1 mg/kg I/V or 2.2 mg/kg S/C often causes bradycardia (with up to a 60 per cent drop in heart rate), first degree heart block and a fall in cardiac output. If this drug is contraindicated in an individual dog, a mixture of *acepromazine* and *oxymorphine* (0.11 mg/kg I/V for each) can be used, but is much less effective in abolishing movement artifacts and may be more suppressive to the detrusor reflex. *Atropine* may be used to overcome the deleterious effects of the *xylazine,* but itself has a dose-dependent effect on the detrusor reflex. At 0.06 mg/kg S/C, it should have no effect, whereas a higher dose or intravenous administration causes some interference. The subcutaneous dose above has been shown not to affect CMG in young healthy dogs, but this may not be the case in older patients or those with neurological dysfunction. It has been recommended that *atropine* not be used during CMG if possible and we would support this view.

Method.

Following sedation, a suitable sized catheter is placed into the empty bladder and connected via a 4-way valve to:

 a. A pressure transducer with strip chart recorder.

 b. An infusion pump.

The bladder can either be filled with air or CO_2 (rate 150 ml/min), or sterile saline (rate 40—80 ml/min) by the infusion pump. As filling occurs, intravesicular pressure is measured simultaneously on the strip chart recorder. A Foley catheter with bulb inflated is necessary in the female and in the male, the tip of the penis may need to be pinched off around the catheter to prevent leakage of fluid and resultant loss of pressure.

A normal bladder with intact innervation initially responds to an increased intravesicular volume with only a minimal rise in pressure (usually less than 20 cm H_2O). Beta adrenergic stimulation facilitates this by causing detrusor smooth muscle relaxation. After a certain capacity is reached, the bladder is no longer able to accomodate to the volume increase. At a threshold pressure volume relationship, a detrusor reflex is initiated causing a normal pressure peak of 70—80 cm H_2O. Bladder wall fibrosis would be expected to reduce both capacity and threshold volume, whereas a sacral spinal cord lesion would affect one or both arms of the detrusor reflex and pressure peak. A normal CMG trace is shown in Figure 4.10.

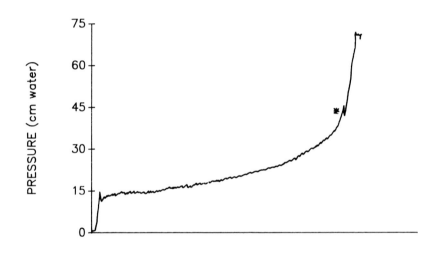

Figure 4.10
Normal cystometrogram (CMG) trace.
Threshold volume/pressure relationship for this dog is indicated by the asterisk

Complications

In man, up to 2% of CMG's result in urinary tract infection (UTI). These probably result from bladder distension, which increases its susceptibility to infection by the bacteria introduced during the catheterisation procedure. Catheterisation not associated with distension (e.g. UPP) is not associated with the same infection rate. In one study, nine out of twenty dogs developed UTI following CMG. Scrupulous attention to sterile technique and routine cleaning of the tip of the penis with betadine are important. A single dose of intravenous antibiotic just prior to starting the procedure should be considered. Haematuria is another common result of the distension produced during CMG and was seen either grossly or microscopically in twelve of the same twenty dogs. Haematuria depends on the maximum pressure reached and is independent of the time for which this is maintained. For additional information see Barsanti *et al* (1981).

URETHRAL PRESSURE PROFILE

Urinary continence has been described as a condition in which intra-urethral pressure exceeds intravesicular pressure. As long as pressure in the urethra is greater than that in the bladder, continence will exist. The UPP is measured as a recording (urinary) catheter is pulled distally from the bladder into the urethra, and along its length. As such, the UPP only measures resting urethral tone. It is, therefore, good for investigation of urine leakage occurring during the storage phase, e.g. a deficient urethral closure mechanism, or for obstructions along the length of the urethra such as a prostatic mass or a stricture. It is of less value for dynamic problems occurring during the voiding phase for which uroflowmetry is more useful. Depending on the patient, sedation may or may not be required for the UPP. In contrast to CMG, however, *xylazine* at 1.1 mg/kg I/V or 2.2 mg/kg S/C, although still the agent of choice, does have significant depressive effects on the UPP. This is because the urethral smooth muscle is affected by the sympatholytic action of *xylazine* (whereas the detrusor smooth muscle of the bladder wall is not). The striated muscle of the urethra (urethralis muscle) is also depressed by *xylazine*. Therefore, appropriate reference values need to be utilised depending on whether or not sedation is used (Table 4.3). *Atropine* does not affect the UPP and can, therefore, be combined with *xylazine* if necessary. We prefer to use no sedation if possible for the UPP, which is the first technique performed in a general urodynamic study. We then go on to perform the CMG using *xylazine* sedation.

Method

A suitable sized, side hole urethral catheter is used (diameter has no effect on UPP) and is again connected via a 4-way valve to:

    a.   A pressure transducer and strip chart recorder.

    b.   An infusion pump.

In addition to this equipment, which is the same as that used for CMG, the exposed portion of the catheter is held in a special catheter withdrawing device to slowly pull the catheter tip from the bladder along and out of the distal end of the urethra. As the tip is withdrawn, the transducer simultaneously records the pressure at the catheter side hole. This pressure is generated by the response of the urethra to a slow distension generated by simultaneous continuous slow infusion (2 ml/min) of sterile saline into the catheter via the infusion pump.

The catheter withdrawal rate should be the same as the chart speed, in order to allow correlation of events on the pressure trace to their exact anatomical locations along the urethral length. The resultant pressure profile is made up by contributions from three components:

    a.   Connective tissues and vascular tone of the urethra.

    b.   Urethralis skeletal muscle located just distal to the prostate in the male and just distal to the urethral midpoint in the female. As well as receiving innervation via the pudendal nerve, this muscle also receives some sympathetic innervation via the hypogastric nerve.

    c.   Urethral smooth muscle which provides the most important overall contribution. This is predominantly under α adrenergic sympathetic control.

Thus, it can be seen that there is no specific anatomical urethral sphincter, but rather a combination of structures which together result in a sphincter mechanism.

	Maximal urethral pressure (MUP) (cm H_2O)			Maximal urethral closure pressure (MUCP) (cmH_2O)	
	MUP + Xylazine	MUP − Xylazine		MUCP + Xylazine	MUCP − Xylazine
Male	46−58	100−120	Male	35−47	90−110
Female	28−37	85− 95	Female	19−27	75− 85

Table 4.3

Normal values for canine urethral pressure profiles (UPP) taken with (+) and without (−) xylazine.

From Richter KP and Ling GV (1985). Effects of xylazine on the urethral pressure profile of healthy dogs. *American Journal of Veterinary Research,* **46** : 1881.

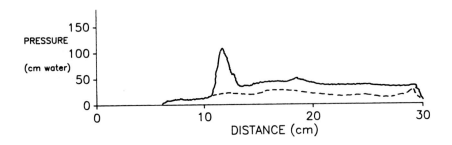

Figure 4.11
Diagram to show normal canine urethral pressure profile.
Values obtained without *xylazine* — solid line; values obtained with *xylazine* — dotted line

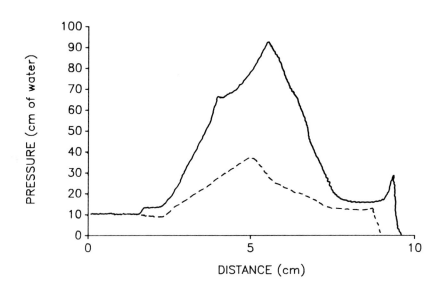

Figure 4.12
Diagram to show normal female canine urethral pressure profile.
Values obtained without *xylazine* — solid line; values obtained with *xylazine* — dotted line.

Normal dog and bitch UPP's are shown in Figures 4.11 and 4.12. The peaks, termed the maximal urethral pressure (MUP), correlate with the location of the skeletal muscle sphincter in both sexes. In the male, there is often another peak at the tip of the penis due to engorgement of the glans during catheter withdrawal. The MUP is said to decline with age in bitches. Maximum urethral closure pressure (MUCP) is the difference between the pressure in the bladder and the MUP. Functional profile length is the length of the urethra over which the MUP exceeds the pressure in the bladder. Of these values, the MUCP has the most important relationship to continence. Virtually all these parameters are reduced in both sexes by *xylazine* as shown by the dotted lines in Figures 4.11 and 4.12. Table 4.3 gives the range of normal values both with and without *xylazine.*

If the catheter is fitted at the tip with small bipolar recording electrodes, the exact location of the urethralis muscles can be identified by its resting electrical activity, which is displayed alongside the UPP trace. *Xylazine* again, however, tends to significantly reduce this activity.

78

The UPP, therefore, can provide data on any increase or decrease in the patient's urethral tone, which may then be rationally modified by pharmacological manipulation.

Sources of error:-

— Air bubbles in the system will dampen the pressure trace and should be avoided.

— *Xylazine* will reduce most parameters, which should be allowed for.

— The orientation of the catheter side hole can cause error, and it is advisable to repeat each UPP once or twice for greatest accuracy.

— The pressure transducer should be calibrated at the level of the urethra.

— The bladder should be empty initially.

URODYNAMICS IN THE CAT

In the cat, *xylazine* (1.1 mg/kg IV) is necessary to perform a UPP. The MUP tends to be at the distal urethra in the queen and the postprostatic urethra in the male cat, which again correlates to the location of striated muscle sphincters. No difference in MUP is found between spayed and entire females.

OTHER TECHNIQUES

The use of an EMG needle in the anus during CMG records the co-ordination of detrusor muscle and external urethral sphincter, because the external anal sphincter contracts synchronously with the skeletal muscle component of the urethral sphincter (urethralis muscle).

Electromyelography is an evaluation of the bulbs spongiosus reflex. Stimulation of sensory nerves in the bladder wall via electrodes placed in the tip of a urinary catheter is performed while recording events in the external anal sphincter muscle (which again contracts synchronously with the urethralis muscle). This checks the integrity of pelvic and pudendal nerves, as well as the sacral cord segments. A similar stimulation device can be used to record either cortical or spinal cord evoked potentials.

Uroflowmetry measures urine flow and, therefore, urethral function during the emptying phase of micturition. It can be combined with a percutaneous CMG technique and has been adequately described (Moreau *et al*, 1983).

FURTHER READING

BARSANTI, J. A., CROMWELL, W., LOSONSKY, J., *et al* (1981). Complications of bladder distension during retrograde urethrography. *American Journal of Veterinary Research* **42**, 819.

GREGORY, C. R. (1984). Electromyographic and urethral pressure profilometry. Clinical application in male cats. *Veterinary Clinics of North America* **14**, 567.

GREGORY, C. R. and WILLITS, N. H. (1986). Electromyographic and urethral pressure evaluations: assessment of urethral function in female and ovariohysterectomised female cats. *American Journal of Veterinary Research* **47**, 1472.

MOREAU, P. M., LEES, G. E. and GROSS, D. R. (1983). Simultaneous cystometry and uroflowmetry (micturition study) for evaluation of the caudal part of the urinary tract in dogs; studies of the technique. *American Journal of Veterinary Research* **44**, 1769.

OLIVER, J. E. and LORENZ, M. D. (1983). Disorders of Micturition. In *Handbook of Veterinary Neurologic Diagnosis,* (Eds. J. E. Oliver and M. D. Lorenz) W. B. Saunders Co., Philadelphia.

OLIVER, J. E. (1987). Disorders of Micturition. In *Veterinary Neurology,* (Eds. J. E. Oliver, B. F. Hoerlein and I. G. Mayhew) W. B. Saunders Co., Philadelphia.

RICHTER, K. P. and LING, G. V. (1985). Effects of xylazine on the urethral pressure profile of healthy dogs. *American Journal of Veterinary Research* **46**, 1981.

ROSIN, A. and BARSANTI, J. A. (1981). Diagnosis of urinary incontinence in dogs: role of the urethral pressure profile. *Journal of American Veterinary Medical Association* **178**, 814.

CHAPTER 4
Part 5

NERVE AND MUSCLE BIOPSY

Simon J. Wheeler B.V.Sc., Ph.D., M.R.C.V.S.

Both the peripheral nervous system and the musculature of animals are amenable to biopsy in many situations, but careful consideration is required before performing these procedures. It is not adequate to remove a piece of tissue, either surgically or otherwise, place it in formalin and submit it to a diagnostic laboratory. Such specimens are most unlikely to provide diagnostic information and the procedure is likely to have a detrimental effect on the patient. Thus, careful planning of the procedure, correct handling and fixation of the tissue and expert interpretation are all required in performing a biopsy.

NERVE BIOPSY

The general principles regarding nerve biopsy have been reviewed by Dyck *et al* (1984) and apply to animals as much as humans. Whilst the examination of a biopsy is useful in selected cases of peripheral neuropathy, it is not a procedure which should be performed in all cases and should probably be restricted to those with a special interest in the subject who have access to the correct processing methods and who can interpret the findings with confidence.

The indication for nerve biopsy is in cases where the presence of a neuropathy has been confirmed by clinical and electrophysiological testing and where further information regarding the nature of the neuropathy is desired. Nerve biopsy should not be performed where neurological dysfunction is considered to be a possibility but no other tests have been performed to confirm this. Biopsy of nerve will lead to the development of neurological deficits and possibly have painful sequelae and this must be remembered prior to performing the procedure, which is done under general anaesthesia.

Peripheral nerve may be collected from a number of sites in the body, the appropriate one being determined by the neurological findings and the results of electrophysiological testing. The following are suitable sites for biopsy:

Sensory nerves:	Lateral cutaneous radial
	Medial cutaneous radial
	Saphenous
	Superficial peroneal
Mixed nerves:	Ulnar (at elbow)
	Tibial (above hock)
Nerve root:	Cranial lumbar
Plexus:	Brachial

In collecting a biopsy of sensory nerves, it is possible to remove the entire thickness of nerve and similarly, in the cranial lumbar region ($L_1 - L_3$), a whole nerve root may be harvested. Where a mixed nerve or plexal nerve are being collected, only a fascicle may be removed.

The nerve is approached and isolated with great care being taken to avoid handling the nerve. The nerve or fascicle is sectioned at the proximal end and a 2—3 cm portion dissected free with either sharp pointed scissors or a No. 11 scalpel blade. The distal end is cut free and the nerve removed. The portion of nerve should only be held by the ends, not by the middle portion. The nerve must be maintained in its longitudinal orientation during fixation, this being most easily achieved by placing it on a piece of dry filter paper or card. Some method of denoting which end of the nerve is proximal is useful. The biopsy is fixed in phosphate buffered glutaraldehyde.

Processing of the biopsy involves the preparation of semi-thin and thin sections for light and electron microscopic examination respectively. A portion of the nerve is retained for single fibre teasing and subsequent examination. Details of the histological methods are given by Dyck *et al* (1984).

Evaluation of the nerve requires a qualitative appreciation of the structure and any pathological change in both the sections and the teased fibres and a quantitive analysis of the fibre composition and of internodal length. Using these methods, comparisons may be made between normal, age matched individuals and the patient.

MUSCLE BIOPSY

Muscle biopsy is also readily performed, but similar considerations apply here as in nerve biopsy. There should be good supportive evidence of myopathy before a biopsy is collected. In selecting a muscle to sample, it is wise to choose one which is neither free from the disease process or one which is most severely affected. The triceps, biceps femoris and cranial tibial muscles are most frequently selected. If motor end plates or terminal nerve branches are to be examined, the lateral digital extensor muscle may be removed intact and the area where the intramuscular nerves enter then processed for examination.

The muscle to be sampled is exposed surgically and the direction of the muscle fibres identified. It is necessary to maintain the muscle sample in its longitudinal orientation following removal. This is achieved by applying a muscle clamp to the fibres and dissecting the portion of muscle free around this clamp. This ensures that the piece of muscle to be evaluated is not damaged and that contraction artifacts are avoided. The muscle section, still in the clamps, is frozen in liquid nitrogen. (Sprinkling talc on the muscle prior to immersion is advocated to prevent the formation of ice crystals in the preparations). Other portions of muscle are immersed in glutaraldehyde for electron microscopy and possibly in formalin.

Processing of the muscle involves preparation of sections for light and electron microscopy. Also, the frozen muscle is stained histochemically to allow muscle fibre type identification and subsequent morphometric evaluation. Biochemical analysis of the frozen muscle may also be undertaken (Swash and Schwartz, 1981; Kakulas and Adams, 1985). If motor point evaluation is to be made, the muscle is stained with methylene blue.

The collection, processing and evaluation of muscle and nerve material by biopsy requires careful planning and expertise. The relatively non-specific collection of samples fixed in formalin is unlikely to prove diagnostic and may be detrimental to the patient. These procedures should probably be restricted to situations where suitable expertise is available.

REFERENCES

DYCK, P. J., KARNES, J., LAIS, A., LOFGREN, E. P. and STEVENS, J. C. (1984). Pathological alterations in the nervous system of humans, In *Peripheral Neuropathy,* Vol.1 2nd edn. (Eds. P. J. Dyck, P. K. Thomas, E. H. Lambert and B. Bunge), W. B. Saunders Co., Philadelphia.

KAKULAS, B. A. and ADAMS, R. D. (1985). *Diseases of Muscle,* 4th edn. Harper & Row, Philadelphia.

SWASH, M. and SCHWARTZ, M. S. (1981). *Neuromuscular Diseases.* Springer-Verlag, Berlin.

CHAPTER 5 # NEURORADIOLOGY

Jeremy V. Davies B.Vet.Med., Ph.D., M.R.C.V.S., D.V.R.

INTRODUCTION

This section is devoted to the techniques involved in creating images of the axial skeleton, the relevant radiographic anatomy and the radiological recognition of conditions affecting the nervous system. Some special techniques relevant to neurological disease are also discussed.

Whilst examples are given of the commonly encountered neurological conditions, the reader will be encouraged to adopt a systematic approach to the evaluation of radiographs.

GENERAL UNIVERSAL DESCRIPTION OF RADIOPATHOLOGICAL CHANGE

Radiographic changes can be classified in almost all instances in the following way: —

Changes in

POSITION

SIZE

NUMBER

CONTOUR

ARCHITECTURE

OPACITY

In the light of these changes the type of pathological process can be determined and a probability list of differential diagnoses offered.

HEAD
(Cranial vault, calvarium)

TECHNIQUES

The anatomy of the calvarium is complex and breed variations diverse. Fortunately, the number of recognised conditions is small and their complexity minimal. However, it is essential to achieve accurately positioned radiographs as even small degrees of misalignment may lead to erroneous interpretation.

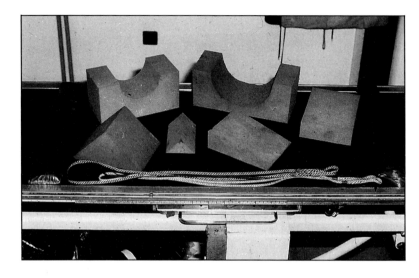

Figure 5.1.
Useful positioning aids:-
lucent foam shapes, ties (football boot laces, calving ropes), floppy sandbags (must not be overfilled)

Lucent foam blocks and ties, mouth gags and tongue forceps are required (Figure 5.1.).
At NO TIME should the head be positioned manually with or without lead protection. To facilitate accurate positioning general anaesthesia is essential. It must be remembered that the endotracheal tube may obscure certain parts of the radiograph, especially in the VD/DV projections and so temporary extubation must be considered.

At all times plain films must be taken before any contrast studies commence.

Each of the projections that may be employed are mentioned with practical tips as to how to avoid common errors. Positioning details can be found in standard atlases of radiographic positioning (see Further Reading).

Plain Lateral Projection (LAT)

Axial rotation of the skull and downward tilting of the mandible are the most likely faults. These can be overcome by judicious use of lucent wedges under the mandible. The beam should be centred on the lateral canthus of the eye.

Plain Ventrodorsal/Dorsoventral Projection (VD/DV)

There is no great advantage in the use of either view except in the brachycephalic breeds and cats where only the DV view is appropriate. Axial rotation of the animal is the most likely fault. Every effort should be made to align the animal from the tip of the nose to the tip of the tail in an accurately vertical position. The beam should be centred on the midline between the eyes.

Plain Lateral Oblique Projection (OBL)

Oblique projections of the skull are of limited value in neurological cases. However, they will overcome superimposition of bilateral symmetrical structures and are of especial use in the evaluation of temporomandibular joints, tympanic bullae and teeth. Most often they will be employed in the evaluation of the bullae. The animal is placed in lateral recumbency with the area of interest closest to the film. The skull is rotated through 20° along its long axis so that its dorsal midline approaches the table. The beam is centred on the base of the skull. A comparison view of the contralateral bulla is essential. Bullae should also be evaluated on the VD projections and/or the VD (open mouth) projection.

Plain Ventrodorsal Open Mouth Projection (VD [open mouth])

The animal is placed in dorsal recumbency with no axial rotation. The mouth is drawn open by the tongue which is pulled well forward between the lower canines by a pair of tongue forceps and a tie. Retraction of the tongue prevents a soft tissue opacity being cast over the bullae. The maxilla is retracted by a second tie ensuring that it creates an angle of 90° with the film. The beam is centred along the hard palate. Minor alterations in the angle of the beam from the vertical will overcome anatomical variations in the brachycephalic breeds. The animal must be extubated. (Figure 5.2).

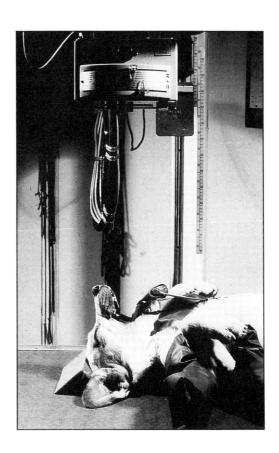

Figure 5.2
Positioning for
VD (open mouth) view

Plain Skyline Projection (SKYLINE)

Skyline projections of any lesion that disfigures the outer contour of the skull are essential to evaluate the involvement of deeper structures. Lucent positioning blocks are necessary for these views. The lesion is aligned at right angles to the beam and the beam centred on the midpoint of that lesion.

Plain Foramen Magnum Projection

The animal is placed in dorsal recumbency with no axial rotation. The jaws are kept closed and the neck is flexed so that the hard palate creates an angle of 25° − 40° to the vertical. The angle is dependent upon the breed/type. The beam is centred at the mid point between the eyes and exits through the foramen magnum. It is not necessary to extubate the animal but severe kinking of the endotracheal tube can be overcome by employing special tubes with reinforced walls that resist kinking.

Angular Venography

The animal is placed in sternal recumbency and positioned as for DV views of the calvarium. Both angularis oculi veins are catheterised. This is not feasible in the brachycephalic breeds. The catheters are sutured or taped in place and three-way taps attached. Both jugular veins need to be occluded at the time of injection. This is best achieved by applying a rolled bandage to the jugular grooves on each side of the neck. An elasticated bandage around the neck will compress the rolls onto the jugular veins at the appropriate moment. Extension tubes should be attached to each three-way tap to prevent unnecessary X-ray exposure of the operator. Prior to the contrast injection, a plain film should be taken for comparison.

It is essential that the skull remains in exactly the same position during the contrast study especially if subtraction techniques are to be employed. Whilst the jugular veins are occluded 3—6 ml of a water soluble contrast agent (150—300 mg I/ml) are administered simultaneously via both catheters. The film is exposed immediately at the end of the injections. The contrast film can be studied in comparison with the plain film but, ideally, subtraction will allow the preparation of a radiograph on which only the contrast filled cavernous venous sinuses at the base of the brain can be seen. Asymmetry of the vessels suggests the presence of a space occupying lesion (Griffiths & Lee, 1971). Subtraction techniques require special film and copying facilities and are only likely to be carried out in specialist centres.

Pneumoventriculography

Techniques involving the direct injection of air into the cranial ventricles have been described but are rarely employed. Recent non-ionic water soluble contrast agents such as Iohexol are frequently seen to enter the subarachnoid spaces of the cranium during myelography with no ill-effects to the patient. Deliberate injection of these compounds into the ventricles has not been advocated.

RADIOGRAPHIC ANATOMY

Skull

The anatomy of the skull is complex and is further complicated by the wide variation of skull types encountered. These are usually divided into dolichocephalic ('long nosed'), mesaticephalic and brachycephalic ('short nosed') types. Extremes of miniaturisation also influence skull conformation. Interpretation of skull radiographs is certainly facilitated by frequent reference to anatomical texts, radiographic atlases and, best of all, anatomical specimens.

Foramen Magnum

In cases of occipital dysplasia, abnormal dorsal extension of the foramen magnum is seen and is a common variant in toy and miniature breeds and may be of little clinical significance.

RADIOLOGY

Alterations in:-

Position

As nearly all radiographs will be taken of anaesthetised animals changes of position will not be evident. Clinical evaluation of head carriage is essential.

Size

Reduction in size (microcephaly, anencephaly) may occur as fatal congenital anomalies but are unlikely to be the focus of radiographic attention.

Symmetrical enlargements of the calvarium will occur in cases of hydrocephalus (Figure 5.3).

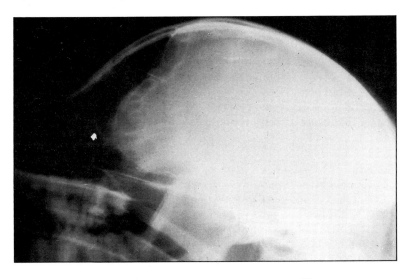

Figure 5.3
Hydrocephalus in this dog shows an enlarged, domed calvarium. Normal skull symmetry has been retained. The skull appears to have an almost homogeneous appearance, the normal convolutional markings that resemble beaten copper, having been lost.

Number

Teratogenic anomalies are unlikely to be the focus of radiographic attention.

Contour

Congenital loss of the integrity of the calvarium does occur. Persistent fontanelles are not uncommon, especially in the Chihuahua, but are unlikely to alter the external contour of the skull. A craniofacial anomaly of the Burmese cat may result in protrusion of the brain through the defect (exencephaly) but this is unlikely to present as a radiological case. Alterations in the shape of the foramen magnum have already been discussed.

Acquired alterations in contour are most likely to be of traumatic or neoplastic origin (Figure 5.4) and may assume an infinite number of appearances. When this alteration in contour involves the calvarium it may impinge upon neural tissue. Fractures of the canine skull are less frequent than in man because of the relatively thicker bone. When looking for fractures, a careful assessment of the soft tissues for focal areas of swelling may well draw the eye to the bony lesion. Similarly protrusions of the eyeball may well signal retrobulbar lesions.

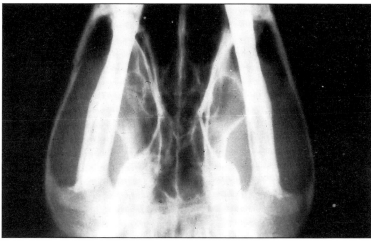

Figure 5.4
The contour of the right zygoma has been lost because of a fracture in this dog following a fight. A focal lucency is evident at the fracture site.

Architecture

Both the internal and marginal architecture of the skull are probably impossible to assess and so changes in opacity and contour can only be evaluated.

Diffuse Decrease in Opacity

Generalised decrease in bony opacity is most likely to occur in cases of hyperparathyroidism (Figure 5.5). This may be primary or as a result of hyperplasia or neoplasia of the parathyroids or, more commonly, secondary as a result of dietary mismanagement or chronic renal disease. Changes in the skull are particularly prevalent in renal secondary hyperparathyroidism.

The hydrocephalic skull will be enlarged ('stretched') and will appear to have a decreased density with loss of the convolutional markings of the calvarium (Figure 5.3.).

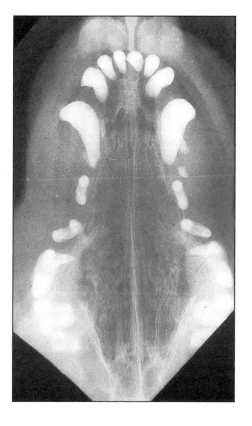

Figure 5.5
There is a generalised decrease in mineral density in the skeleton. Dorsal spines and vertebral bodies would be especially lucent and pathological fractures might occur in the ribs and the lumbar dorsal spines. These changes are typical of hyperparathyroidism. Changes affecting the skull are more often seen in those cases associated with renal disease ('Rubber jaw'). Because of the loss of mineralisation within the skull, the fine turbinate pattern appears exaggerated and the teeth appear to be 'floating in mid air' as the alveolar bone is almost invisible. This is typical of a case of renal secondary hyperparathyroidism.

Focal Decrease in Opacity

Focal decreases in opacity may be encountered in congenital anomalies, fractures, osteomyelitis and neoplasia.

Multiple Decrease in Opacity

Multiple lucencies are characteristic of multiple myeloma but are likely to be obvious in thinner areas of the skeleton before the skull. Other neoplasms, particularly soft tissue tumours invading bone, and osteomyelitis may result in multiple lucencies.

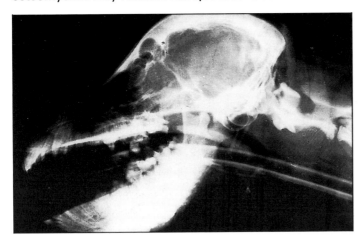

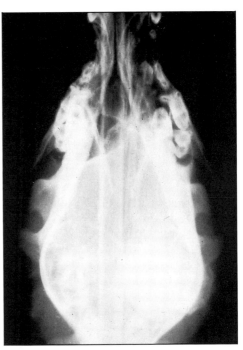

Figure 5.6a (above), 5.6b (right)

a. In this lateral view of the skull of a West Highland white terrier with craniomandibular osteopathy, there is a diffuse thickening of the dome of the calvarium and the mandibles but in this case little change in the tympanic bullae.

b. In this VD view of a different dog, new bone deposited on the left bulla particularly, is typical of craniomandibular osteopathy.

Diffuse Increase in Opacity

Osteopetrosis, a rare hereditary condition affecting the axial and appendicular skeleton, has been reported but probably the most common cause of a diffuse increase in opacity is craniomandibular osteopathy (Figure 5.6). This disease, seen in young West Highland white terriers, other small terriers and a few other breeds, is unlikely to accompany neurological signs. Metaphyseal osteopathy, a metabolic bone disease of the long bones of large growing dogs, can affect the skull causing diffuse increase in opacity. The skeletal pain associated with the condition may lead the clinician to believe that he is dealing with a quadriparetic animal.

Focal Increase in Opacity

Osteosarcoma, osteoma and osteochondroma, may all lead to focal areas of increased opacity. More advanced cases of otitis media will lead to a bony reaction to the chronic infection within the middle ear.

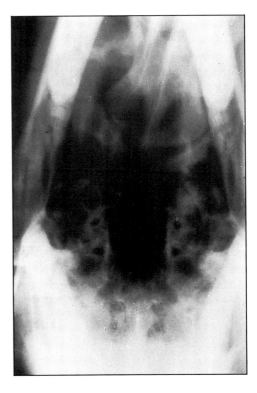

Figure 5.7
A VD (open mouth) view of the tympanic bullae show the left bulla to have an increase in soft tissue density within it due to the presence of granulation tissue and/or exudate. A slight increase in thickness of the bony wall is also noted.

The walls of the affected bulla and the adjacent petrous temporal bone may become sclerotic. Additionally, the air contrast within the bulla may be lost, being replaced by a soft tissue opacity indicating the presence of exudate or granulation tissue. (Figure 5.7).

Multiple Increase in Opacity

Osteoblastic metastases may result in multiple areas of increased opacity.

SPINE

TECHNIQUES

Only bony structures are visible and to minimise the difficulty arising from the complex anatomy, accurately positioned lateral and ventrodorsal films are essential. Myelography and other contrast techniques help in the evaluation of the spinal cord and spinal nerves. Occasionally, discography is performed. The reader is referred to atlases of positioning but practical tips for each of the projections are given.

Plain Lateral Cervical Projection (LAT)

The animal is placed in lateral recumbency with the fore legs tied back tight against the sternum. The neck is partially extended. Axial rotation must be avoided, usually by wedging the sternum and the skull. Dipping of the cervical spine over the film is best avoided by placing a small lucent wedge under the mid part of the neck (Figures 5.8 and 5.9). The beam is centred on the area of interest. It is necessary to take at least two lateral views (C_{1-4} and C_{4-7}) to overcome geometric distortion and the different exposure factors needed for the cranial and caudal portions of the neck. Coned views of the area of interest may also be made. This is the best projection for evaluation of the intervertebral disc spaces.

Plain Lateral Flexed Cervical Projection (LAT-FLEX)

Lateral views of the neck in the force flexed position may exaggerate malalignment of adjacent vertebrae. Extreme care should be taken if atlantoaxial instability is suspected or fracture dislocations are present as further soft tissue damage may be caused during radiography.

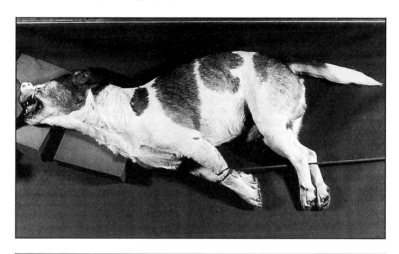

Figures 5.8 and 5.9

Positioning for lateral views of the cervical spine.
Foam wedges ensure that the whole of the cervical spine is horizontal to the table. There should be no axial rotation. The forelegs are drawn caudally and the neck extended to prevent superimposition of the scapulae and associated soft tissues on the caudal cervical vertebrae.

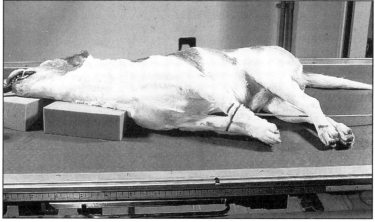

Plain Lateral Extended Cervical Projection (LAT-EXT)

This projection may also exaggerate malalignment and the caveats mentioned above stand.

Plain Ventrodorsal Cervical Projection (VD)

The animal is placed in dorsal recumbency with no axial rotation and the neck extended over the film. Appropriate angulation of the beam will allow accurate penetration of the disc spaces but this is often an unhelpful view in cases of disc disease.

Plain Odontoid Peg Projection

The positioning described for the plain ventrodorsal open mouth projection (see above) is used but it may be necessary to angle the beam at about 10° in a dorsoventral directon to the hard palate.

Plain Lateral Thoracic Projection (LAT)

The animal is placed in lateral recumbency with the legs forcibly tied cranially and caudally. Axial rotation must be prevented, any natural dips in the spine must be padded and the legs are best separated by foam pads so that they remain parallel to each other and parallel to the table (Figures 5.10 and 5.11). Several views will be necessary to evaluate the whole of the thoracic spine.

Plain Ventrodorsal Thoracic Projection (VD)

Ventrodosal films of the thoracic spine are difficult to interpret because of the superimposition of the sternum and mediastinal structures. However, they should not be ignored routinely because of this. The fore and hind limbs are tied cranially and caudally so that they are parallel to each other and axial rotation of the whole spine prevented with the judicious use of lucent foam wedges and pads.

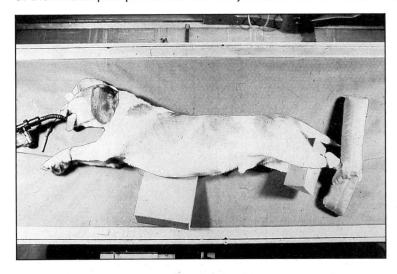

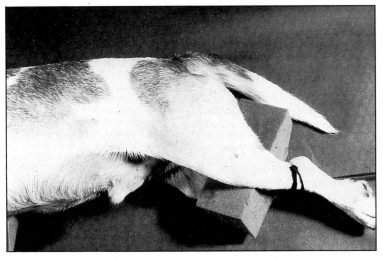

Figures 5.10 and 5.11
Positioning for lateral views of the thoracic, thoracolumbar and lumbar spine. The spine is forcibly extended with ties. Axial rotation is corrected by padding the sternum. Foam pads between the hind legs help overcome rotational distortion.

Plain Lateral Thoracolumbar and Lumbar Projection (LAT)

Positioning is as for the lateral thoracic spine with appropriate centring.

Plain Ventrodorsal Thoracolumbular and Lumbar Projection (VD)

Positioning is as for the ventrodorsal thoracic spine (see above) with appropriate centring. The absence of radiodense overlying structures makes these useful films.

Plain Lateral Lumbosacral Projection (LAT)

Positioning as for the lateral thoracic spine (see above) with the beam severely collimated and centred on the lumbosacral joint.

Myelography

Myelography is now a safe procedure providing the operator is able to penetrate atraumatically the subarachnoid space. The new nonionic water soluble contrast media *(metrizamide, iopamidol, iohexol)* are all extremely safe. *Iohexol* is the safest and the cheapest. Short bevel spinal needles are best for making the injection, though ordinary hypodermic needles will suffice. Contrast containing 300-350 mg Iodine per ml is used in doses varying from 1.0 − 10 ml depending on the size of the animal and the expected location of the lesion. Puncture of the subarachnoid space can be made in the mid to low lumbar area or via the cisterna magna. The safety of the new media and the effective flow of these materials means that the cisternal route is preferred. Only if the lower limit of an obstructive lesion needs to be determined is it necessary to additionally make a lumbar puncture. As with all contrast examinations it is essential to precede myelography with a satisfactory set of plain films. Cisternal puncture is described in Chapter 4. During cisternal puncture it is necessary to forcibly flex the neck, thus kinking the endotracheal tube. It is possible to employ tubes with specially reinforced walls that resist kinking. Alternatively, releasing the inflatable cuff during neck flexion allows the animal to breathe around the tube.

Vertebral Sinography (Lumbar sinus venography, interosseous vertebral venography)

Techniques involving the filling of the lumbar venous sinuses in order to evaluate spinal canal structures in the lumbosacral area have been described. Most commonly an injection of contrast is made via a bone marrow needle inserted into one of the cranial coccygeal vertebrae. If the caudal vena cava is compressed during the injection the vertebral sinuses will fill with contrast. It has been noticed during routine intravenous urography that if a rapid bolus injection is made using a wide bore catheter inserted in the saphenous vein the vertebral sinuses will often be opacified. It is seldom necessary to consider these techniques now as the new non-ionic water soluble contrast media such as *Iohexol* penetrate the sacral canal well when administered via a cisternal puncture.

Epidurography

During subarachnoid injection of contrast media an epidural injection may inadvertently occur. The images thus derived are often confusing. Deliberate epidural injection has been described but it is a technique with limited applications.

Discography

Direct injection of positive contrast media into discs has been described but it is a technique with limited applications.

RADIOGRAPHIC ANATOMY

Atlas (C_1)

The atlas is a short vertebra with prominent lateral processes. In ventrodorsal projection the lateral foramina, through which the spinal arteries pass, are present in the lateral processes.

Axis (C_2)

The axis is the largest cervical vertebra. It is an elongate bone with a thin, relatively lucent dorsal spinous process. Projecting from the cranial margin of the axis in the midline is the odontoid peg. This is sometimes visible on lateral views but more often has to be inspected on the ventrodorsal or special views. There is no intervertebral disc between C_1 and C_2.

Cervical Vertebrae (C_{3-7})

The remainder of the cervical vertebrae are all similar. The dorsal spinous processes increase in size caudally. The lateral processes project cranially often intersecting with the preceeding intervertebral disc space. These are often confused as mineralised disc material or bony fractures. The lateral processes of C_6 are especially large. The C_{2-3} disc space is the largest, the others are of similar size to each other, though $C_7 - T_1$ normally is smaller. Linear lucencies occasionally are seen in the cervical vertebrae and are thought to be the passage of nutrient vessels. In ventrodorsal projection, the shadow cast by the laryngeal cartilages may give a false impression of the presence of a radiodense foreign body. The ventral column of a myelogram normally 'kinks' and narrows over the C_{2-3} intervertebral disc space. Linear lucencies seen in the myelographic shadow represent the origin of spinal nerve roots. There is a natural expansion of the spinal cord at the level of the brachial plexus. (C_{6-7}).

The cranioventral borders of the bodies of vertebrae C_{5-7} are frequently deformed in those breeds that are prone to cervical spondylopathy. The cranioventral margin has a 'step like' appearance leading to poor support of the disc annulus. Not suprisingly, the associated discs often rupture later in life.

Thoracic Vertebrae (T_{1-13})

The thoracic vertebrae are all similar, possessing specialised facets for the articulation of the rib heads. The dorsal spinous processes are prominent and project caudally from $T_1 - T_{10}$, the dorsal spine of T_{11} (the anticlinal vertebra) projects dorsally and the dorsal spines of the remainder project cranially. It must be remembered that between the heads of ribs 2 to 10 a radiolucent intercapital ligament exists. This reinforces the longitudinal ligament making dorsal disc protrusion unlikely.

Lumbar Vertebrae (L_{1-7})

The lumbar vertebrae are all similar and relatively simple to evaluate. Myelographically there is a natural enlargement of the spinal cord at the site of the lumbosacral outflow ($L_4 - L_5$ vertebrae). From this point on, the diameter tapers and elongate lucencies represent the 'tails' of the cauda equina.

Sacrum

The sacrum comprises three fused vertebrae that articulate with the ilia. Its shape and position is variable. A normal myelographic column will penetrate the sacral canal.

RADIOLOGY

Changes in:-

Position

The position of various segments of the vertebral column may be altered in congenital and acquired luxations and in fractures (Figure 5.12).

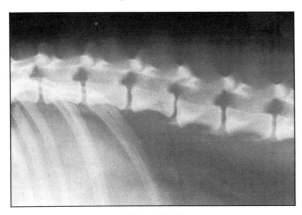

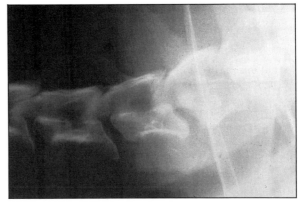

Figure 5.12	Figure 5.13

Figure 5.12
An intervertebral luxation at L_{2-3} has resulted in a step deformity in the alignment of these vertebral segments. Also noticeable are a narrowing of the disc space, a reduction in size of the intervertebral neuroforamen and an increase in the width of the associated apophyseal joint.

Figure 5.13
At C_7 the vertebral body length has reduced giving the vertebra a more square shape. The internal architecture of the body has also been disrupted. Collapse of this vertebra is occurring because of an osteodestructive neoplasm (osteosarcoma).

Size

Vertebrae may collapse in osteodestructive disease such as metabolic osteopaenias and neoplasia. Trauma and infection may also lead to an apparent reduction in size (Figure 5.13).

Number

The archetypal number of vertebrae in the dog and cat are:- cervical: 7, thoracic: 13, lumbar: 7, sacral: 3 and coccygeal: 6—20. There may be an apparent change in number as congenital transitional vertebrae occur. At the junction of one section of spine to another, a vertebra may assume characteristics of both sections, e.g. a first lumbar vertebra with vestigial ribs, a lumbarised sacral vertebra with transverse processes (Figure 5.14). At first glance it will appear as if there is an abnormal number of vertebrae. This is unlikely to have any clinical significance but may cause some alteration in the overall alignment of the spine. Lumbosacral transitional vertebrae will occasionally make it difficult to accurately align the pelvis for a ventrodorsal view of the hips.

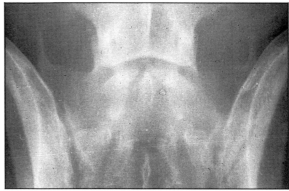

Figure 5.14
In this dog a vertebral segment within the pelvis has short curved transverse processes. The dog had seven normal lumbar vertebrae and so this is probably a lumbarised sacral segment — a transitional vertebra. These are usually of no clinical significance. However, asymmetric lumbosacral transitional anomalies will often be associated with some pelvic asymmetery rendering accurate positioning for VD hip films difficult, if not impossible.

Contour

Spine

Curvature of the spine may occur in any one of three directions or sometimes a combination of these. Scoliosis is a lateral curvature in the horizontal plane when viewed from above (Figure 5.15). Kyphosis is a dorsal curvature in the vertical plane when viewed from the side (Figure 5.16). Lordosis is a ventral curvature in the vertical plane when viewed from the side (Figure 5.17). These deviations may be so severe that the neonate is not viable but, more often than not, they are subclinical. As the animal gets older and heavier, they may be accompanied by degenerative changes that lead to clinical signs.

Figure 5.15
Curvatures in the horizontal plane, here at the thoracic inlet and over the base of the heart, are called SCOLIOSIS.

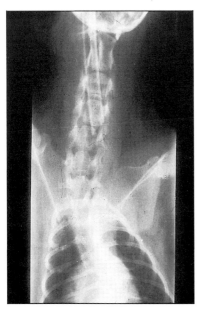

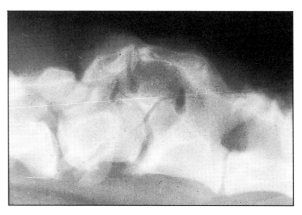

Figure 5.16
A gross deformity of L_4 and to a lesser extent the adjacent vertebrae, has led to a kinking of the spine (convex dorsally). This deformity has resulted from a hemivertebra and is called KYPHOSIS.

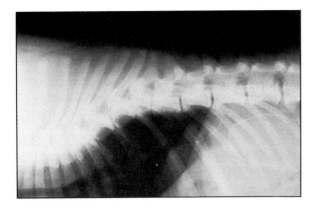

Figure 5.17
Vertebral anomalies in mid and lower thoracic vertebrae have led to an overall dipping of the spine (convex ventrally). This deformity is called LORDOSIS.

Vertebrae

Individual vertebrae may have an altered shape, they may be transitional (see above) or block (two segments congenitally fused) but asymptomatic (Figure 5.18). However, congenital malformations of the hemivertebra type ('wedge', 'butterfly', spina bifida, congenital absence of the odontoid peg) may be associated with neurological deficits.

Acquired alterations in contour may arise from fractures, osteomyelitis or neoplasia.

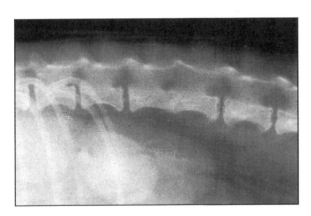

Figure 5.18
An incidental finding during a urinary investigation revealed a congenital 'fusion' of L_2 and L_3. These malformations are usually of no clinical significance.

Architecture

Both the internal and marginal architecture of the vertebrae are difficult to assess, so changes in opacity and contour are of greater significance. Osteodestructive changes associated with neoplasia and osteomyelitis are the most likely to alter the architecture (Figure 5.19).

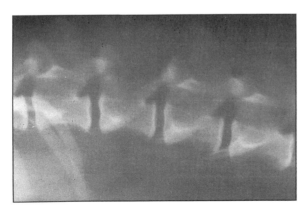

Figure 5.19
The marginal architecture of L_2 has been lost in as much as the dorsal spine and dorsal part of the neural arch have been destroyed. The internal architecture has also been affected as the remnants of the lateral aspects of the neural arch are being eroded as a result of an osteodestructive neoplasm.

Opacity

Diffuse Decrease in Opacity - Generalised decrease in bony opacity may be associated with disuse osteoporosis, primary and secondary hyperparathyroidism, hyperadrenocorticalism, steroid overdosage and mucopolysaccharidosis (Figure 5.20).

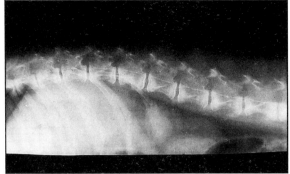

Figure 5.20
Generalised loss of mineral opacity occurs in hyperparathyroidism, in this case secondary to inappropriate diet. The radiograph, at first sight, appears poorly exposed or processed. This is because there is little contrast between soft tissues and the poorly mineralised skeleton.
(See also Figure 5.5).

Focal Decrease in Opacity

Focal infective or neoplastic lesions may lead to a decrease in opacity. The lesion may be primarily within bone or may be extending into the vertebra from the surrounding soft tissues (Figures 5.21 and 5.22)

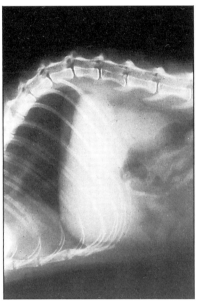

Figure 5.21
There is some loss of opacity in the mid portion of the vertebral body of L_3. Some marginal proliferation of fluffy new bone has also occurred ventrally. These changes are associated with a focal osteomyelitis.

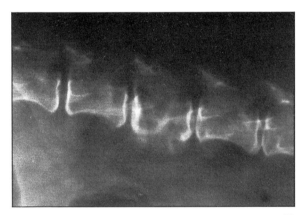

Figure 5.22
Focal lucencies within the vertebral body and neural arch of L_4 in this West Highland White Terrier have been caused by myeloma. An amorphous mineralisation of soft tissues is evident ventral to the vertebral body.

Multiple Decrease in Opacity

Multiple lucencies are likely to arise from multiple myeloma (Figure 5.23).

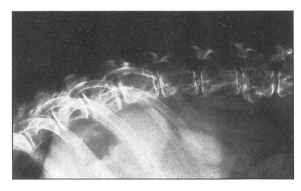

Figure 5.23
Multiple punched out focal lucencies are seen throughout the spine in this dog as a result of multiple myeloma.

Diffuse Increase in Opacity

Osteopetrosis has already been mentioned (see above). A more common cause of diffuse increase in opacity is hypervitaminosis A in the cat, where massive, proliferative bony deposits may affect any part of the axial or appendicular skeleton, but especially the cervical spine (Figure 5.24).

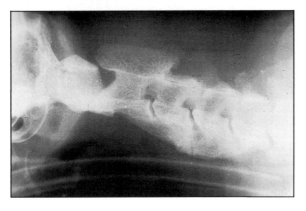

Figure 5.24
Diffuse, well defined deposits of new bone are present along the ventral aspects of the cervical vertebrae in this cat. This has resulted from a diet rich in liver (hypervitaminosis A).

Focal Increase in Opacity

Focal increases in opacity arise from osteoblastic activity resulting from neoplasia or in response to infection. The primary lesion may be within the vertebra but the sclerosis could well be an attempt by the vertebra to keep out a neoplastic or infective process (Figure 5.25).

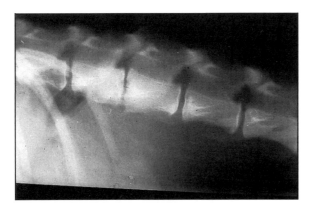

Figure 5.25
In this dog the L_{2-3} disc space has collapsed as a result of a septic focus (discospondylitis). In an attempt to wall off the infection, the vertebral end plates either side of the affected disc have become more dense (sclerotic).

Multiple Increase in Opacity

Osteoblastic metastases may result in multiple areas of increased opacity.

INTERVERTEBRAL JOINTS

There are essentially two types of joint in the vertebral column - the intervertebral joints and the apophyseal (synovial) joints. Similar criteria can be used to evaluate these joints as have already been discussed in the introduction.

Decrease in size of the intervertebral disc space and/or the intervertebral neuroforamen

If the disc deforms and protrudes or prolapses, the disc space or neuroforamen will narrow (Figure 5.26). Comparison of immediately adjacent segments of the spine is necessary. Often, in more subtle cases, it is easier to appreciate a change in shape of the neuroforamen than the disc space itself. Fractures and dislocations may lead to a decrease in size. It must be remembered that quite gross displacements of the spine in one plane may be almost invisible on the right angle view. Chronic infection centred on the disc (discospondylitis) will eventually lead to a reduction in the size of the disc space. However, the most common reasons for an apparent reduction in size is an oblique or inaccurately centred radiograph.

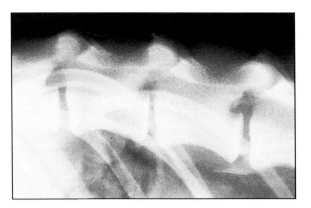

Figure 5.26
The $T_{13} - L_1$ disc space is narrower than the adjacent disc spaces. The associated neuroforamen has also reduced in size and has lost its characteristic Scottie's head shape. Mineralised discs are noted at T_{10-11} and T_{11-12}. These may well be clinically quiescent and only confirm the presence of degenerative disc disease. The narrowed disc space is much more likely to be clinically significant.

Increase in size of the intervertebral disc space and/or the intervertebral neuroforamen

In the early stages of discospondylitis, lysis of the adjacent end plates of the two vertebrae will lead to an increase in the size of the disc space (Figure 5.27). Fractures and dislocations can increase size.

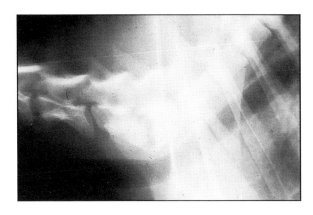

Figure 5.27
In this dog an aggressive and active septic focus in the C_{6-7} intervertebral disc space has led to destruction of the adjacent vertebral end plates. This gives an impression of an increase in size of the disc space. Note that the margins are ragged and ventrally and dorsally new bone is trying to contain the infection.

Alterations to the Apophyseal Joints

Degenerative joint disease affecting the apophyseal joints (synovial joints) will lead to typical signs of a degenerative arthritis, that is, loss of joint space and loss of sharpness of opposing joint surfaces due to the deposition of periarticular new bone (Figure 5.28). These joints can be affected by a septic arthritis where the changes will be both destructive and proliferative. The joints may be involved in vertebral neoplasia. Comparison of pairs of these joints on the ventrodorsal view is of value.

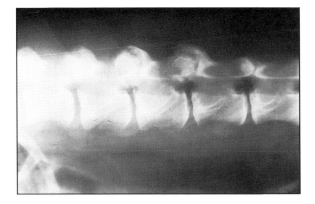

Figure 5.28
Major depositions of new bone and loss of the joint spaces are evident in this case of degenerative joint disease affecting the apophyseal joints in the lumbar spine (vertebral arthritis).

Spinal Soft Tissue

Unless there is a change in radiographic opacity these tissues are not visible.

Disc Annulus and Nucleus

Degenerating discs undergo a process leading to mineralisation. This process tends to start in the centre of the nucleus and radiate outwards. The partially degenerate disc is more vulnerable to deformation than a fully mineralised one. The presence of mineralised disc material often does little more than demonstrate the presence of degenerative disc disease (Figure 5.29). As yet unopacified or only partially opacified discs warrant the closest scrutiny.

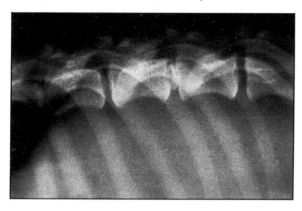

Figure 5.29
A fully mineralised disc is present at T_{12-13}. It remains *in situ* and is probably of no clinical significance other than to confirm that the dog has degenerating discs.

Spinal Cord, Meninges and Meningeal Spaces

Lesions may be extradural, intradural/extramedullary or intramedullary (Figure 5.30). Their presence can only be determined with the aid of myelography.

Figure 5.30 (a., b. and c)
Radiolucent lesions that are demonstrated during myelography can be considered as extradural (a), intradural but extramedullary (b) or intramedullary (c)

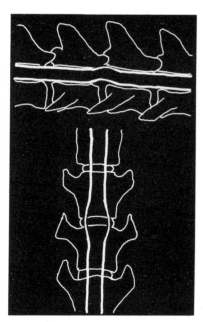
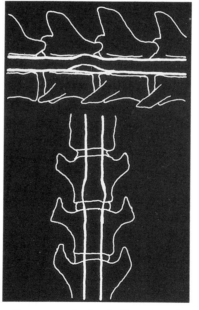
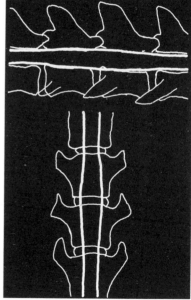

a. The ventral column is deviated dorsally, the dorsal column is slightly attenuated and, in ventrodorsal projection, the columns appear to diverge because of the presence of a space occupying lesion ventral to the cord.

b. The presence of an intradural mass is causing the ventral contrast column to bisect and pass either side of it. It is also causing the dorsal column to deviate and in ventrodorsal projection the columns diverge.

c. An intramedullary mass is causing the contrast columns to diverge in all planes.

N.B. The exact location of the lesion around the cord will determine which of the columns is so affected and so two views at right angles are essential for interpretation.

Extradural lesions include: intervertebral disc protrusion or prolapse, thickening of the longitudinal ligament, thickening of the ligamentum flavum, haematoma, extradural fat deposits, vertebral body deformation, cervical and lumbosacral spondylopathy, extradural tumours (vertebral, metastases) (Figure 5.31).

Intradural, extramedullary lesions, include: intradural tumours (neurofibroma, meningioma) (Figure 5.32).

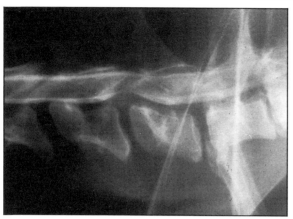

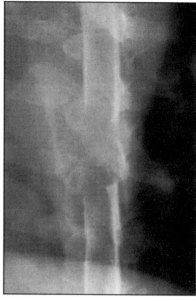

Figure 5.31
A massive disc protrusion at C_{6-7} is a good example of an extradural lesion. In this case the protruding disc material is faintly opacified.

Figure 5.32
In this case an intradural lesion has caused the subarachnoid space to widen and the accumulation of contrast at this point has caused a classical 'golf tee sign'. Because of the size of the lesion, the contralateral column has been obliterated but beyond the lesion both columns are restored.

Intramedullary lesions include: intramedullary haemorrhage or oedema, intramedullary tumours (ependymoma, astrocytoma) (Figure 5.33). It must be remembered that the normal expansions of the cord at the brachial and lumbosacral outflows will mimic intramedullary enlargements.

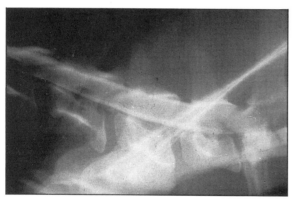

Figure 5.33
An intramedullary mass at the cervicothoracic junction in this dog is causing the contrast columns to diverge, attenuate and finally arrest.

MISCELLANEOUS TECHNIQUES

PORTAL VENOGRAPHY

Technique

Cases presented with non specific central nervous signs, possibly attributable to hepatic encephalopathy, may require a contrast study to eliminate the possibility of a congenital or acquired venous shunt.

Percutaneous splenic injection of contrast is possible. It is said that most humans lose up to one unit of blood following this procedure. In small animals it is most likely that the procedure will be performed under general anaesthesia and so administration of the contrast via a laparotomy is probable. Again, direct splenic injection is possible and haemorrhage can be monitored and controlled. However, the insertion of a catheter into a mesenteric vein allows repeated injections to be made particularly if shunt occlusion is to be performed at the same time. The possibility of injecting contrast following partial ligation offers the radiologist/surgeon an accurate means of assessing the success of the procedure.

Portal venography is best carried out on a couch with a fluoroscopic facility. Under general anaesthesia and routine asepsis, a small mid line incision is made just caudal to the umbilicus.

Through this a small length of jejunum is delivered and an 18G (1.2 mm) or 20G (0.9mm) catheter inserted into a mesenteric vein and tied in place. A 3-way tap is attached to the catheter. Through this, and via an extension tube to keep the operator's hand out of the primary beam, contrast can be delivered. Three to ten mls of water soluble contrast medium (300 – 400 mg l/ml) are delivered as a rapid bolus. If fluoroscopy is available, the timing of the passage of contrast through the portal system can be assessed prior to making spot films. If not, an exposure made just at the end of injection usually will suffice. Whilst in the VD orientation for the laparotomy, it may be possible to determine the presence or absence of a shunt. However, it is usually necessary to make a further injection in lateral recumbency to be sure of the location of the shunt. If a shunt is demonstrated the laparotomy is extended toward the xiphisternum. It is then worth isolating the vessel and temporarily occluding it with a bulldog clamp. A further injection of contrast will now demonstrate, first, that the correct vessel has been isolated and, secondly, the extent of hepatic vascular architecture. Partial ligation can be performed and further test injections made to evaluate the relative flow through the shunt and the liver. The vessel is usually ligated with silk suture. As a rule of thumb, overligation results in the intestines becoming congested and blue. Appropriate ligation seems to be at a point just short of this colour change. Those cases which show a diffuse, branching hepatic vasculature, undoubtedly carry the best prognosis. It is advisable to take a liver biopsy before routine closure of the abdomen.

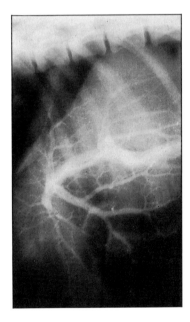

RADIOLOGY OF PORTAL VENOGRAPHY
Normal Vascular Anatomy

Blood from the pancreas, spleen and all the gastrointestinal tract, save for the anal canal, reaches the liver via the hepatic portal vein. This accounts for some 80% of the total supply to the liver. Blood is distributed throughout the liver by a system of afferent and efferent vessels. A small supply arrives via the 'true' hepatic arteries which are separate from the portal supply. A normal liver venographically will have a diffuse branching system of vessels which extend from the hilus to the periphery in all lobes (Figure 5.34).

Figure 5.34
A mesenteric vein has been catheterised and water soluble contrast medium (WSCM) administered. The contrast medium is seen to pass via the portal system into normal arboreal pattern of hepatic vessels. Some contrast is just entering the caudal vena cava (normal portohepatic venogram).

Acquired Shunts

Acquired shunts occur as a result of portal hypertension usually in response to severe liver disease. They are easily recognised by the proliferation of multitudes of tortuous, anomalous vessels (Figure 5.35).

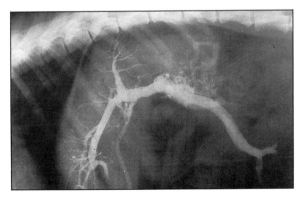

Figure 5.35
Contrast is seen to pass via the portal system and into the substance of the liver where a sub-normal arboreal pattern of vessels is present (c.f. Figure 5.34). The caudal vena cava has not yet opacified. An amorphous, tortuous collection of collateral vessels are developing dorsal to the portal vein and extend over the renal shadows towards the spine. These are typical collateral vessels resulting from portal hypertension (acquired shunt).

Congenital Shunts

These shunts may be intra (Figure 5.36) or extra (Figure 5.37) hepatic (i/h, e/h) and can occur between the portal inflow and the caval outflow (i/h, right patent ductus venosus or i/h left patent ductus venosus); e/h portocaval via the gastroduoedenal vein; e/h portocaval via the gastrosplenic vein; e/h portoazygos via the azygos system. The presence of a shunt is easily suspected when the hepatic vessels fail to opacify and contrast is seen to pass directly into the caudal vena cava or azygos system. The precise location of the shunt may be difficult to determine without multiple views. However if ligation is to be attempted under X-ray control then this is not vital.

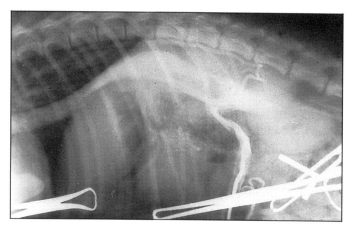

Figure 5.36
The portal system and hepatic vessels have not opacified. Contrast has shunted directly into the caudal vena cava and the azygos system (congenital extrahepatic shunt).

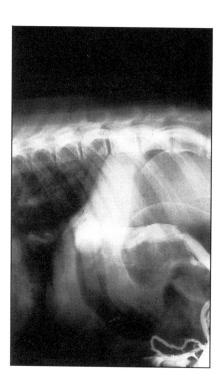

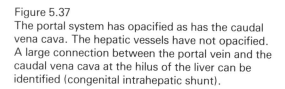

Figure 5.37
The portal system has opacified as has the caudal vena cava. The hepatic vessels have not opacified. A large connection between the portal vein and the caudal vena cava at the hilus of the liver can be identified (congenital intrahepatic shunt).

COMPUTED TOMOGRAPHY

The most useful method for the identification of brain lesions which is now available in veterinary neurology is **computed tomography** (CT). This technique is used widely and has been reported extensively in the veterinary literature. Its use has transformed the diagnostic approach to intracranial lesions in all species (see Further Reading). Not only will CT scanning identify the presence of a lesion within the brain, but it is possible to make some evaluation of the type of lesion based on the CT characteristics. Computed tomography also has a role in the evaluation of the spine in certain circumstances.

Technique

Performance of a CT scan requires general anaesthesia in dogs and cats. The CT scan makes images of the brain by slices, usually 3—5mm in thickness. In animals, it is usual to make the images in a dorsoventral plane, compared with the coronal views which are standard in man (Figure 5.38). Following an initial scan, a second is made after the intravenous injection of a water soluble iodine containing contrast medium. Some lesions will be apparent on the plain CT images, but usually the findings of the non-contrast study are restricted to identifying anatomical abnormalities such as hydrocephalus, haemorrhage and secondary effects of tumours. Brain oedema, deviation of the midline as reflected by displacement of the falx cerebri and abnormalities of the ventricular system, may be consequences of the presence of a tumour (Figure 5.38d).

Figure 5.38
Computed tomography, adenocarcinoma of nasal cavity
and forebrain of dog.

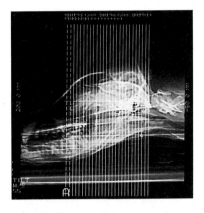

a. Scout film (lateral view of skull). Vertical lines show planes of section of CT images.

b. — g. Transverse images at various levels of skull. The images are those made following intravenous administration of water-soluble radiographic contrast medium.

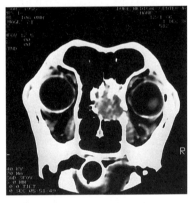

b. Note soft tissue density in right nasal cavity.

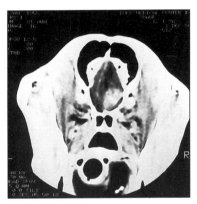

c. Note dense white area of enhancement in brain parenchyma and deviation of midline from the right side.

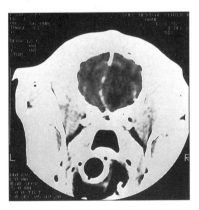

d. Note marked deviation of the midline and reduced opacity of brain parenchyma on right side due to brain oedema.

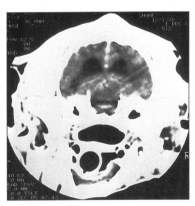

e. Note lateral ventricles (the oblique lines are artifacts).

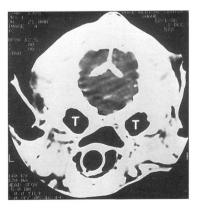

f. The inverted 'Y' in upper part of the cranial vault is part of the osseous tentorium. Note also the paired tympanic bullae (T) ventro-lateral to the cranial vault.

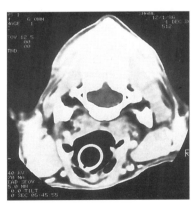

g. Image at the level of the foramen magnum.

Contrast medium administration leads to enhancement of the image of many tumours due to alterations in the blood-brain barrier by the tumour and changes in vascularity in the peritumoural tissues with subsequent contrast uptake (Figures 5.38c).

Evaluation of CT images is based on the principles of radiology, that is, observation and interpretation of changes in density, shape, position, size, and architecture of the brain.

There are occasional cases of spinal disease where the information provided by myelography can be further deliniated with the use of CT. Routine plain and contrast enhanced views are made. Interpretation of the images provided may further define the relationship between the spinal cord and the lesion.

Whilst the availability of the equipment required for CT scanning is limited in veterinary neurology to larger teaching institutions, efforts to secure the services of a CT unit in a hospital often prove successful and are to be encouraged.

OTHER IMAGING TECHNIQUES

Other imaging techniques may prove useful in brain disorders. Scintigraphy may provide information in some cases, but the resolution of this imaging method is rather poor and limits the usefulness. However, SPECT scintigraphy (Single Photon Emission Computed Tomography), a combination of scintigraphy and CT has proved useful in the detection of brain lesions in some circumstances, though veterinary applications have been limited.

Magnetic resonance imaging (MRI) also has been employed in the diagnosis of brain lesions. MRI has the advantage of being able to differentiate tissue types, potentially avoiding the need to biopsy lesions (Figure 5.39).

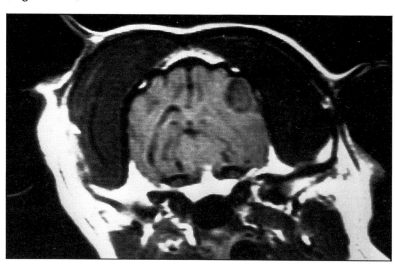

Figure 5.39
Magnetic resonance imaging. Meningioma in right cerebral cortex. Note lesion, slight midline deviation and collapse of right lateral ventricle.

FURTHER READING

DOUGLAS, S. W., HERRTAGE, M. E. and WILLIAMSON, H. D. (1987). *Principles of Veterinary Radiography,* 4th edn. Balliere Tindall, London.

GRIFFITHS, I. R. and LEE, R. (1971). Ophthalmoplegia in the dog and the use of cavernous sinus venography as an aid to diagnosis. *Journal of the American Veterinary Radiological Society* **12**, 22.

TURREL, J. M., FIKE, J. R., LeCOUTEUR, R. A. and HIGGINS, R. A. (1986). Computed tomographic characteristics of primary brain tumours in fifty dogs. *Journal of the American Veterinary Medical Association* **188**, 851.

WHEELER, S. J., CLAYTON JONES, D. G. and WRIGHT, J. A. (1985). Myelography in the cat. *Journal of Small Animal Practice* **26**, 143.

WHEELER, S. J. and DAVIES, J. V. (1985). Iohexol myelography in the dog and cat: a series of one hundred cases, and a comparison with metrizamide and iopamidol. *Journal of Small Animal Practice* **26**, 247.

WRIGHT, J. A., BELL, D. A. and CLAYTON JONES, D. G. (1979). The clinical and radiological features associated with spinal tumours in thirty dogs. *Journal of Small Animal Practice* **20**, 461.

CLINICAL PHARMACOLOGY AND THERAPEUTICS OF THE NERVOUS SYSTEM

Peter M. Keen B.V.Sc., Ph.D., M.R.C.V.S.

PART 1. CLASSIFICATION OF DRUGS BY MODE OF ACTION

An understanding of mechanisms of drug action is necessary to appreciate the effects, uses and interactions of the various drugs dealt with in Part II of this chapter. These drugs act almost exclusively through the various neurotransmitter systems of the brain. Because of the functional complexity of these systems, this account must necessarily involve considerable generalisation and the reader is referred to the texts listed under 'Further Reading' for a more detailed treatment.

A. DRUGS INTERACTING WITH THE NORADRENALINE SYSTEM

The functions of the noradrenaline system include regulation of:-

mood

arousal

blood pressure

Drugs that activate the noradrenaline system

a   Release noradrenaline

Amphetamine releases noradrenaline and also 5-hydroxytryptamine and dopamine. It is thus a psychomotor stimulant and is dealt with below.

b.   Inhibit noradrenaline activation

Amitriptyline, among other effects, inhibits re-uptake of noradrenaline into nerve endings, while monoamine oxidase inhibitors such as *iproniazid* delay breakdown of noradrenaline and so each in its own way increases the concentration of noradrenaline in the synaptic cleft thus causing arousal and elevation of mood. These drugs are hence known as 'antidepressants'.

Drugs that inhibit the noradrenaline system

a. α_2 stimulants

Xylazine and *detomidine* selectively activate the α_2 receptors through which noradrenaline inhibits its own release and thus produce sedation, analgesia and a fall in blood pressure. *Yohimbine* selectively blocks these α_2 receptors and so may be used to antagonise the action of *xylazine*.

b. β-blockers

Propranolol blocks the action of noradrenaline at β-receptors and so reduces tension and produces a fall of blood pressure, the latter by its actions in the peripheral nervous system.

B. DRUGS INTERACTING WITH THE DOPAMINE SYSTEM

The functions of the dopamine system include regulation of:-

motor activity

behaviour

vomiting

prolactin secretion

Prolactin secretion

Dopamine inhibits secretion of prolactin from the lactotrophes of the anterior pituitary gland. Thus drugs such as *bromocriptine* (Parlodel) which stimulate dopamine receptors reduce prolactin secretion and are used to treat pseudopregnancy. Conversely, the phenothiazine tranquillisers such as *acepromazine* (see below) which are dopamine antagonists are contraindicated in pseudopregnancy.

Vomiting

Dopamine is an excitatory neurotransmitter in the vomiting pathway. *Apomorphine* stimulates these dopamine receptors and is a powerful emetic and conversely the dopamine antagonist *metoclopramide* (Emequell) is used as an anti-emetic. (Dopamine inhibits gastric motility and so *metoclopramide* also increases gastric emptying by a peripheral action.)

Acepromazine

Acepromazine and other phenothiazine tranquillisers are dopamine antagonists and are classed as neuroleptics or major tranquillisers. They lower reactivity to external stimuli, modify behaviour, are antiemetic and increase prolactin secretion. Prolonged use in man may give rise to a motor dysfunction (tardive dyskinesia) characterised by involuntary movements.

Amphetamines

Dexamphetamine (now a Controlled Drug) releases noradrenaline and dopamine and so increases motor activity, produces wakefulness, psychic stimulation and anorexia and is classed as a psychomotor stimulant.

C. DRUGS INTERACTING WITH INHIBITORY AMINO ACIDS

1. GABA (γaminobutyric acid)

GABA. the chief inhibitory neurotransmitter, is contained in short inhibitory neurones throughout the brain.

Drugs that activate the GABA system

The GABA receptor is closely linked to a chloride channel in the neuronal membrane. Occupation of the receptor opens the chloride channel which inhibits cells firing.

Benzodiazepines potentiate GABA by facilitating its binding to the receptor. Thus members of this group are to varying degrees sedative, anticonvulsant and reduce anxiety and aggression. They are known as anxiolytic sedatives or minor tranquillisers.

Barbiturates also facilitate the binding of GABA to its receptor, although the relevance of this to their overall depressant effects is not clear.

Sodium valproate is anticonvulsant by virtue of its ability to inhibit GABA breakdown.

Ivermectin activates the GABA system by releasing GABA from nerve terminals. Mammals, unlike the parasites on which *ivermectin* acts, do not use GABA as a neurotransmitter in their peripheral nervous system and *ivermectin* is unable to enter the brain. Hence, *ivermectin* does not normally produce nervous effects in mammals. In Collie dogs, however, the blood-brain barrier is permeable to the drug so that unlicensed use of *ivermectin* in these animals may lead to severe and particularly prolonged CNS depression.

Drugs that oppose the GABA system

Picrotoxin combines directly with the GABA-controlled chloride channel which it closes thus opposing the effect of GABA. *Picrotoxin* is thus a general CNS stimulant. When used to stimulate respiration it may cause convulsions and so has been superseded by the safer *doxapram*. *Picrotoxin* has been used to treat *ivermectin* overdose.

2. Glycine

Glycine is an inhibitory neurotransmitter in the spinal cord. *Strychnine* is a glycine antagonist and so causes enhancement of spinal reflexes, and, in high doses, spinal convulsions.

D. DRUGS INTERACTING WITH THE OPIOID SYSTEM

The opiate analgesics interact with the receptors for a range of endogenous opioid peptides including the endorphins, the enkephalins and dynorphin. Acting through the mu receptor, *morphine* gives analgesia and cough suppression, but also respiratory depression and physical dependence. More recently developed agents such as *butorphanol* and the longer-lasting *buprenorphine* act partly at least through kappa receptors and so produce less respiratory depression and physical dependence than *morphine* but tend to be more sedative.

E. DRUGS INTERACTING WITH EXCITATORY AMINO ACIDS

The amino acid glutamate, or a closely-related substance, is thought to function as a widespread excitatory transmitter in the brain and spinal cord. The dissociative anaesthetics such as *ketamine* block one class of glutamate receptor, the NMDA receptors. Other glutamate antagonists may find application in the treatment of epilepsy and in the prevention of ischaemic brain damage but none is yet in clinical use.

F. DRUGS THAT INTERACT WITH SODIUM CHANNELS

Some drugs act, not through neurotransmitter systems, but directly through the sodium conductance channels of neuronal membranes which open during cell firing.

1. Drugs that block sodium channels

Lignocaine acts as a local anaesthetic by blocking sodium conductance channels and the same mechanism accounts for its anticonvulsant activity (and its anti-arrhythmic activity in the myocardium).

Phenytoin also blocks sodium channels but only during rapid firing. It thus suppresses the spread from an epileptic focus but has relatively little effect on normal cortical function and so is less sedative than other anticonvulsants such as the barbiturates.

2. Drugs that open sodium channels

The chlorinated hydrocarbon insecticides (e.g. Gammexane) and also pyrethroids (e.g. *cypermethrin*) act to prolong the opening of sodium conductance channels and so cause CNS excitement in overdose.

PART II. USE OF DRUGS IN SPECIFIC CONDITIONS

SEIZURES

STATUS EPILEPTICUS

Convulsions are best controlled by intravenous injection of a *benzodiazepine*. *Diazepam* (Valium) 0.25 – 1.0 mg/kg I/V, is most commonly employed but it is rapidly redistributed following I/V injection and has a short half-life of elimination (Table 6.1) and so may require repeated injection. An alternative is *clonazepam* (Rivotril) 0.05 – 0.2 mg/kg slowly I/V.

If *benzodiazepines* fail to control the convulsions recourse must be had to the barbiturates. *Phenobarbitone* is available in injectable form (Phenobarbitone Injection; Gardenal Sodium), 2 – 4 mg/kg I/V, but has a long latency of effect and is slowly eliminated (Table 6.1). Alternatively, *pentobarbitone* can be used, 4 – 20 mg/kg I/V to effect, although this is a less selective anticonvulsant than *phenobarbitone* and so may cause considerable sedation.

GENERALISED TONIC/CLONIC SEIZURES ('GRAND MAL')

Therapeutic principles

The overall aim of therapy is to control the seizures with a minimum of sedation. For this reason, if medication is given once daily, it should be given in the evening.

A pre-requisite of successful therapy is to maintain a constant level of the drug in the body. For this we require drugs with relatively long half-lives of elimination. A rapidly-eliminated drug requires frequent administration and is likely to produce unacceptable fluctuations in blood levels.

Anti-convulsant drugs need to be administered over considerable periods of time and this introduces a number of complications:-

If a constant dose is given at regular intervals the drug will accumulate in the body. As a rule of thumb, if a dose is administered at intervals of one half-life, then plateau levels will be reached after five half-lives (see Table 6.1 for representative half-lives). Note that a similar period will elapse between changing the dose of a drug and stabilisation at the new level.

Many anti-convulsant drugs induce the hepatic microsomal enzyme systems which are responsible for their metabolism. Thus, after a period of continuous medication, the animal will become tolerant not only to the drug itself but also to other drugs metabolised by the same pathway. *Phenobarbitone* and *phenytoin* show cross tolerance of this kind.

The longer a drug is given the more likely it is to cause long term adverse effects.

During treatment care must be taken not to precipitate status epilepticus in any of the following ways:

by abruptly withdrawing medication

by abruptly changing from one drug to another; the effect of the first may be lost before that of the second is established.

Acepromazine, chlorpromazine and other dopamine antagonists should be avoided as they may precipitate seizures in a susceptible animal.

Chloramphenicol should also be avoided because it inhibits the hepatic microsomal enzymes, greatly enhancing the effect of those anticonvulsants which are metabolised by this route.

Table 6.1
Elimination half-lives of anticonvulsants in the dog*

Generic Name	Brand Name	Half-life (hours)
diazepam	Valium	2−5
phenobarbitone	Gardenal, Luminal	64
primidone	Mysoline	9−12**
phenytoin	Epanutin	4½
ethosuximide	Zarontin	17
carbamazepine	Tegretol	1−2
sodium valproate	Epilim	2

*   Data adapted from Frey & Loscher (1985) and Frey (1986)
** Half-life is of parent drug which is metabolised to phenobarbitone (see text)

Drugs used

a.   Phenobarbitone (Gardenal, Luminal)

Phenobarbitone is the drug of choice for the long term control of generalised seizures in both the dog and cat. It acts to suppress spontaneous discharges with little effect on spread to other areas. In the naive animal *phenobarbitone* is slowly eliminated, partly by hepatic metabolism and partly through renal excretion of unchanged drug.

The initial oral dose in the dog is 1.5 — 2.5 mg/kg twice daily (b.i.d) and in the cat 0.5 — 1.5 mg/kg b.i.d. This dose may initially cause sedation and ataxia but these effects soon disappear due to development of tolerance and the dose may then have to be increased several-fold bearing in mind that following each change in dosage a period of more than a week must elapse before the drug reaches its new plateau. It is hoped that in this way control of seizures may be achieved without an unacceptable degree of sedation/ataxia.

Phenobarbitone may give rise to a number of minor side-effects including polyphagia, polydipsia and polyuria (the latter due to inhibition of ADH release). It has also been reported to cause whining in toy breeds.

b.   Primidone (Mysoline)

Primidone would seem to carry no advantages over *phenobarbitone* to which it is, in fact, metabolised and to which its effect is almost entirely due. Moreover, *primidone* is potentially more toxic than *phenobarbitone* and so it is best kept as second choice for those animals which do not respond to *phenobarbitone*. *Primidone* itself has anticonvulsant activity and is broken down in the liver to *phenobarbitone* and a second metabolite PEMA, which is relatively inactive. Since the half-life of *phenobarbitone* is much longer than that of *primidone* (see Table 6.1) it accumulates, so that when steady state conditions are reached 14 days after initiation of therapy, plasma levels of *phenobarbitone* are nearly five fold higher than those of *primidone* so that 85 per cent of the anticonvulsant activity can be attributed to the *phenobarbitone*.

In the dog, *primidone* is initially given at 15-30 mg/kg orally daily in two or three divided doses increasing to 30-50 mg/kg daily as tolerance develops. *Primidone* is not suitable for use in the cat because conversion to *phenobarbitone* is much less efficient than in the dog.

As is to be expected, *primidone,* like *phenobarbitone,* may produce sedation/ataxia, polyphagia, polydipsia and polyuria. It may also, however, cause liver damage, a problem not encountered with *phenobarbitone.*

c.   Phenytoin (Epanutin)

Unlike barbiturates, which act to suppress the epileptic focus, *phenytoin* stabilises membranes and so prevents the spread of seizure activity. As a result of this different mechanism of action, *phenytoin* is less sedative than *phenobarbitone.* It is broken down by the same hepatic enzyme that metabolises *phenobarbitone* and is a potent inducer of this enzyme.

The major limitation of *phenytoin* is its very short half-life (Table 6.1). Doses as high as 35 mg/kg t.i.d. orally must be given to attain therapeutic levels in plasma and this makes it unsuitable for use as an anticonvulsant in the dog.

Reports of *phenytoin* toxicity in the dog are rare, possibly because of the low plasma levels normally achieved. Potential toxic effects are: i) hepatic insufficiency; ii) conditioned folate deficiency *(phenytoin* induces the enzyme which breaks down folate) leading to megaloblastic anaemia and iii) gingival hyperplasia.

Phenytoin is more slowly metabolised in the cat than in the dog (half-life 24-108 hours) and so may be given at 2-3 mg/kg/day orally but accumulation to toxic levels, heralded by sedation, ataxia and anorexia, may occur.

d.   Other Drugs

Carbamazepine (Tegretol) and *sodium valproate* (Epilim) are not suitable for long-term control of seizures owing to their very short half lives (Table 6.1). *Benzodiazepines* are also rapidly eliminated and, in addition, tolerance to their anticonvulsant effect develops rapidly. *Ethosuximide* (Zarontin) has been used in man for absence seizures ('petit mal') but there is no clear indication that this condition occurs in the dog or cat.

BEHAVIOURAL DISORDERS

DRUGS USED

Progestagens

The progestagens, *megoestrol acetate* and *medroxyprogesterone acetate* act via the hypothalamus to reduce gonadotrophin secretion and hence reduce testosterone levels. They thus find their chief application in those behavioural disorders which are related to male sexual drive. In addition they, and particularly *megoestrol,* act directly on the CNS to influence mood and general tractability and so also find application in a number of stress-related disorders.

The toxicity of progestagens given over a period of time is by no means negligible. They may cause hyperglycaemia, glucose intolerance and raised growth hormone levels — the so-called 'diabetes/acromegaly syndrome'. They may also cause polydipsia, polyuria and polyphagia leading to increased weight gain. More rarely, progestagens may cause mammary hyperplasia.

Megoestrol acetate is given by regular oral administration. *Medroxyprogesterone acetate* is given intramuscularly (i.m.) or subcutaneously (s.c.) as a repository injection. Dosage rates are:-

> *Megoestrol acetate:* Dog: initially 2 mg/kg per day orally for 2 weeks, gradually reducing the dosage thereafter. If no response after a further week the dose may be briefly increased to 4 mg/kg/day. Cat: 2mg/kg daily orally for 1 – 3 weeks, reducing the dose thereafter.

> *Medroxyprogesterone acetate:* Dog: 10-20 mg/kg i.m. or s.c. every 3 – 6 months. Cat: 10 mg/kg every 3 – 6 months.

In general, *megoestrol* is preferred to *medroxyprogesterone* for most behavioural conditions on account of its greater direct effect on the brain and the fact that oral administration allows the dosage to be more accurately controlled.

Minor tranquillisers

Minor tranquillisers such as the benzodiazepines *diazepam* (Valium) and *nitrazepam* (Mogadon) find application in a number of behavioural disorders including phobias (e.g. thunderstorms), anorexia and spraying in cats. They may also be used to reduce sexual drive while progestagens are taking effect.

Dosage rate is 0.25 mg/kg three times daily (t.i.d.) in both dogs and cats.

Anti-anxiety drugs

The tricyclic antidepressant *amitriptyline,* 1 – 2 mg/kg orally daily, may be used to reduce the anxiety which underlies behavioural disorders such as excessive grooming in cats and separation anxiety in dogs.

Psychomotor stimulants.

Paradoxically low doses of the psychomotor stimulant *dexamphetamine* (Dexedrine) are effective in hyperkinesis in dogs. Care must be taken not to give an overdose which may cause hyperactivity and stereotyped (repeated, pointless) behaviour. Dose in dogs is 0.2 – 1.3 mg/kg orally daily.

Major tranquillisers

Major tranquillisers such as *chlorpromazine,* so called because they are effective in a range of human psychoses, reduce reactivity to external cues and so find little application in the therapy of behavioural conditions in dogs and cats.

CLASSIFICATION OF CONDITIONS BY PREFERRED THERAPY

Class 1

Related to male sex drive hence progestagens are first choice. Benzodiazepines are reserved for use if progestagens fail or to suppress symptoms while progestagens are taking effect.

> Aggression
> Urine-marking
> Mounting
> Sexual perversion
> Roaming
> Spraying

> In the last case *benzodiazepines* may be preferred.

Class 2

Stress-related conditions in which *benzodiazepines* are the agents of first choice and progestagens second choice.

> Phobias
> Anorexia

Class 3

Anxiety-related syndromes in which *amitriptyline* is first choice and progestagens are used if this fails:

> Excess grooming
> Separation anxiety

Class 4

Hyperkinetic syndromes in which *dexamphetamine* is specifically indicated.

ACUTE TRAUMA TO BRAIN AND SPINAL CORD

BRAIN TRAUMA

Corticosteroids are widely accepted as the standard treatment for brain trauma, their chief effect being to reduce brain oedema. If, depending on the circumstances of the case, shock is present then large doses of corticosteroids (e.g. 2—5 mg/kg *dexamethasone* i.v. t.i.d. for 2 days) are usually given. If the animal is not in shock then lower doses of corticosteroids (e.g. 0.25 mg/kg *dexamethasone* i.v.) should be given to reduce brain oedema while avoiding the side effects of larger doses of corticosteroids.

Fluid intake should be restricted to minimise oedema.

The osmotic diuretic *mannitol* (Osmitrol) 1—2 g/kg iv every 4—6 hours for 3 days has also been given to reduce oedema, although recent work suggests that doses of 0.25 g/kg may reduce intracranial pressure while avoiding the risks of severe dehydration and renal dysfunction. *Mannitol* should **not** be used if there is hypovolaemic shock or ongoing haemorrhage.

BLUNT TRAUMA TO SPINAL CORD

A great deal of experimental work has been done on mechanisms of nervous tissue damage in blunt injury to the spinal cord. Briefly, it seems that apart from the initial direct damage to spinal cord pathways caused by the trauma, there are also indirect mechanisms whereby mediators released from damaged cells cause secondary cellular damage and reduce spinal cord blood flow which in turn causes ischaemic necrosis. Currently, the number of postulated mechanisms is matched by an equal number of suggested remedies.

Corticosteroids are the treatment of choice for spinal cord trauma and have been shown to improve spinal cord blood flow and increase functional recovery. One trial showed that soluble corticosteroid (in this case *methyl-prednisolone sodium succinate*) produced best results. The suggested dose of *methyl-prednisolone* was 30 mg i.v. on days 1 and 2 followed by 5 mg i.m. t.i.d. on alternate days for a total of 9 days.

A major consideration when using corticosteroids in spinal cord trauma is that both corticosteroids and trauma to the spinal cord may separately lead to gastrointestinal ulceration so that a combination of the two is particularly dangerous in this respect. For instance, corticosteroids have caused fatal colonic perforation in dogs undergoing surgery for intervertebral disc protrusion. A lower dosage regime designed to avoid this complication is *dexamethasone* 0.25 mg/kg i.v. then 0.1 mg/kg i.m. t.i.d. for 3 days then 0.1 mg/kg at increasing intervals.

Oedema does not play a major part in the reaction of the spinal cord to trauma and so, in contrast to trauma of the brain, there is no place for osmotic diuretics such as *mannitol* in the management of this condition.

INTERVERTEBRAL DISC PROTRUSION

With severe pain.

> *Prednisolone* 0.5 mg/kg orally b.i.d. for 72 hours reduces inflammation of nerve roots, increases blood flow and hence reduces pain. The risk of gastrointestinal ulceration mentioned above should be borne in mind.

With total paralysis.

> *Dexamethasone* 2 mg/kg iv repeated 4 hours later, then 0.1 mg/kg i.m. b.i.d. for 2—3 days may improve the prognosis.

HEAT STROKE

The priority must be to reduce body temperature. This is best done by total body immersion in cold water. Antipyretic analgesics are **not** indicated since the thermoregulatory centre is not the source of the hyperthermia.

Glucocorticoids or *mannitol* (see Brain Trauma above) may be used to reduce cerebral oedema.

NARCOLEPSY

Agents of choice in this condition are the psychomotor stimulants (see above). *Dexamphetamine* (Dexedrine) 0.2—1.3 mg/kg daily orally may be used. This is now classified as a Controlled Drug. An alternative is *imipramine* (Tofranil) 0.5—1.0 mg/kg daily orally. This may take some time to establish its effect and should not be suddenly withdrawn. Monoamine oxidase inhibitors are contraindicated.

HEPATIC ENCEPHALOPATHY

AETIOLOGY

Hepatic encephalopathy occurs in advanced liver disease and/or portal systemic shunting and is largely due to failure of the diseased liver to remove toxic products of gut metabolism from the portal circulation. These toxic products include:

Ammonia produced by bacteria in the colon would normally be converted to urea in the liver. This no longer occurs and so plasma ammonia rises, plasma urea falls and ammonium biurate crystals may be formed in the urine. Dietary protein is a substrate for ammonia-producing bacteria and so exacerbates the condition.

Amino acids. There is a rise in plasma aromatic amino acids (tyrosine, phenylalanine, tryptophan) which are normally metabolised in the liver. These may enter the brain to interfere with amine neurotransmitter mechanisms. There is a concurrent fall in branched-chain amino acids (valine, leucine, isoleucine) which are metabolised in muscle rather than in liver and, as these compete with aromatic amino acids for uptake into the brain, the uptake of the latter into brain tissue is further increased. Plasma concentrations of mercaptans, which are produced by gut bacteria from methionine, also increase and may enter the brain. One of the mercaptans, dimethyl sulphide, gives the breath its characteristic odour.

TREATMENT

Cease protein intake, as dietary protein is the major source of ammonia.

Empty the colon by an enema or a cathartic. This removes colonic bacteria and their products.

Lactulose (Duphalac) 5 – 15 mls orally t.i.d. daily. *Lactulose* is a semisynthetic disaccharide which is split by gut bacteria to yield lactic and acetic acids. The consequent fall in intestinal pH suppresses ammonia production and reduces ammonia absorption.

Gut sterilisation. In human medicine *neomycin* is given orally to sterilise the bowel. *Neomycin* (20 mg/kg orally b.i.d.) has been found of little use in dogs in this respect and carries the potential disadvantage that it may alter the bacterial flora of the bowel and so interfere with the degradation of lactose.

An i.v. infusion of 5% dextrose may be used as a way of raising blood glucose and promoting conversion of ammonia to glutamate.

Thiazide diuretics should be avoided as they may cause an hypokalaemic alkalosis and hence promote renal synthesis of ammonia and ammonia absorption.

INFECTIONS OF THE CENTRAL NERVOUS SYSTEM

VIRAL INFECTIONS

No specific treatment is available for viral infections of the central nervous system such as canine distemper or feline infectious peritonitis. In cases where there is evidence of cerebral oedema, anti-oedema doses of *dexamethasone* (2.2 mg/kg) may be used but should not be repeated frequently on account of its side effects.

BACTERIAL MENINGOENCEPHALITIS

General principles

In the treatment of infections of the nervous system, as in bacterial infection in general, the choice of antibacterial agent is governed by two main criteria: that the agent chosen should be active against the organism(s) concerned and that it should attain effective concentrations over a period of time at the site of infection. The latter presents a particular problem in the case of the brain because of the blood brain barrier which limits access of drugs to the brain from the systemic circulation. In most body tissues drugs are able to diffuse from the blood into tissue fluid through gaps between the capillary endothelial cells. In the brain, however, the endothelial cells are joined by tight junctions so that drugs can enter the brain only by the transcellular route, that is only if they are sufficiently lipid-soluble to diffuse across the membranes of the endothelial cells. The blood-brain barrier may be bypassed by intrathecal injection, although this technique is rarely employed in veterinary medicine. When the meninges are inflamed, permeability to certain drugs is increased and on this basis antibiotics may be grouped into three classes as shown in Table 6.2.

Table 6.2
Classification of antibacterials according to the ease with which they enter the brain

	Bactericidal	Bacteriostatic
Group A Reach adequate concentrations in the brain	*potentiated sulphonamides;* *certain cephalosporins* *(e.g. cefotaxime)*	*chloramphenicol*
Group B Reach adequate concentrations **only** in presence of inflammation	*penicillins*	*certain tetracyclines (e.g.* *doxycycline, erythromycin)*
Group C Do not reach adequate concentrations even in presence of inflammation	aminoglycosides other cephalosporins	other tetracyclines other macrolides

There is some debate as to whether drugs of Group B may be inferior to those in Group A because, as inflammation subsides, they may no longer be able to penetrate to clear the infection. Whichever antibacterial agent is used it may be beneficial to give the first dose by the intravenous route to ensure high initial tissue levels.

Bacteriostatic or bactericidal

The immune system of the brain is deficient relative to many other tissues and as a result a bactericidal agent is to be preferred for the treatment of brain infections. To this end the agents in Table 6.2 have also been classified as bacteriostatic or bactericidal.

Organisms involved.

The organisms most commonly found in cases of bacterial meningoencephalitis in the dog and cat are streptococci, staphylococci, pasteurella and, occasionally, coliforms.

Agents of choice

In the absence of precise identification of the organisms concerned, *ampicillin* would appear to be the agent of choice. Alternative agents are: for staphylococci and streptococci — *benzylpenicillin* or *cefotaxime;* for pasteurella — *benzylpenicillin* or *potentiated sulphonamides;* for coliforms — *potentiated sulphonamides* or *chloramphenicol.*

Ancillary treatment

Bacterial meningoencephalitis is often accompanied by cerebral oedema and, to limit the extent of this, excessive fluid intake should be avoided. Corticosteroids reduce cerebral oedema and other inflammatory changes but in so doing impair host defences and, by reducing inflammation, retard entry of group B antibiotics into the brain. Controlled trials have failed to show any benefit of corticosteroids in bacterial meningitis.

The same does not apply to brain abscesses. Trials in cats have shown that in this condition combined use of corticosteroids and antibiotics is superior to antibiotics alone.

Bacterial meningoencephalitis in dogs is frequently accompanied by a marked fever which may be reduced by administration of *acetylsalicylic acid* (Aspirin).

MYCOTIC INFECTION

The most common mycotic infection of the CNS of dogs and cats is Cryptococcus. Table 6.3 lists the agents most commonly used for the treatment of systemic mycoses in domesticated animals.

Amphotericin acts by damaging the cell membrane and in so doing increases permeability to *flucytosine* so that the two are synergistic and the therapy of choice for systemic cryptococcosis is *flucytosine* (Alcobon) 100 – 150 mg/kg/day orally in divided doses together with *amphotericin* (Fungizone) 0.25 – 0.5 mg/kg i.v. 3 times weekly. BUN should be monitored regularly to detect any renal damage caused by *amphotericin*. Unfortunately, while flucytosine enters the CNS, *amphotericin* does not, and so the latter is not effective against intracranial organisms.

Flucytosine must be given until remission occurs. Toxic hazards following long-term flucytosine administration include oral and cutaneous ulceration, enterocolitis and depressed bone marrow function.

The alternative treatment is *ketoconazole* (Nizoral) 10 mg/kg/day orally, but this may cause liver damage.

Corticosteroids are positively contraindicated in mycotic infections which are most commonly seen in immunocompromised animals, often following corticosteroid therapy.

GRANULOMATOUS MENINGOENCEPHALITIS (PRIMARY RETICULOSIS)

Prednisolone 1 – 2 mg daily orally may bring about a temporary improvement in this condition but does not affect the long term outcome.

Table 6.3
Agents for the treatment of systemic mycoses

Generic Name	Brand Name	Activity	Comments
amphotericin	Fungizone	Fungi (e.g. Aspergillus) and yeasts (e.g. Cryptococcus, Candida)	i.v. only, renal toxicity
ketoconazole	Nizoral		oral, hepato-toxicity
flucytosine	Alcobon	Yeasts (e.g. Cryptococcus, Candida) only	oral

FURTHER READING

FENNER, W. R. (1984). Treatment of central nervous system infections in small animals. *Journal of the American Veterinary Medical Association,* **185,** 1176.

FREY, H. -H. and LOSCHER, W. (1985). Pharmacokinetics of anti-epileptic drugs in the dog: a review. *Journal of Veterinary Pharmacology and Therapeutics* **8,** 219.

FREY, H. -H. (1986). Use of anticonvulsants in small animals. *Veterinary Record,* **118,** 484.

HOERLEIN, B. F., REDDING, R. W., HOFF, E. J. and McGUIRE, J. A. (1985). Evaluation of naloxone, crocetin, thyrotropin releasing hormone, methylprednisolone, partial myelectomy and hemilaminectomy in the treatment of acute spinal cord trauma. *Journal of the American Animal Hospital Association,* **21,** 67.

KORNEGAY, J. N. (1986) *'Neurologic Disorders',* Churchill-Livingston, New York.

KRUCK, Z. L. and PYCOCK, C. J. (1985). *'Neurotransmitters and Drugs',* 2nd Edn., Croom Helm, London.

CHAPTER 7

DIAGNOSIS AND MANAGEMENT OF SEIZURES

John Barker B.Vet.Med., M.R.C.V.S.

INTRODUCTION

Seizures are a common neurological problem in small animals and their correct diagnosis and management are of considerable importance. Many clinicians are frequently called upon to manage an 'epileptic' dog, but whilst many such cases will be suffering from **idiopathic** epilepsy there are other causes of seizures which must be considered before this diagnosis can be reached.

DEFINITIONS

Epilepsy is any disorder characterised by repeated seizure activity, of whatever cause.

Idiopathic epilepsy is a seizure disorder in which no cause can be delineated and for which no causative lesion can be identified. Idiopathic epilepsy occurs generally in pedigree animals with low seizure threshold.

Partial epilepsy is characterised by involvement of only a limited area of the animal's brain, clinically manifesting itself as a minor behavioural or motor abnormality without alteration of consciousness.

Complex partial epilepsy is accompanied by some clouding of consciousness.

Secondary generalisation is the evolution of a partial seizure into a full scale attack.

Generalised-at-onset epilepsy has no partial component.

Ictus is the seizure itself.

CAUSES OF SEIZURES

Seizures may broadly be classified as being extracranial and intracranial in origin. **Extracranial** causes of seizures include metabolic, toxic and nutritional disorders and systemic disease. **Intracranial** causes include any where there is an epileptic focus within the brain, either where a pathologically identifiable lesion is present or in animals without such a lesion. This latter group of **idiopathic epileptics** form by far the largest group of cases.

PROBLEM SOLVING

The clinician faced with the owner of an animal which has suffered seizures is in an unique clinical situation and has unique clinical problems. This is a result of the episodic nature of the disorder and the likelihood that the animal will not be examined during a seizure. Unless these problems are recognised and addressed logically, the clinician will be faced at a later date with a dissatisfied client and an inadequately controlled patient. It is essential that the case receives the attention it deserves (and no more) and the owner receives a realistic, accurate prognosis.

In order to arrive at the optimum resolution of the case, the clinician must control tightly the history taking as this is the only insight into the clinical state of the animal during the seizure, and sequentially elicit accurate data on which to base appropriate investigation and logical therapy.

PROBLEMS AND SOLUTIONS — THE CLINICIAN

HISTORY TAKING

Clinicians in general practice only very rarely see animals having epileptic attacks and must depend entirely on the story told by an anxious and frightened owner. Differential diagnosis of transient signs described by a subjective lay observer taxes clinical acumen and cannot be adequately dealt with in a brief consultation. The impact of even a single seizure on an owner can be profound and merits sympathy from the lay staff first dealing with the case and from the clinician.

Breed.

Accurate figures for seizure incidence do not exist, but data suggesting that one in 200 mongrel dogs suffer from idiopathic epilepsy have been published. The incidence in cats is much lower. Superimposed on the species incidence in dogs are breed incidences. Care must be taken in assessing these, since undoubtedly some 'epileptic' breeds have only mongrel incidence but have suffered undue attention. In others, there exists within the breed a genetically defined population with an inherited low threshold for seizures, a factor superimposed on the basic mongrel incidence of idiopathic epilepsy. This inheritance may be multifactorial and thus concentrated by inbreeding in the affected line; there is some evidence for a single autosomal mode in early-onset epilepsy in some breeds (Keeshond, Welsh springer).

Breeds with low seizure threshold in certain lines include the German shepherd dog, golden retriever, Labrador retriever, German shorthaired pointer, and Border collie. Clinical seizure type and prognosis may be stereotypic of the breed and it is essential to be aware of this when taking the history, as it provides a valuable indication of seizure origin in individual members of these breeds. Other breeds rarely suffer from idiopathic epilepsy, notably terriers, boxers, Rottweilers, Afghan hounds and Dobermans.

Age.

Myelination of the dog brain is not usually complete until six months of age and idiopathic epilepsy is not seen before this time. Age of onset of seizures in idiopathic epileptics of susceptible breeds correlates well with inbreeding coefficients and is evidence of the multifactorial mode of inheritance in these breeds. The more inbred, the earlier the onset. Animals less than six months of age or over six years of age should be suspected of having extracranial disease or acquired lesions causing the seizures and should be thoroughly investigated in this respect, before diagnosing idiopathic epilepsy.

Sex.

Male animals appear to have an increased incidence of idiopathic epilepsy and are more likely to respond to brain insults by a clinical seizure than are their female littermates. This is not a sex-linked factor but a hormonal effect modified by castration and hormone therapy. Similarly, seizure threshold in bitches may vary with the oestrus cycle, decreasing in pro-oestrus and oestrus and increasing in pseudocyesis and pregnancy.

Clinical History.

The following points are of diagnostic and prognostic value:

Household	—	presence of small children
	—	in-contact animals
	—	access to toxins
	—	emotional upset.
Patient	—	pedigree and litter history
	—	vaccination history
	—	feeding and excercise routines
	—	medical, surgical and trauma history prior to onset of seizures.
Seizures	—	time, date and place of first attack
	—	prodromal signs in previous hours and days
	—	pre-ictal signs
	—	ictal description
	—	post-ictal recovery
	—	changes in subsequent seizures
	—	changes in seizure frequency
	—	patterns with place, time, feeding, excercise etc.
	—	changes in inter-ictal personality

Household.

In large breeds, which may be aggressive in the post-ictal period, the presence of small children must be considered by the veterinarian at this stage. The author has known tractable animals to be actively dangerous after a seizure and owners should be made aware of this possibility.

In-contact animals may have suffered from intercurrent illness, for example, toxoplasmosis, canine distemper, feline infectious peritonitis. Also, there may have been access to toxins, for example, lead, pesticides etc. Emotional upsets or stress may precipitate attacks on particular occasions, this being seen especially in very attached German shepherd dogs and Labradors.

Patient.

Details such as pedigree and litter history elucidate inheritance, neonatal hypoxia, encephalitis and similar causes. Vaccination history is self evident. Medical history may point to traumatic, viral, parasitic or neoplastic origins for attacks. Feeding and excercise details may reveal 'timelocking' of seizures to metabolic changes.

Seizure.

The first seizure is always the most difficult to elucidate as the owner is ill-prepared, but it is the most significant. Partial onset acquired attacks may rapidly become secondarily generalised in low threshold animals, thus their acquired origin is obscured. Prodromal and pre-ictal signs such as care-seeking or anxiety should be noted. Lateralising or localising clinical signs suggest a focal and hence acquired cause, whereas acute onset generalised signs are typical of idiopathic or metabolic origins. The ictal phase may be so brief that the owner and the clinician fail to recognise the attack as a seizure or confusion may exist with syncope (see Chapter 13). Typically, the idiopathic epileptic is relaxed and drowsy at onset, whereas the syncopal dog may be active or coughing and then suffers a relaxed 'floppy' attack, sometimes with later seizure activity if the hypoxia is prolonged.

From the owner's description, a mental picture of the seizure should allow distinction of partial, complex partial, partial with secondary generalisation or generalised-at-onset attack. These classifications are of prognostic value and all others ('petit mal', 'grand mal', 'absence' etc) should be avoided. Partial attacks without generalisation are seen in acquired epilepsy in animals with high seizure thresholds. Complex partial attacks in Labradors are typical of the breed and may not require therapy. Partial attacks with secondary generalisation are seen in deteriorating patients. Generalised-at-onset attacks are seen in idiopathic epilepsy in several breeds in a well-defined, structured form, but are more confused if of metabolic origin. Post-ictal recovery indicates the severity of the seizure and its length is of prognostic value. An animal suffering a partial seizure may well have a rapid and complete recovery in minutes with no sequelae, whereas, after a generalised attack there may be brain oedema, hypoglycaemia, hyperpyrexia and gross cerebral dysfunction for some hours or even days. Lengthening recovery periods with subsequent seizures and deterioration of personality between attacks carries a poorer prognosis than increased seizure frequency alone. Animals with space-occupying lesions frequently pace, nod or head press between attacks.

EXAMINATION

On presentation, idiopathic epileptic animals are either clinically normal or, if post-ictal, may display misleading neurological disturbances which can lead to gross diagnostic errors as to the severity of their problem. Profound but transient neurological signs after seizures are usually of no diagnostic or prognostic value. However, minor, persistent signs are very significant.

Clinical Examination.

Animals with a history of seizures should have a full clinical and neurological examination which must be objective and without presumption. The general clinical examination by sytems will provide valuable clues to the origin of acquired seizures and may even reveal that the origin is not neurological, but that the patient is suffering from cardiac syncope, vaso-vagal attacks etc. Metabolically disturbed patients, patients with primary malignancies or focal infections should also be noted at this stage.

A detailed neurological examination, as outlined in Part 1, should never be omitted, since acquired epileptics frequently have persistent deficits which are noted between seizures. Cranial nerve function must be evaluated and of particular importance are the menace response, pupillary light reflexes, cover test and vestibular responses (Chapters 2 and 9). The limbs and body should be examined with emphasis on conscious proprioception, placing response, hemistanding, hemiwalking and the spinal reflexes. In the author's experience, animals with space occupying lesions of the brain usually have neurological abnormalities in addition to the seizures, though in occasional animals with such lesions, only seizures may be seen early in the course of the disease. Idiopathic epileptic patients are usually completely normal between seizures, but caution should be employed in the animal found in a post-ictal state where the seizure has passed unobserved, or in the hepatoencephalopathic case, either of which may display profound localising neurological signs, which turn out to be transient.

Evaluation of an animals state of consciousness is often neglected. In the absence of focal signs, apathy to examination, torpor, delirium or mindless pacing suggest cortical depression in toxic or metabolic states. In encephalitic cases, depression may be the only presenting sign. Animals being treated with *primidone* may show limited attention span and whine or fidget persistently on examination.

ANICILLARY DIAGNOSTIC AIDS

(See Chapter 4)

In order to accurately prognose to the owner of a seizuring animal, attempts have to be made to define the cause of the seizures. This may involve complex and expensive diagnostic tests which may yield little useful information. Careful and intelligent test selection should adequately cover the likely possibilities, whereas slavish application to a fixed gamut of tests may lead to no elucidation.

Reaching a diagnosis of idiopathic epilepsy, depite the fact that this is the most frequent cause of seizures in dogs, is largely dependent on characterising the clinical signs and ruling out other potential causes. Where the clinical signs indicate a focal neurological lesion or the signalment falls out with what is normally expected, then attempts to identify a cause should be vigorously perused.

Laboratory evaluations.

In general, urinalysis, haematology and biochemical profiling is mandatory, if only to provide a data base for assessing the effects of future anticonvulsant therapy. If indicated, estimation of blood lead concentration can be valuable. The author carries this out routinely on animals of inner city origin and considerable lead burdens can be demonstrated. Canine distemper and toxoplasma serology, hepatic clearance tests, blood ammonia, glucose tolerance tests and glucose/insulin ratios may be indicated.

Cerebrospinal fluid evaluation.

Routine CSF sampling is not indicated in the majority of cases where idiopathic epilepsy is the most likely diagnosis. However, if other intracranial causes of seizures are considered, or in cases unresponsive to anticonvulsant therapy, CSF evaluation is potentially valuable.

Electroencephalography.

EEG may be useful in assessing clinical epileptic animals as it is of value in revealing acquired epileptic focal lesions, post-traumatic scarring, generalised cortical damage in encephalitis, hydrocephalus, cortical depression in hepatic and toxic syndromes, etc., especially if provocative techniques are used. Serial recordings are of particular value. The EEG is of no use in screening clinically normal animals for potential epilepsy and its use for this is to be deplored. In general, idiopathic epileptics have normal inter-ictal EEG's.

THERAPY

(See Chapter 6)

Therapy is directed to the primary cause of acquired epilepsy and also to the control of seizures from whatever cause. The latter is further divided into anticonvulsant therapy and adjuvant techniques. Any seizure of any cause facilitates subsequent attacks and even if the original cause of the attacks is controlled, the animal may become a self-perpetuating epileptic requiring continued therapy.

Where a focal lesion is identified, therapy may be aimed at that lesion, for example, surgical removal or chemotherapy of tumors. Where a metabolic cause is noted, the derangement must be corrected if possible.

Idiopathic epileptic animals fall into two groups: the easily controllable, which respond well to cheap anticonvulsant therapy and the apparently refractory, which demand disproportionate input with frustrating results and dissatisfied clients.

Simplicity in treatment is the watchword and clinicians should confine therapy to compounds in which they have experience and faith. Failure of expectations in therapy leads to owners who 'drift' from practice to practice, a situation which can be avoided if a realistic assessment of expectations is explained at the outset. It is frequently stated that the best degree of 'control' which can be expected in idiopathic epileptics is a halving of the seizure frequency, that is, a doubling of the inter-ictal period. This must be made clear to clients, some of whom may find such a prospect unsatisfactory.

ANTICONVULSANT THERAPY FOR CHRONIC SEIZURES

Despite the plethora of anticonvulsants available for the control of epilepsy in man, the use of the dog as a model for human epilepsy has served largely to reduce drastically the number of compounds for rational therapy for epilepsy in our species. The development of many anticonvulsants in the past depended on the clinical response of human patients and the transfer of use of these compounds was uncritical.

The decision whether or not to treat an individual should be determined from the seizure type, recovery and frequency. There is evidence that the success of control of generalised-at-onset idiopathic epilepsy is related to the time of starting adequate therapy and that any such cases should be treated after **one** attack. Animals with prolonged recovery periods, or with a seizure frequency of more than **one per month** should also be treated, whatever the seizure type. In general, veterinarians are too slow in initiating and too inclined to withdraw therapy from their patients. Seizure free periods of a year or more are indications for cautious and gradual withdrawal.

Benzodiazepines

Carbamazepine (Tegretol), *clonazepam* (Rivotril) and *diazepam* (Valium) all have pharmokinetic properties which render them unsuitable as **chronic** anticonvulsants in the dog and cat. They are very rapidly metabolised and adequate therapeutic blood concentrations are rarely demonstrable in chronic therapy. Tolerance to their pharmacological effects develop rapidly, but they may be of short term value.

Phenobarbitone

This drug is the mainstay of anticonvulsant therapy in our species. It is cheap and available as an elixir (30mg/ml) or tablets (15,30,60, and 100mg). It produces seizure control with acceptably low levels of sedation and has minimal side effects on appetite or weight gain. The initial dose should be 1.5—2.5mg/kg twice daily (b.i.d.) orally in dogs and 0.5—1.5mg/kg (b.i.d) orally in cats. Drug assays* should be carried out 10—28 days following commencement of treatment to allow adjustment of oral doses. The therapeutic range is 15—45µg/ml.

Primidone

Primidone (Mysolin) is effective largely as its main metabolite, *phenobarbitone*, and thus is a more expensive way of administering this drug. Dosage is initiated at 15—30mg/kg per day as three equal, divided doses. Therapeutic blood levels of 15—45µg/ml of *phenobarbitone* are desirable. *Primidone* has few advantages over *phenobarbitone* as it offers little or no increase in control over the latter and is more hepatotoxic.

Phenytoin

Critical clinical analysis and studies of the pharmokinetics of *phenytoin* (Epanutin) suggest that it is not suitable for use in the dog, because of its poor absorption and short half life. In the cat, delayed excretion leads to toxicity. Drug assays rarely reveal adequate blood concentrations.

Valproic acid

Valproic acid (Epilim) is active as its metabolites in man. In the dog it is excreted rapidly and unmetabolised.

* JSPS Laboratories, 81 Harley Street, London W1.
  T.G. Yarrow Laboratories Ltd, 249-251 Mile End Road, London E1 4BJ.
  Grange Laboratories, P.O. Box 4, Wetherby LS22 5JU.

ADJUVANT THERAPY

The owner's history may suggest supplementary therapy to aid in seizure control. Thus the use of oral *diazepam* or *clonazepam* for brief periods when emotion-induced attacks are predictable; *acetazolamide* (Diamox) in oestral bitches; hormones (Tardak, Perlutex) or physical castration of dogs may be of value. Owners can be supplied with injectable *diazepam* and taught to give intramuscular injections (20-40mg) in dogs with cluster attacks. Soluble *dexamethasone* (2mg/kg intravenously) is indicated in post-ictal brain oedema cases with prolonged, confused recoveries.

THERAPY OF STATUS EPILEPTICUS

Status epilepticus is a twenty minute emergency and requires vigorous treatment to alleviate it and to avoid prolonged, distressing sequelae. Owners of animals having generalised seizures must be made aware of this and instructed to seek urgent veterinary attention if any seizure appears prolonged.

Animals in 'status' are hyperpyrexic, hypoglycaemic and have grossly disturbed blood flow and brain oedema. They should be admitted and given an immediate intravenous bolus of *diazepam* at 1mg/kg. If this does not allow adequate handling they should be given intravenous *phenobarbitone* or *pentobarbitone* to effect and an intravenous catheter inserted. Maintenance of a patent airway and adequate respiration should be ensured. Blood is collected for biochemical profiling and a bolus of 5ml of 50% glucose solution and *dexamethasone* (2mg/kg) is given intravenously. Fluids are given at maintenance levels. Intravenous or, preferably, oral *phenobarbitone* is given as the animal's condition improves and steps are taken to determine the precipitating factor for the 'status', particularly if the animal is previously unknown to the clinician. Remember that the findings of any neurological evaluation made after such an episode are to be treated with great circumspection.

PROBLEMS AND SOLUTIONS - THE OWNER

NATURE OF THE CONDITION

Any disturbance to the consciousness and personality of a domestic pet is traumatic to the owner and the unpredictability of an epileptic attack enhances the anxiety. Gross changes in family relationships to the animal occur with the larger and more aggressive idiopathic epileptic breeds and owners will seek advice on and request euthanasia. It behoves the clinician to appreciate the reality of this anxiety and advise accordingly, especially in households with small children at real risk. Post-ictal aggression in some golden retrievers and German shepherd dogs is rarely seen by the clinician in practice but is frightening in the extreme in the confines of a small house. Inter-ictal deterioration in the personality of the ill-controlled epileptic is no less a problem. Animals may lose their individual quirks and association with the owners and, with subsequent attacks, suffer progressive dementia. On recovery from clusters of attacks, or status epilepticus, some have totally changed personalities and may fail to relate to their human companions for some days or months. Detailed and time-consuming counselling may be demanded from the veterinarian during this period.

APPARENT FAILURE OF THERAPY

Expectation of total seizure control is high in both owner and clinician, a situation encouraged by lay and professional human and veterinary literature. Such expectations are often destined for disappointment. Successful therapy in idiopathic epilepsy implies selection of adequate dosage of suitable anticonvulsants by the veterinary surgeon, full compliance by the owner with the dosage regimes (the commonest cause of failure of therapy in human epileptics is non-compliance), acceptance of side effects (especially sedation and increased appetite) and adequate drug absorption and response from the patient. The use of routine drug assay of blood concentrations will allow monitoring of both compliance and absorption and has much to recommend it.

In the case where seizures are not controlled adequately, a number of steps should be taken. A detailed neurological examination should be made to ensure that focal diseases are not being overlooked. The serum *phenobarbitone* concentration should be checked to ensure that therapeutic doses are being administered. The dose may be increased such that the serum concentration reaches the top of the therapeutic range. If the dog still experiences seizures, additional therapy may be administered, for example, *clonazepam*. It is vital that the regular anticonvulsant is not ceased abruptly or the dose reduced. Despite these measures, a significant number of dogs will not be controlled adequately and some which are, will experience side effects, particularly sedation.

The unpredictable nature of the epileptic attack and the frequency of naturally occurring refractory periods to overt seizures, often of several months duration, leads to unsubstantiated claims for the efficacy of compounds, herbal or otherwise, as effective anticonvulsants. Very stereotyped, misleading and optimistic therapeutic regimes are published, quoted and believed, and this alone has led to many difficulties, since expectations of success are heightened above reasonable levels. The adoption of the naturally epileptic dog as a test bed for anticonvulsant drugs in recent years and the publication of the findings has served to severely define the limits of our therapeutic armory and, one hopes, correspondingly increase our efficacy.

THE BREEDER AND THE STIGMA OF 'EPILEPSY'

Breeders of pedigree animals who willingly accept physical problems in their products will rarely discuss epilepsy openly or accept its genetic nature in some breeds. Conversely, in some breeds, simplistic theories of the inheritance, with the establishment of 'carrier' detection using the EEG and elimination programmes, are simply not facing the reality of the situation and are to the detriment of the breeds concerned. The stigma of idiopathic epilepsy further leads to refusal to discuss the problem with the pet owners of epileptic dogs, whose own anxiety is thus increased. The veterinary surgeon is uniquely positioned to overcome this impasse.

FURTHER READING

BUNCH, S.E. (1986) Anticonvulsant drug therapy in companion animals. In *Current Veterinary Therapy IX.* (Ed. R.W. Kirk) W.B. Saunders Co., Philadelphia

FARNBACH, G.C. (1984) Serum concentrations and efficacy of phenytoin, phenobarbitone and primidone in canine epilepsy. *Journal of the American Veterinary Medical Association,* **184,** 117

FREY, H.H. and LOSCHER, W. (1985) Pharmokinetics of anti-epileptic drugs in the dog. *Journal of Veterinary Pharmocology and Therapeutics,* **8,** 219

HOLLIDAY, T.A. (1980) Seizure disorders. *Veterinary Clinics of North America,* **10, (1),** 3

PARENT, J.M. (1988) Clinical management of canine seizures. *Veterinary Clinics of North America,* **18, (3),** 605

CHAPTER 8

BRAIN DISORDERS IN DOGS AND CATS

Geoff C. Skerritt B.V.Sc., F.R.C.V.S.

The diagnosis of disorders of the central nervous system always involves the procedure of localisation. This is the interpretation of the observable clinical signs and of the results of the neurological examination in order to determine the likely site of a CNS lesion. Table 8.1. summarises the clinical signs likely to occur due to lesions at specific sites within the brain. In human neurology the facility of computerised tomography (CT scan) has virtually completely superseded localisation by clinical signs. Unfortunately, few veterinarians are able to benefit from this advance in neurodiagnosis because of the great expense of the equipment. Sometimes even gross localisation to the brain is not straightforward either because the disease process is diffuse throughout the CNS or because concurrent systemic signs complicate the interpretation of the CNS symptoms. Certain signs can, however, be clearly attributable to lesions within the brain and may be regarded as characteristic:-

SEIZURES — seizure activity always has its origin within either the forebrain or the diencephalon, even though the pathogenesis may be associated with an extracranial cause.

BEHAVIOURAL CHANGES — sudden or episodic changes in temperament, or the occurrence of unusual behavioural traits are invariably due to disease affecting the frontal or temporal lobes of the cerebrum, the limbic system, or the diencephalon.

VISUAL DEFICITS — which occur in the presence of intact pupil responses (see Chapter 9 on neuro-ophthalmology) result from lesions involving either the optic radiation or the occipital lobe of the cerebrum.

CRANIAL NERVE DEFICITS — the existence of deficits of cranial nerve function should always alert the clinician to the possibility of cranial nerve nuclei involvement, especially if several different nerves seem affected. It should be remembered that damage to the motor nuclei will yield lower motor neuron signs even though the lesion is central. Chapter 2 describes the disorders affecting cranial nerve function.

CEREBELLAR SIGNS — dysmetria, intention tremor, ataxia and nystagmus may all suggest involvement of the cerebellum in the disease process.

VESTIBULAR SIGNS — head tilt, rolling, leaning, circling and nystagmus are all signs that occur in vestibular disease. The distinction between peripheral and central vestibular syndromes relies on the presence of the postural, proprioceptive or motor deficits associated with a lesion of the caudal brainstem (see Chapter 2).

Table 8.1
Summary of the Clinical Signs Associated with Single Focal Lesions
at Specific Sites within the Brain (See Fig. 8.1)

Region	Clinical signs	Cranial nerves affected
Cerebral cortex	Behavioural changes seizures depression postural deficits (contralateral) mild hemiparesis (contralateral) circling head aversion	May be loss of facial sensation (contralateral), visual deficits (may be homonymous hemianopia) with intact pupil responses
Diencephalon	Behavioural changes hemiparesis (contralateral) — but gait can be normal postural deficits (contralateral) endocrine disorders autonomic dysfunction	II — optic chiasma — visual deficits with pupil response deficits
Midbrain	Depressed or loss of consciousness, hemiparesis (either side) or quadriparesis, postural deficits (either side)	III — pupil dilation (ipsilateral) ventrolateral strabismus (ipsilateral) IV — dorsomedial strabismus (contralateral) V — loss of facial sensation (ipsilateral) loss of corneal and palpebral reflexes (ipsilateral) paralysis of muscles of mastication (ipsilateral) VI — medial strabismus (ipsilateral)
Pons	Hemiparesis (either side), ataxia, postural deficits (either side), voluntary micturition affected	
Cerebellum	Dysmetria, intention tremor, ataxia (ipsilateral), nystagmus, hypertonia	May be deficit of menace response, may be vestibular signs (e.g. paradoxical head tilt)
Medulla	Hemiparesis (ipsilateral), postural deficits (ipsilateral), falling to one side, circling, head tilt	VII — paralysis of facial muscles (ipsilateral) VIII — central vestibular signs, deafness IX and X — dysphagia and laryngeal paralysis XI — paralysis and atrophy of trapezius, brachiocephalicus and sternocephalicus muscles (ipsilateral) XII — paralysis and deviation of the tongue (towards affected side)

LOSS OF CONSCIOUSNESS — lesions within the ascending reticular activating system, extending from the midbrain, via the thalamus and hypothalamus to the cerebral cortex result in altered states of consciousness. The classic examples are intracranial trauma and narcolepsy, although hydrocephalus, hepatic encephalopathy and lysosomal storage diseases are further examples.

This is not an exhaustive list of clinical signs of brain disease but the existence of any of these signs should alert the clinician to the likelihood of brain involvement. Too often the realisation that the lesion is in the brain results in a reluctance to pursue the investigation, presumably because of the complexity of the organ. In fact, a methodical approach can be most rewarding and many cases are far from hopeless.

The approach adopted here is by clinical signs, reflecting the manner in which a case is presented. It is assumed that the usual routines of history-taking and physical examination have been completed.

SEIZURES AND BEHAVIOURAL CHANGES

The investigation of the seizure case is described in Chapter 7. However, the presence of neurological dysfunction during the interictal period will suggest that an organic lesion is present.

Behavioural changes commonly accompany seizure activity during the prodromal and post-ictal phases of idiopathic (true, primary, inherited) epilepsy. Psychomotor seizures are characterised by recurrent episodes of bizarre and abnormal behaviour, e.g. fly-catching, tail-chasing, flank-sucking. Large areas of the cerebral cortex (frontal and temporal lobes, hippocampus) and diencephalon (thalamus, hypothalamus) are concerned with temperament and behaviour, and lesions in these sites yield predictable changes.

Compulsive pacing and circling may occur during the interictal period especially when a lesion is present in a prefontal lobe. Circling is not a very helpful localising sign since it can result from lesions elsewhere in the brain and may be directed towards or away from the lesion.

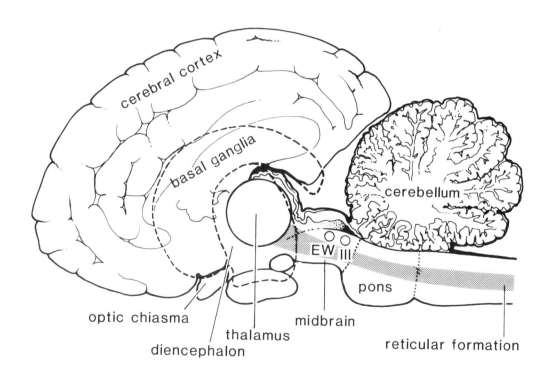

EW — Edinger-Westphal nucleus (parasympathetic supply to the eye)
III Oculomotor nerve somatic motor nucleus

Figure 8.1
The main functional regions of the brain

Rather surprisingly, lesions in the cerebrum do not result in much alteration of gait. However, involvement of the primary motor area will affect the animal's ability to negotiate obstacles. The commonest concurrent finding when seizures are due to an organic lesion is a deficit in postural reactions: proprioceptive positioning, hemiwalking and hopping tests may all reveal an abnormality.

Visual deficits, as detected by the menace test, cotton wool ball test and the ability to avoid obstacles, may be due to lesions affecting the occipital cortex. Normal pupillary responses are present with a lesion at this level.

DIFFERENTIAL DIAGNOSIS

When one or more localising signs are present in a patient suffering from recurrent seizures, the signs correlate with the site of the lesion in the cerebrum or diencephalon. Focal lesions in this part of the brain are relatively rare and can usually be identified as (i) neoplastic; with an insidious progression; (ii) traumatic; acute onset and may progress or seizures may occur up to two years later, or (iii) cerebrovascular; acute onset but non-progressive.

Neoplasia

Primary and metastatic neoplasia can occur at any age but the incidence is very rare in animals less than five years old. Seizures are not usually the first sign of neoplasia in the cerebrum; postural and visual deficits are apparent for some time before seizures occur.

Trauma

Seizures may follow intracranial trauma immediately or commence up to two years after the injury. When seizures occur soon after the incident there are usually other neurological signs present. Depression and coma may develop due to haemorrhage and oedema causing an increase in intracranial pressure.

Cerebrovascular accidents

Whilst the incidence of spontaneous intracerebral haemorrhage is very rare in animals, as compared with man, haemorrhage is an occasional complication of inflammatory and degenerative disease of the CNS. A syndrome of spontaneous cerebral infarction of unknown aetiology, however, does occur in cats. Adult cats of any breed may be affected; the onset is peracute and is characterised by behavioural changes (often towards aggression), compulsive circling and seizures. Contralateral postural and visual deficits are common.

VESTIBULAR SIGNS

The vestibular system controls the position of the eyes, trunk and limbs in response to changes in head position and maintains a balanced body posture. Vestibular function is co-ordinated with visual and proprioceptive information to provide the animal with spatial orientation.

The vestibular apparatus comprises the labyrinth of the inner ear, the vestibular nerve, the vestibular nuclei in the medulla oblongata and the flocculonodular lobe of the cerebellum. The labyrinth consists of five membranous compartments:- the three semicircular canals, the utricle and the saccule. The membranous labyrinth contains a fluid, the endolymph which excites receptors with its movements. The osseous labyrinth of the petrous temporal bone surrounds and protects the membranous labyrinth. The receptors in the labyrinth can detect gravitational forces (utricle and saccule), linear acceleration and deceleration (mainly utricle), and angular acceleration and deceleration (semicircular canals).

The axons of the receptor endings in the inner ear comprise the vestibular nerve which enters the brainstem at the cerebellopontine angle. The vestibular ganglion along the course of the vestibular nerve is the equivalent of a dorsal root ganglion. Most of the vestibular nerve fibres synapse in the vestibular nuclei with neurons whose axons either project rostrally to the somatic motor nuclei of cranial nerves III, IV and VI, or caudally to enter a vestibulospinal tract in the spinal cord. Some vestibular nerve fibres go past the vestibular nuclei and enter the cerebellum via the caudal cerebellar peduncle; these fibres synapse in either the flocculonodular lobe or a fastigial nucleus.

These central connections of the vestibular system allow eye, trunk and limb movements to occur in response to changes in head position. In addition this same sensory information is supplied to the cerebellum so that it can be included in whatever co-ordinating activity is required.

The movements of the eyes in response to head movement provide important clinical information. When the head is turned the eyes move slowly away from the direction in which the head is turning but then rapidly jerk back in the same direction as the head. This eye movement occurs several times whilst the head changes position and is known as normal positional nystagmus. The spontaneous nystagmus that usually occurs in vestibular disease is due to an imbalance between the normal active side and the less active affected side; the result is a nystagmus with its fast phase towards the active side. Spontaneous nystagmus is usually horizontal, and occasionally rotatory; vertical nystagmus is rare and is always associated with a central lesion. Nystagmus can be induced by the caloric test which involves irrigating the external ear canal with either hot or ice cold (safer!) water. Nystagmus is a normal response to caloric stimulation and an absence of response usually indicates vestibular disturbance. Unfortunately, this test is not completely reliable but can be helpful for assessing brainstem function in a comatose animal.

The other characteristic signs of vestibular disease are head tilt, compulsive rolling or circling, and leaning. These signs all result from an imbalance of activity along the vestibulospinal tracts. Normally, these pathways are strongly facilitatory to ipsilateral extensor muscles. In vestibular disease there is an ipsilateral decrease in extensor muscle tone and a contralateral increase.

A head tilt is a rotation of the head about its longitudinal axis with the lower ear usually indicating the side on which the lesion is located. A head aversion is a rotation of the head, together with a deviation of the nose downwards and to one side. This is an important distinction between head positions since an aversion may occur with a cerebral lesion but a tilt always suggests vestibular or cerebellovestibular involvement. The interpretation of head tilt is further complicated by the occasional occurrence of a paradoxical head tilt when the lower ear is on the side opposite to the lesion. A paradoxical situation frequently arises with tumours at the cerebellomedullary angle, causing compression of the supramedullary part of the caudal cerebellar peduncle.

DIFFERENTIATION OF PERIPHERAL FROM CENTRAL VESTIBULAR DISEASE

The peripheral part of the vestibular system comprises the labyrinth and the vestibular nerve; the central part consists of the vestibular nuclei and the flocculonodular lobe of the cerebellum. Since the therapy and prognosis are different for diseases occurring in these two locations it is important to distinguish between peripheral and central vestibular disease. Both result in various degrees of head tilt, rolling, circling and leaning. Nystagmus can occur in either syndrome but is only vertical in central disease. The most reliable difference is concerned with the proximity to the vestibular nuclei of the motor and proprioceptive tracts within the brainstem. Thus, in central vestibular disease there is invariably disturbance of gait and postural reactions. In addition, a brainstem lesion may involve the nuclei of other cranial nerves resulting in a variety of deficits. (Chapter 2).

Although lesions of the middle ear alone will not result in vestibular signs, it is often involved with the inner ear in disease processes. Since both the facial nerve (cranial nerve VII) and the sympathetic nerve to the eye pass through the middle ear, it is not uncommon for an ipsilateral facial paralysis and a Horner's syndrome to accompany the signs of vestibular disease.

DIFFERENTIAL DIAGNOSIS

Congenital and Idiopathic Vestibular Disorders

An acute onset of peripheral vestibular signs can occur in dogs of any age, adult cats and in kittens of certain breeds.

Young Animals

A syndrome of varying degrees of head tilt, circling, rolling and mild ataxia has been reported in a number of breeds (e.g. German shepherd, Doberman, miniature schnauzer). Usually, several puppies in the litter are affected by an acute onset of clinical signs at 3—12 weeks of age. Ancillary tests do not reveal any abnormality in these cases, and no lesions have been detected at post mortem. Most animals make a 100% recovery by 16 weeks of age, although a slight head tilt may persist. Deafness can occur and does not usually resolve. A similar syndrome has been recorded in Siamese and Burmese kittens.

Adult Cats

Cats of any age may suffer an acute onset of severe vestibular signs. Laboratory tests in these cases are normal, no lesions have been detected and the cause of the syndrome is unknown. A horizontal or rotary spontaneous nystagmus is present at first but often disappears by 72 hours. There is no logical therapy in these cases and affected animals are usually normal after 2—3 weeks.

Adult Dogs

An acute vestibular syndrome of unknown aetiology, very similar to the disease in cats, can occur in dogs of any age. The signs are often so dramatic and sudden in onset that the condition is wrongly diagnosed as 'stroke', especially in older dogs. In fact, there are no signs of either cerebral or brainstem involvement and at post mortem, haemorrhages and infarcts have not been present. These dogs usually recover over 1—2 weeks.

Infections of the Vestibular System

Infection of the inner ear leading to a peripheral vestibular syndrome can occur through (i) extension of a middle ear infection, arising either from otitis externa or via the auditory tube, or (ii) through haematogenous spread from an infectious focus elsewhere in the body.

Any breed or age of dog or cat can be affected, the signs developing acutely or over several weeks and often as a sequel to chronic otitis externa. On otoscopic examination, the tympanic membrane may be seen to be ruptured, or it may appear grey and bulging due to exudate in the middle ear.

Radiological examination may reveal a radiopaque tympanic bulla or, in severe cases, actual lysis of adjacent bone.

Conservative treatment of inner and middle ear infections involves the administration of antibiotics both orally and topically. *Chloramphenicol* is the antibiotic of choice, especially for topical use where the tympanic membrane is ruptured. It is important that the oral medication be continued for at least 4—6 weeks. *Dexamethasone* at 0.1 mg/kg daily in two divided doses may be given for a few days to reduce the inflammation around the vestibular nerve.

Surgical treatment is available for more severe or persistent cases of middle ear infection. Drainage through the tympanic membrane (myringotomy) is adequate in most cases with bulla osteotomy as a more radical approach when necessary. The bulla can be palpated in most dogs and cats but the surgical approach is complicated by the proximity of the external carotid artery and the hypoglossal nerve. A Steinmann pin can be used to enter the bulla and the cavity should then be drained and irrigated. Swabs should be taken for bacterial examination, and then a drainage tube sutured in place for 4—5 days.

Toxic and Nutritional Vestibular Disease

High doses of certain antibiotics given for a prolonged period are known to produce degenerative changes in both the vestibular and auditory systems. The antibiotics mainly incriminated are *streptomycin, neomycin* and *gentamycin.* Either unilateral or bilateral vestibular signs, together with deafness, may be seen. The damage is irreversible but some compensation for the vestibular disturbance is possible.

Central vestibular symptoms are an early sign of thiamine deficiency in cats fed exclusively on fish, or following long-term anorexia. Seizures and coma are later signs in thiamine deficiency but dramatic reversal is possible with early therapy.

Neoplasia

A slow progression (over 6—9 months) of peripheral vestibular signs that are refractory to medical therapy is suggestive of a tumour involving the inner ear or the vestibular nerve. Tumours of nervous tissues are rare at this site in dogs and cats but adjacent osteosarcomas or fibrosarcomas are reported.

Unilateral slowly progressive central vestibular signs may be due to a primary CNS tumour in the brainstem, or an adjacent meningioma. Gliomas and 4th ventricle choroid plexus papillomas are not uncommon, and the incidence is highest in the brachycephalic breeds. A head tilt, which may be paradoxical, ataxia, hemiparesis and postural deficits are the usual clinical signs of central vestibular neoplasia. The prognosis is always grave in these cases with progression to complete debility within 12 months.

CEREBELLAR SIGNS

The cerebellum is not capable of initiating motor activity. Its function is to coordinate and refine muscle actions, and to regulate muscle tone in the maintenance of body posture. It receives information about intended motor activity from the higher centres of the brain (e.g. cerebrum, basal ganglia, red nucleus), and compares this with proprioceptive information from active muscle and tendons.

The structure and organisation of the cerebellum is complex. The Purkinje neurons of the cerebellar cortex exert an inhibitory influence on the neurons of the cerebellar nuclei, which in turn facilitate the brainstem neurons at the origin of the downgoing motor pathways. The activity of the Purkinje neurons is regulated by the mossy fibres which bring afferent information along the spinocerebellar, pontocerebellar, reticulocerebellar and vestibulocerebellar tracts. The Purkinje neurons are also influenced by the climbing fibres from the olivary nuclei, a relay along the route of most of the extrapyramidal pathways.

Cerebellar disease does not, therefore, cause paresis or paralysis. The effect on movement is rather an incoordination, or ataxia. Typically, the ataxic gait is seen as a dysmetria, or inability to measure and regulate motor activity. Usually, the gait is hypermetric, the animal taking greater strides than necessary. The postural responses of the affected animal are present but delayed and exaggerated. Muscle tone tends to be increased. There is a broad based stance and a tendency for the trunk to sway from side to side. A slight head tremor is often seen in cerebellar disease; it is usually more obvious when voluntary movements of the head are made, as in eating and drinking. In these circumstances it is referred to as an intention tremor. The nystagmus seen in some cases of cerebellar disease is really an intention tremor of the extraocular muscles. The failure of the menace test in animals with extensive cerebellar disease is probably due to a loss of facilitation of the facial nerve nucleus.

Most cases of cerebellar disease will show various combinations of these characteristic signs. Unilateral lesions produce ipsilateral deficits. It may be possible to localise a focal cerebellar lesion to a specific site since there are three functional regions of the cerebellum, (i) the flocculonodular lobe — vestibular signs, (ii) the rostral vermis and adjacent parts of the cerebellar hemispheres — spinocerebellar function and postural tone, and (iii) the caudal vermis and the rest of the cerebellar hemispheres — skilled movements.

DISEASES OF THE CEREBELLUM

Focal lesions of the cerebellum do occur, although involvement of adjacent structures oten complicates the clinical picture. Primary or metastatic neoplasms are usually unilateral, located at the cerebellomedullary angle, and produce ipsilateral cerebellovestibular signs. Abscesses sometimes occur within the cerebellum; *Toxoplasma gondii* can be responsible for a focal granulomatous lesion.

Congenital cerebellar disease

A number of congenital diseases of the cerebellum have been described in dogs and cats. They can be divided into neonatal syndromes, in which the clinical signs are present at birth, and postnatal syndromes which are not apparent until some weeks after birth.

Neonatal syndromes — These conditions are the result of abnormal development of the cerebellum of the foetus. The clinical signs do not progress but they do persist and apparent improvement can be due only to compensatory mechanisms.

The virus of feline panleucopenia can be transmitted in utero and destroys actively mitotic cells in the cerebellum during the last week of gestation and the first two weeks after birth. The cells principally affected are the granule neurons; at post mortem the cerebellum shows grossly visible hypoplasia. Kittens with cerebellar hypoplasia are obviously ataxic and dysmetric as soon as they begin to walk, at 3—4 weeks of age.

Canine herpes virus has been shown to produce a similar syndrome in puppies. So far no cases of cerebellar hypoplasia in puppies have proved to be due to canine parvovirus infection.

Postnatal syndromes — In contrast to the neonatal syndromes, young animals with postnatal development of cerebellar disease are normal for some weeks, or even months, after birth. Typical signs of diffuse cerebellar disease then begin to be apparent and there is either rapid or slow progression, or no further deterioration.

The pathogenesis of postnatal cerebellar degeneration is broadly of two types, (i) abiotrophies, in which there is an intrinsic metabolic defect of cells, mainly Purkinje neurons, and (ii) lysosomal storage diseases. Abiotrophies are inherited diseases that have been reported in a number of breeds including Kerry blue terriers, Gordon setters, Airedale terriers, Bernese mountain dogs and Jack Russell terriers. The clinical signs are ataxia, dysmetria and intention tremor. Storage diseases affect neurons throughout the CNS but cerebellar signs of ataxia and hypermetria reflect cerebellar involvement. The commonest example is globoid cell leucodystrophy seen in the cairn and West Highland white terrier. The onset of clinical signs is usually at 4—6 months and progression occurs over a period of up to 12 months.

LOSS OF CONSCIOUSNESS

The ascending reticular activating system (ARAS) is responsible for maintaining the cerebral cortex in a state of arousal in the normal conscious animal. The part of the ARAS regulating consciousness is mainly located in the midbrain and thalamic regions of the brainstem. The ARAS receives input from all the somatic sensory and special sense pathways (e.g. touch, pain, vision, hearing), and in turn stimulates the cerebral cortex via its projections to the frontal lobe. Reduced stimulation of the ARAS results in drowsiness, and lesions within the ARAS lead to altered states of consciousness, e.g. stupor and coma.

In contrast to loss of consciousness through depression of the ARAS, sleep is actively induced through a complex mechanism involving several sleep centres located in the diencephalon, mid brain, pons and medulla.

When an altered state of consciousness occurs acutely and shows progression, the most likely reason is intracranial trauma. If the circumstances make this diagnosis unlikely, then the owner should be carefully questioned about possible ingestion of toxins (e.g. ethylene glycol). If coma develops slowly and follows other clinical signs, e.g. behavioural changes, seizures, systemic signs, the reason may be metabolic disease, neoplasia, or CNS viral or bacterial infections.

INTRACRANIAL TRAUMA

Head injuries in animals often result in intracerebral or subarachnoid haemorrhages, with or without skull fractures. Invariably, such injuries are accompanied by an accumulation of tissue fluid within the cerebral parenchyma. The development of cerebral oedema leads to a slowly progressive increase in intracranial pressure which, if left uncontrolled, will result in tentorial herniation. In this situation the cerebrum protrudes beneath the tentorium cerebelli and compresses the midbrain. The progression of the clinical signs is characteristic; a slowly deepening coma accompanied by progressively dilating pupils. Urgent attention is required to reduce the cerebral oedema and check the rising intracranial pressure, otherwise secondary haemorrhages will occur and the cerebellum may herniate through the foramen magnum causing fatal compression of the medulla oblongata.

The first priority in the management of a case of intracranial trauma is to ensure that there is a patent airway; endotracheal intubation or a tracheostomy may be necessary. A decrease in the arterial partial pressure of carbon dioxide reduces the cerebral blood flow and this helps to reduce intracranial pressure. This effect can be enhanced by either hyperventilation or ventilation with oxygen, although there is a danger of reducing the PCO_2 so far that alkalosis is induced.

Although the value of corticosteroid therapy in intracranial trauma has recently been questioned, there is still good evidence that *dexamethasone* given intravenously (i/v) at a dose of 2 mg/kg is effective in reducing cerebral oedema; second and third dosages of 0.2 mg/kg i/v at 6—8 hour intervals may be given, if necessary.

Dexamethasone takes about 6 hours to be effective so that an intravenous hyperosmolar fluid may be indicated where a more immediate effect is required. *Mannitol* (20% w/v) at a dosage of 0.25 gm/kg i/v is the most suitable osmotic diuretic for reducing cerebral oedema. However, *mannitol* should be used with caution as leakages through ruptured blood vessels will lead to further transfer of fluid from the circulation to the tissues.

In addition to these measures to reduce cerebral oedema, lactated Ringer's solution may be administered for shock therapy, taking care to avoid overhydration. The patient should not be overheated since this will exacerbate the cerebral oedema.

A response to medical therapy should be seen within 4 or 5 hours. Serial assessments should be made every 30 minutes to confirm that the progression of clinical signs has been halted. If there is negligible response to conservative treatment surgery may be considered; elevation of skull fractures and even craniectomy may help to reduce brain compression. If a response to therapy is apparent within 6 hours of commencement, the prognosis is good. A rapid and unresponsive deterioration suggests brainstem haemorrhage and carries a much poorer prognosis than cerebral involvement.

NARCOLEPSY

The underlying cause of narcolepsy is believed to be a disturbance of neurotransmitters within the brainstem sleep centres. Narcolepsy is a condition of excessive sleepiness. In animals, the commonest presentation is of frequently occurring short episodes of collapse (cataplexy). Affected animals lose consciousness very briefly, become flaccid and areflexic, and recover quickly; the whole episode may only last seconds.

Cataplectic episodes may occur as frequently as 20—30 times a day and seem to be particularly precipitated by excitement. Narcolepsy is an inherited disorder in the Doberman but is recorded in many other breeds and crossbreeds; the onset of clinical signs is usually before 12 months of age but can be later.

During cataplectic episodes, the affected dog can generally be aroused by shaking or making loud noises. *Imipramine* has proved to be successful in reducing the number of cataplectic episodes in dogs.

MULTIFOCAL AND DIFFUSE BRAIN LESIONS

Although it is clearly helpful in both diagnosis and prognosis to be able to localise a lesion to a specific region of the brain, there are many occasions when brain disease in small animals presents as a collection of apparently unrelated signs. In these circumstances it is necessary only to recognise that clinical signs are present that characterise a disorder of the brain. Factors such as the speed of onset, the age and breed of the animal, and the existence of systemic signs will aid the diagnosis.

There are many examples of diseases producing multifocal or diffuse lesions within the brain or central nervous system. They can be classified under the usual headings of inflammation, degeneration and neoplasia.

INFLAMMATION

Inflammation of the brain is called encephalitis; usually the close association of the brain with the meninges results in concurrent inflammation of the meninges and thus meningoencephalitis.

The usual route of infection is via the bloodstream, although occasionally infectious agents reach the brain through the cerebrospinal fluid (CSF) or along cranial nerves. The clinical signs of encephalitis are acute in onset and progressive. The lesions are irritative rather than depressive so that abnormal neurological activity is seen rather than neurological deficits.

Diagnosis of encephalitis and meningitis may be helped by an analysis of cerebrospinal fluid. Moderate increases in CSF protein are seen in chronic viral diseases and very high levels occur with bacterial and fungal infections. Increased numbers of white cells are seen in CSF in most infectious diseases of the CNS; mononuclear cells predominate in viral diseases and neutrophils are the commonest cell type in bacterial diseases. Fluorescent antibody techniques can be very helpful in the diagnosis of canine distemper. (See Chapter 4.)

Canine Distemper — Three distinct syndromes of canine distemper encephalitis are recognised.

The classic disease in immature animals is characterised by conjunctivitis, oculonasal discharges, diarrhoea, vomiting and coughing. The disease usually progresses to involve the central nervous system, inducing signs of multifocal neurological disease. Cerebral involvement results in seizures and behavioural changes. Incoordination, dysmetria and nystagmus are all seen as the cerebellum becomes involved. Rhythmic contractions of groups of muscles in the limbs or face are characteristic of distemper encephalitis.

In mature dogs of 4—8 years of age, canine distemper virus can produce a more chronic syndrome. Vaccinated dogs can be affected and systemic signs of distemper are usually absent. There is a slow development of hindlimb paresis and incoordination, with progression to involve the forelimbs. Menace test deficits, abnormal pupil responses, nystagmus and head tremors may all develop as the disease progresses. The lesions are not usually found in the cerebral cortex so that seizures and behavioural changes are not features of this syndrome. The disease becomes static in some dogs.

The third syndrome is so-called old dog encephalitis. This disease affects mature dogs, usually over 6 years of age. The clinical signs are a reflection of the predominant site of the lesions within the cerebral cortex. A progressive development of visual deficits, behavioural changes, head-pressing, compulsive circling, etc., is characteristic.

Rabies — The rabies virus reaches the CNS via peripheral nerves. The multifocal lesions are found in the brainstem, basal ganglia, hippocampus and spinal cord.

The clinical signs of rabies in the dog are usually apparent 2—8 weeks after a bite from an infected animal, the incubation period depending on the site of inoculation and the amount of virus introduced. Virus is excreted in saliva for 3 days before the clinical signs are shown. There is a progression of clinical signs over 3—8 days; restlessness, anxiety, vomiting and temperament change precede complete paralysis and death.

Feline Infectious Peritonitis — There are two distinct variations of this fatal viral disease of young cats, depending on the immunocompetence of the infected cat. Fibrinous peritonitis with ascites, pyrexia and anorexia occurs in cats with little cell-mediated immunity. In cats with partially depressed cell-mediated immunity and adequate humoral immunity, a syndrome exists without peritoneal or pleural involvement but with a likelihood of developing neurological signs due to meningoencephalitis such as fever, hyperaesthesia, cranial nerve dysfunction, hindlimb paresis, convulsions, head tremor and nystagmus.

In both forms of the disease greatly increased values of total serum protein and globulin are almost diagnostic. Leucocytosis and increased CSF protein are also seen.

Toxoplasmosis — The CNS is particularly susceptible to infection with *Toxoplasma gondii,* although most of the acute inflammatory response that develops is a hypersensitivity reaction on the part of the host.

Cats are fairly resistant to the organism and rarely show clinical signs, even though they are infected and shedding oocysts into the environment. Prenatal infection of puppies causes diarrhoea, dyspnoea and ataxia before 10 days of age. In postnatally infected dogs the clinical signs of CNS infection are often complicated by the lower motor neuron signs of polymyositis, which may occur without CNS involvement. Chorioretinitis is common in cases of toxoplasmosis.

Histologically, Toxoplasma causes a multifocal necrosis of the CNS with mononuclear infiltration and foci, or cysts, of tachyzoites. Muscle biopsies in cases showing polymyositis will usually demonstrate the organisms. CSF analysis may reveal increased numbers of mononuclear cells and elevated protein levels. Antibody titres in serum should show at least a fourfold rise during active infection, although they may be low due to immunosuppression resulting from concurrent infection, e.g. distemper virus.

Oral therapy with a combination of *pyrimethamine* (0.5-2 mg/kg) and *sulphadiazine* (60 mg/kg) is recommended. Also *clindamycin* (10-100 mg/kg per day in divided doses) has been shown to be efficacious. Therapy should always be continued for at least 14 days.

Cryptococcosis — CNS infection with *Cryptococcus neoformans* can occur through haematogenous spread or directly through the cribriform plate. The organism is a yeast which is spread by inhalation.

Most affected dogs and cats show clinical signs of a multifocal CNS infection with ocular involvement. Blindness, seizures, circling, ataxia, head-pressing, head tilt and nystagmus are just a few of the signs that may be seen. Chorioretinitis and optic neuritis are common findings. Organisms may be found in CSF samples, with or without cultures. Serology is not very helpful in diagnosis.

Amphotericin B and *flucytosine* are the drugs of choice for cryptococcal infections, although their efficacy in CNS infection is in some doubt.

DEGENERATION

There have been many recorded cases of degenerative disease of the CNS in dogs and cats. The essential features of these diseases are that their onset is usually several months after birth and they then show gradual progression.

Some of these diseases have been described in the section on cerebellar conditions because their lesions are restricted to the cerebellum; others affect the spinal cord primarily and are described in Chapter 10.

The lysosomal storage diseases represent a large group of degenerative disease of the CNS with a multifocal location. Deficiences of specific lyososomal enzymes lead to intracellular accumulation of a variety of substances. These diseases are classified as either neuronal storage diseases or leucodystrophies, depending on whether the substance accumulates in either neurons or white matter. Most of the lysosomal storage diseases are inherited through autosomal recessive genes. Table 8.2 lists some of the recorded storage diseases and the breeds affected.

Table 8.2
Lysosomal Storage Diseases in Dogs and Cats*

Disease	Breeds in which disease is recorded	Clinical Signs
Ceroid lipofuscinosis	English setter (1—2 years)† Chihuahua	Personality change, blindness, ataxia, seizures
GM$_1$ gangliosidosis	Beagle (3—6 months) Domestic cat (2—3 months) Siamese and Korat cats (2—3 months)	Head tremors, ataxia, visual deficits
GM$_2$ gangliosidosis	German shorthaired pointer (6—12 months) Domestic cat (2 months)	Dementia, seizures, blindness
Fucosidosis	Springer spaniel (2 years)	Behavioural change, ataxia, dysphonia, dysphagia, seizures
Globoid cell leukodystrophy	West Highland white terrier (2—6 months) Cairn terrrier (2—6 months) Poodle (2 years) Beagle (4 months) Bassett hound (1½—2 years) Domestic cat (5—6 weeks)	Hindlimb ataxia, progressive paraparesis, hypermetria, visual deficits
Mannosidosis	Domestic cat (7 months)	Ataxia, tremors
Sphingomyelinosis	Siamese cat (2—4 months) Domestic cat (2—4 months) Poodle (2—4 months)	Ataxia, hypermetria, tremors

* This is not a complete list of all the recorded storage diseases.

† The age at which clinical signs are apparent is given in brackets.

Because the clinical signs are a reflection of neuronal dysfunction due to accumulation of metabolic substances, the storage diseases are not apparent until the affected animals are several months old, and in some cases 18 months or older. Blindness, intention tremor, behavioural changes, seizures and quadriplegia are all possible clinical signs in storage diseases. There is a gradual progression until euthanasia is necessary.

NEOPLASIA

Most neoplasia in the CNS occur as focal lesions with localising signs appropriate to the site in which they develop. Lymphosarcoma and reticulosis are the only two examples of neoplastic disease which develop diffusely.

Lymphosarcoma occurs in young cats and although lesions may develop in the brain, particularly at the cerebellomedullary angle, epidural tumours in the vertebral canal are more common.

Reticulosis (Granulomatus meningoencephalitis) is characterised by the perivascular accumulation of mononuclear cells within the CNS. There is some variation in the nature of the lesion, however, so that it is not clearly either an inflammatory or neoplastic disease but displays features of both processes. Although an infectious agent is suspected, none has been isolated. Some cases of reticulosis develop focal lesions so that the clinical signs are of a slowly progressive, unilateral space-occupying lesion. In the diffuse form multifocal signs develop. There are no antemortem diagnostic tests, although dramatic, but temporary, improvement on corticosteroid therapy is typical.

CONGENITAL MALFORMATIONS

Gross malformations of the brain can occur in both dogs and cats. Although the lesion is probably single and focal it may be so extensive that the clinical signs reflect multifocal dysfunction. These disorders may be congenital or acquired in origin. The congenital malformations may be inherited or may have arisen through some in utero insult.

The most frequent example of a congenital malformation of the brain is hydrocephalus. This is a dilation of the ventricular system occurring as a result of either overproduction or reduced absorption of CSF, the latter being the most usual mechanism. Acquired hydrocephalus is usually due to obstruction of CSF outflow by a tumour. The congenital form is most common in the small brachycephalic breeds. The clinical signs of congenital hydrocephalus are usually apparent within a few weeks of birth and are then progressive. Affected animals are often dull, may be blind, develop seizures, and may become quadriplegic. The skull is usually large and domed, with open fontanelles and both eyes show a ventrolateral strabismus. Radiography and electroencephalography may be helpful in diagnosis.

The clinical signs of congenital hydrocephalus may be relieved on a long term basis by oral therapy with either *dexamethasone* (0.1 mg/kg) or *acetazolamide* (0.5—1 mg/kg tid). The surgical treatment of hydrocephalus involves the subcutaneous insertion of a tube to shunt CSF from a lateral ventricle to either the right atrium or the peritoneal cavity.

FURTHER READING

AVERILL, D. R. and DeLAHUNTA, A. (1971). Toxoplasmosis of the canine nervous system: Clinicopathologic findings in four cases. *Journal of the American Veterinary Medical Association,* **159**, 1134.

BLAKEMORE, W. F. (1975). Lysosomal storage diseases. *Veterinary Annual,* **15**, 242.

BLAUCH, B and MARTIN, C. L. (1974). A vestibular syndrome in aged dogs. *Journal of the American Animal Hospitals Association,* **10**, 37.

BRAUND, K. G. (1980). Encephalitis and meningitis. *Veterinary Clinics of North America,* **10**, 31.

CHRISMAN, C. L. (1980). Vestibular diseases. *Veterinary Clinics of North America,* **10**, 103.

DeLAHUNTA, A. (1976). Feline neurology. *Veterinary Clinics of North America,* **6**, 433.

DeLAHUNTA, A. (1980). Diseases of the cerebellum. *Veterinary Clinics of North America,* **10**, 91.

FEW, A. B. (1966). The diagnosis and surgical treatment of canine hydrocephalus. *Journal of the American Veterinary Medical Association,* **149**, 286.

GREENE, C. E. Ed. (1984). Clinical Microbiology and Infectious Diseases of the Dog and Cat. W. B. Saunders Co., Philadelphia.

KORNEGAY, J. N. (1978). Feline infectious peritonitis: the central nervous system form. *Journal of the American Animal Hospitals Association,* **14**, 580.

KORNEGAY, J. N., OLIVER. J. E. and GOGACZ, E. J. (1983). Clinicopathologic features of brain herniation in animals. *Journal of the American Veterinary Medical Association,* **173**, 1111.

KORNEGAY, J. N. Ed. (1986). *Neurologic Disorders. Contemporary Issues in Small Animal Practice, Vol. 5.,* Churchill Livingstone, New York.

MITLER, M. M., SOAVE, O. and DEMENT, W. C. (1976). Narcolepsy in seven dogs. *Journal of the American Veterinary Medical Association,* **168**, 1036.

MOLOFSKY, W. J. (1984). Steroids and head trauma. *Neurosurgery,* **15**, 424.

OLIVER, J. E. (1968). Surgical approaches to the canine brain. *American Journal of Veterinary Research,* **29**, 353.

PALMER, A. C., MALINOESKI, W. and BARNETT, K. C. (1974). Clinical signs including papilloedema associated with brain tumours in twenty-one dogs. *Journal of Small Animal Practice,* **15**, 359.

PREVOST, E., McKEE, J. M. and CRAWFORD, P. (1983). Successful medical management of severe feline crytococcosis. *Journal of the American Animal Hospitals Association,* **18**, 111.

SELCER, R. R. (1980). Trauma to the central nervous system. *Veterinary Clinics of North America,* **10**, 619.

VANDEVELDE, M., KRISTENSEN, B. and GREENE, C. E. (1978). Primary reticulosis of the central nervous system in the dog. *Veterinary Pathology,* **15**, 673.

ZAKI, F. A. (1977). Spontaneous central nervous system tumours in the dog. *Veterinary Clinics of North America,* **7**, 153.

CHAPTER 9

ABNORMALITIES OF EYES AND VISION

S. M. Petersen Jones B.Vet.Med., M.R.C.V.S., D.V. Ophthal.

A neuro-ophthalmological examination is simple to perform and should form part of every full clinical examination.

The linking of ophthalmology with neurology can be a daunting prospect. However, it is very useful in the investigation of disorders of the nervous system.

This chapter is divided into two parts:-

Part 1 — A suggested routine for a neuro-ophthalmological examination.

Part 2 — Neuro-ophthalmological problems are dealt with by presenting signs, this part being arranged into five sections:-

Section I   Visual problems

Section II   Difference in size of pupils - Anisocoria

Section III   Abnormalities of eye position and movement

Section IV   Abnormalities of blink

Section V   Abnormalities of lacrimation which have a neurological basis

The sections are intended to be a guide to the investigation of each presenting sign, rather than an exhaustive dissertation on each subject. Suggested further reading is included at the end of the chapter.

PART 1 — NEURO-OPHTHALMOLOGICAL EXAMINATION

CLINICAL HISTORY

Taking a full clinical history is, as usual, mandatory. The time of onset and rate of progression of signs can be helpful. It is important to know if any medication has been given (by owner or by referring veterinary surgeon). The history may give an indication of any visual impairment, although dogs which gradually lose vision cope very well in familiar surroundings and unilateral blindness is easily overlooked by the owners.

FULL CLINICAL EXAMINATION

A full clinical examination is important. Neuro-ophthalmological signs may also be accompanied by abnormalities far from the eye. An example of this is a patient with a brachial plexus lesion who presents with Horner's syndrome in addition to forelimb paresis.

Table 9.1
Cranial Nerves Influencing the Globe and Adnexa

(a) Sensory (afferent) nerves:-		
Type of Nerve Supply	**Nerve(s) involved**	**Sensory Function**
General somatic afferent	Trigeminal nerve (V) (mainly ophthalmic branch)	Globe and adnexa (touch, pain, temperature, etc.)
Special somatic afferent	Optic nerve (II)	Vision
(b) Motor (efferent) nerves: —		
Type of Nerve Supply	**Nerves(s) involved**	**Motor Function**
General somatic efferent	Oculomotor nerve (III) Trochlear nerve (IV) Adbucens nerve (VI)	Levator palpebrae superioris muscles and extraocular muscles
General visceral efferent a) Parasympathetic branch	(i) Within oculomotor nerve (III)	Pupillary constrictor muscles
	(ii) Within facial nerve (VII)	Secretory control of lacrimal glands
b) Sympathetic branch	Pass via thoracolumbar outflow (T1—T3) and vago-sympathetic trunk	Pupillary dilator muscles Smooth muscle within orbit and eyelids
Special visceral efferent	Facial nerve (VII)	Muscles of facial expression

Table 9.2
Suggested facilities/equipment for examination: —

1. Room capable of being darkened.
2. Area in which obstacle course may be constructed.
3. Obstacles for obstacle course (e.g. chairs, litter bin, etc.).
4. Bandage to use as a blindfold.
5. Focal light sources — such as pen torch.
6. Ophthalmoscope (direct and, if available, indirect).
7. Mosquito artery forceps for testing skin sensation.
8. Wisp of cotton wool for testing corneal sensation.
9. Schirmer tear test strips.
10. Drugs:— *Tropicamide* 1% drops — a parasympatholytic pupillary dilator (for examination of lens and fundus)
    Pilocarpine 1% drops — a direct acting parasympathomimetic (pupillary constrictor)
    Physostigmine 0.5% drops — an indirect parasympathomimetic
    Phenylephrine 10% drops — a direct acting sympathomimetic (pupillary dilator)
11. Further equipment may be desired for ophthalmological examination (e.g. goniolens, magnifying loupes, slit lamp, etc.)
12. Specialised equipment for measuring electroretinogram, evoked visual potentials.

NEURO-OPHTHALMOLOGICAL EXAMINATION

Table 9.1 lists the cranial nerves which influence the eye and their relevant functions and Table 9.2 lists the equipment required for a full neuro-ophthalmological examination. A set routine should be used so that no abnormalities are overlooked.

PRIMA FACIE

Initial observations of the patient before it is restrained can be very useful. Does the animal act as if it is visually impaired? Is there a head tilt? Is nystagmus present?

VISION TESTING

A patient's vision may be assessed by the following tests. The results need careful interpretation, for example some dogs are clumsy and tend to blunder into objects whilst others may be so terrified that they just cower and do not respond normally to the menace test. The extent and localisation of visual field deficits, as assessed by vision testing, can be helpful when deciding where a lesion of the central visual pathways could be located.

Obstacle course. Owner and dog are positioned with an obstacle course between them (Figure 9.1). The owner calls the dog and the ability of the animal to negotiate the obstacles is observed. This test is repeated with each eye blindfolded in turn (Figure 9.2). Some dogs refuse to walk wearing a blindfold - they just try to remove it. Obstacles are moved between tests so the dog does not learn their position. The test should be repeated under subdued lighting as reduced night vision may be an early sign of conditions such as generalised progressive retinal atrophy. Obstacle courses are generally not useful for cats or puppies.

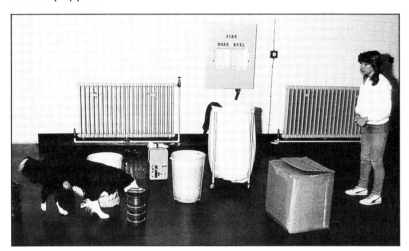

Figure 9.1
Photograph of a dog with one eye blindfolded negotiating an obstacle course

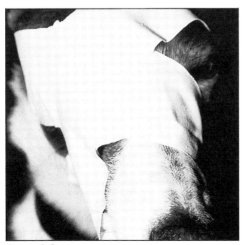

Figure 9.2
Photograph of dog with one eye blindfolded

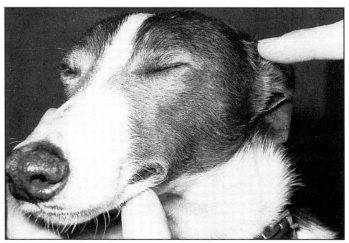

Figure 9.3
Photograph of the menace response

Menace test. A threatening gesture is made within the patient's field of vision. This should result in blinking and possibly withdrawal of the head (Figure 9.3). Each eye is tested individually whilst the other eye is covered by a hand. It should be possible to assess the medial and lateral visual fields of the same eye. Care is taken not to create air currents which the patient feels on its cornea. The menace response is present from about six weeks of age. The pathway is shown in Figure 9.4.

Cotton wool ball test. A cotton wool ball is thrown across the patient's visual field and the reaction noted (Figure 9.5). This is a useful test for cats and puppies. The patient should not be restrained for this test as this may interfere with the reaction.

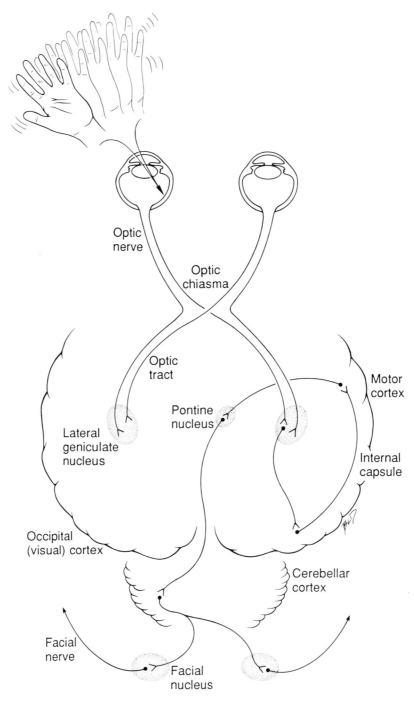

Figure 9.4
Schematic representation of the central pathways involved in the menace response

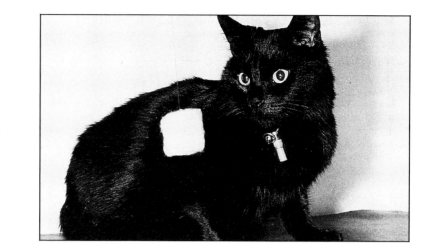

Figure 9.5
Photograph of the cotton wool ball test. The cotton wool ball is thrown across, or swung across (by suspending on a thread) the patient's visual field

PUPILLARY REACTIONS

Comparison of pupil size. The sizes of the pupils are compared (distant direct ophthalmoscopy with a zero dioptre setting may be useful; see Figures 9.6 and 9.7). The room is darkened causing both pupils of a normal animal to dilate fully and evenly (a pen torch held at a distance from the patient and then turned on to illuminate the head will be required to show this). Anisocoria is a condition where a difference exists between the diameter of an animal's two pupils.

Pupillary light reflex (PLR). A light is shone into each eye in turn and the direct pupillary response (ipsilateral pupillary constriction) and consensual pupillary response (contralateral pupillary constriction) of each eye is observed. In cats and dogs, the direct response is slightly greater than the contralateral response, but in practice this is difficult to appreciate. When assessing the PLR there must be enough background illumination to enable one to observe the contralateral pupil. When a constant light is shone into an eye the pupil aperture does not remain exactly fixed, slight alterations in size are normally observed.

The 'swinging flashlight' test. This is a slightly more elaborate way of assessing the PLR. A light source is shone into one eye and the reaction of the pupil noted, the light is quickly swung across to the other eye and the second pupil is seen to constrict slightly or stay at the same aperture.

'Cover test'. The animal is positioned in an evenly lit room and each eye covered in turn. The response of the pupil of the contralateral eye is noted. The pupil size should not alter when the opposite eye is covered.

An evaluation of the briskness and completeness of the pupillary response should be made. The speed of pupillary response is reduced in nervous animals, because circulating adrenaline acts to dilate the pupils though the pupillary responses improve once the animal starts to relax. Older animals may have poorer responses due to iris atrophy.

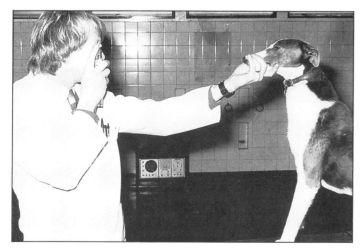

Figure 9.6
Photograph of author comparing the size of a dog's pupils by distant direct ophthalmoscopy

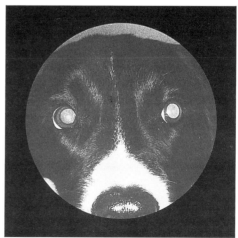

Figure 9.7
Photograph of dog's pupils viewed by distant direct ophthalmoscopy

EYELID POSITION, EYE POSITION AND MOVEMENT

Observe the size of the palpebral fissures, position of the third eyelids, and of the globes. Normal nystagmus is invoked by testing the oculocephalic reflex. This reflex is tested by turning the patient's head laterally, the eyes initially turn in the opposite direction to the direction of rotation and then rapidly re-centre within the palpebral fissure. The process is constantly repeated while the velocity of the animal's head is changing. The speed of the slow phase of the nystagmus matches the speed of rotation of the animal. This reflex must be checked in lateral and dorsoventral planes. The clinician should also look for spontaneous nystagmus, either when the head is held normally or when it is moved to abnormal positions.

SENSATION

Check sensation to the areas supplied by the three branches of the trigeminal nerve (main sensory nerve to head). The skin sensation is tested by squeezing with mosquito artery forceps, or if the animal has long facial hair, just touching these will often result in a wrinkling of the face. Corneal sensation (ophthalmic branch of trigeminal nerve) may be tested using a wisp of cotton wool. The patient blinks when the cornea is touched. Take care not to touch the eyelids as their sensory innervation is partially from the maxillary branch of the trigeminal nerve; this branch may be spared by some lesions which affect the ophthalmic branch. Do not let the patient see your hand when performing this test (Figure 9.8).

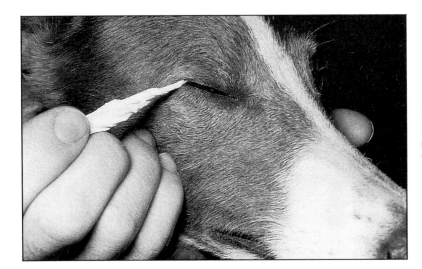

Figure 9.8
Photograph of testing corneal sensation (corneal reflex) with a wisp of cotton wool

MOTOR INNERVATION

The motor innervation to the eyelids should be checked. A blink is induced by the corneal, palpebral or menace reflexes.

DETAILED OPHTHALMOLOGICAL EXAMINATION

This examination should be performed in a darkened room. A focal light source and ophthalmoscope are required. It is normal to start at the adnexa and work systematically towards the posterior part of the eye. This is well described elsewhere (Bedford, 1982).

Note that certain parts of the examination must by necessity be performed before others, e.g. pupillary reactions must be assessed before a mydriatic drug is used, measurement of tear production (Schirmer tear test) should be performed before the eye is moistened by any drops etc.

SPECIALIST EXAMINATIONS

These include electroretinography, measurement of visual evoked potentials and electromyography.

PART 2 — NEURO-OPHTHALMOLOGICAL PROBLEMS

SECTION I. VISUAL PROBLEMS

Visual deficits may result from lesions at any level from the front of the eye to the occipital lobe of the cerebral cortex.

The central visual pathways are shown in Figure 9.9.

VISUAL DEFICITS DUE TO OPHTHALMOSCOPICALLY DETECTABLE DISEASES

A multitude of ocular defects and diseases ranging from corneal opacities to retinal degenerations may result in visual defects. We will only consider lesions occurring within the central visual pathways (Figure 9.9) from the ganglion cells of the retina (Figure 9.10), to the visual cortex.

Optic nerve head abnormalities:-

Papilloedema — this condition itself does not result in visual deficit. In man, swelling of the optic nerve head (papilloedema) is a classical sign of raised intracranial pressure (ICP). In cats and dogs papilloedema is less common in patients with raised ICP, and may occur in patients without an elevated ICP. Anatomical differences between the retinal blood supply of man and animals account for the difference. The

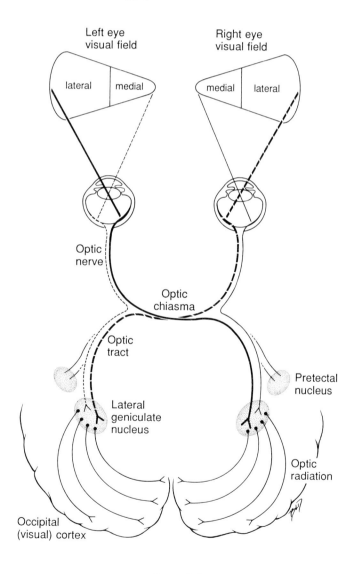

Figure 9.9
Schematic representation of the central visual pathways

147

affected optic nerve head appears enlarged and raised, with engorged superficial blood vessels. The surrounding retina may also appear oedematous. Papilloedema may occur in animals with optic nerve tumours and other intracranial neoplasms and can be a useful indicator of their presence (Palmer *et al,* 1974). It may also occur as a result of other conditions such as acute pancreatitis (Rubin 1974). Papilloedema must not be confused with 'pseudopapilloedema' which is a normal variation of the canine optic nerve head. Dogs with pseudopapilloedema have a prominent, rather than swollen optic nerve head; this occurs when ganglion cell axons gain a myelin sheath a short distance before the lamina cribrosa. German shepherd dogs and golden retrievers commonly exhibit pseudopapilloedema.

Papillitis — this is inflammation of the optic nerve head and results in visual deficits. The optic nerve head is swollen and haemorrhages often are present. Canine distemper virus infections may cause papillitis in dogs, but in many cases the aetiology remains obscure. High levels of systemic corticosteroids may suppress the inflammation and restore vision, but relapses are possible once clinical signs have resolved.

Optic nerve head atrophy — Permanent damage to the optic nerve or optic tracts results in the dying back of axons to their origin at the ganglion cells and eventually to the loss of the ganglion cells themselves. The affected optic nerve head appears shrunken and grey. Again, knowledge of the variation in appearance of the normal optic nerve is required before the abnormality can be detected. Optic nerve head atrophy takes time to develop and will not be present when the animal first suffers from a loss of vision. It is also a feature of advanced generalised retinal degeneration.

Optic nerve head hypoplasia — is occasionally seen. There is accompanying hypoplasia of the central visual pathways. The animal is usually severely visually impaired.

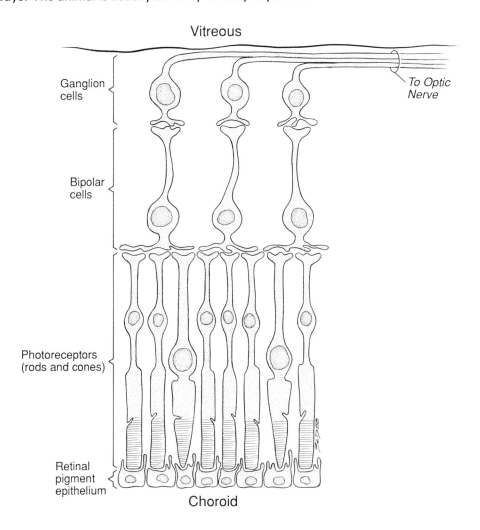

Figure 9.10
Diagram to show the relationships between photoreceptors, bipolar cells and ganglion cells

VISUAL DEFICITS DUE TO NON-OPHTHALMOSCOPICALLY DETECTABLE DISEASES

Vision tests and pupillary responses are used to localise lesions of the central visual pathways.

The central visual pathways.

The details of the central visual pathways (see Figures 9.9) must be understood before attempting to localise lesions within them. Visual information from one side of the body projects to the opposite cerebral cortex. This does not mean that the information from the left eye projects to the right cortex, but that the information from the left visual field of each eye (i.e. things that are seen to the left of the body) project to the right cerebral cortex and vice versa. In domestic animals more than half of the optic nerve fibres cross (decussate) at the optic chisma to the opposite side of the body. In cats 65% of fibres decussate, whereas in dogs 75% of fibres cross over. This is in contrast with man where 50% of the visual fibres decussate. The uneven division between decussating and non-decussating fibres in domestic species explains the slight differences in pupillary responses to light in these species compared to man.

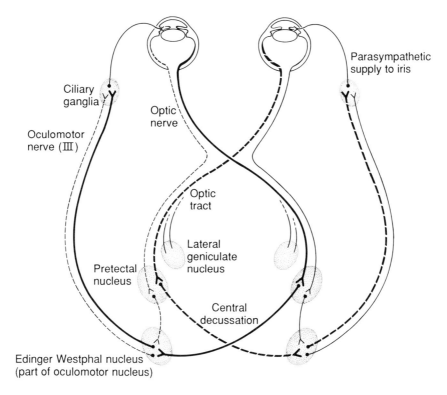

Figure 9.11
Neuronal pathway for pupillary light reflex

Neuronal pathway for pupillary light reflex. (Figure 9.11).

Axons from the ganglion cells of the retina which are involved in the pupillary light reflex (PLR) accompany those concerned with conscious perception of vision to just before the lateral geniculate nucleus. The axons concerned with the pupillary light reflex pass over the lateral geniculate nucleus to the pretectal nucleus, where they synapse with cell bodies of axons which pass on to the contralateral Edinger-Westphal nucleus within the oculomotor nucleus. Parasympathetic nerve fibres from the Edinger-Westphal nucleus initially pass within the oculomotor nerve and then on to the ciliary ganglion where they synapse with cell bodies of post synaptic axons. The post synaptic axons pass via the short ciliary nerves to innervate the pupillary constrictor muscles. The parasympathetic nervous system is the main efferent arm of the pupillary light reflex. (The sympathetic nervous system innervates the pupillary dilator muscle and plays little part in the PLR).

The majority of axons from the ganglion cells concerned with the PLR cross to the contralateral side of the body in the optic chiasma and then a majority cross back to the original side of the body in the central decussation. In practice this means that a light shone in one eye will result in slightly more constriction of the pupil of the same eye than of the contralateral eye.

Linking the results of the tests for visual deficits with those for pupillary responses.

Figure 9.12 shows the effect of lesions on the visual fields. Figure 9.13 is a flow diagram to help link the results of vision testing with the pupillary responses. The central visual pathways may be divided into four regions for our purposes, (a) the prechiasmal section (retina and optic nerves); (b) the optic chiasma; (c) the postchiasmal optic tracts (pre-lateral geniculate nucleus) and (d) the lateral geniculate nucleus, optic radiation and optic cortex.

a.   Prechiasmal lesions (retinal and prechiasmal optic nerve)

Complete lesions affecting the retina or optic nerve will render the eye of the affected side blind. If the lesion is unilateral the owners may not notice the resulting visual deficit. The menace test for the affected eye is absent and the animal will be unable to negotiate an obstacle course with the normal eye covered. A static anisocoria is present, the affected eye's pupil being slightly dilated in comparison with the normal eye's pupil. In darkness both pupils will dilate evenly. The direct pupillary light reflex will be absent from the eye on the side of the lesion, as will the consensual response. The swinging flashlight test is abnormal, when the light swings from the normal to the abnormal eye the pupil of the abnormal eye dilates (the pupil of a normal animal would slightly constrict). In normal room light, if the unaffected eye is covered, the abnormal eye's pupil will dilate. This is defined as a 'positive' (abnormal) cover test result. Bilateral lesions result in fixed, dilated, relatively non-responsive pupils and a blind animal. Even with advanced retinal disease there will often be some degree of pupillary light reflex and cats with bilaterally detached retinas often have some pupillary response.

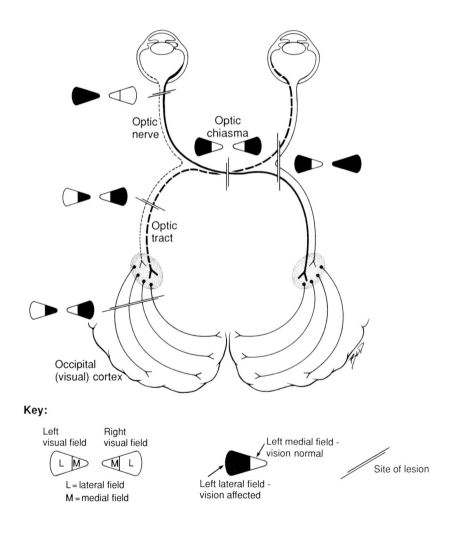

Figure 9.12
Effect on visual fields of lesions within the central visual pathways at various levels.

Fundoscopy and, if necessary, electroretinography will help differentiate between retinal and prechiasmal optic nerve lesions. Retinal lesions may be due to retinal degenerations and detachments. Optic nerve lesions may include optic nerve hypoplasia, optic neuritis (Fischer and Jones, 1972) neoplasia (Williams *et al*, 1961; Barnett *et al*, 1967) trauma, and optic nerve compression.

b. Lesions of Optic Chiasma

Neoplasia involving the chiasma has been reported. It produces bilateral blindness with dilated unresponsive pupils (Braund *et al*, 1977; Skerritt *et al*, 1986). Vascular occlusions may affect the chiasma by causing ischaemia and nerve degeneration. Localised abscesses may also impinge on the chiasma. Pituitary neoplasms in dogs and cats rarely compress the optic chiasma, unlike the situation in man (Palmer, 1974).

c. Post chiasmal optic tract lesions prior to divergence of fibres of PLR

Visual impairment due to unilateral post chiasmal lesions is more difficult to demonstrate than that due to prechiasmal lesions. Careful use of the menace test may show loss of the medial visual field of one eye and the lateral visual field of the other eye, a defect described as homonymous hemianopia. The vision of the eye contralateral to the optic tract lesion will be most affected because more than 50% of fibres in the optic nerves decussate to the opposite side. Pupillary dilation will occur as normal in darkness. The swinging flashlight test and cover tests are relatively normal, except that whichever eye the light is shone into, the pupil on the contralateral side to the lesion will remain more dilated.

The internal capsule and rostral crus cerebri are in close association with the optic tracts, and may also be affected by lesions involving the optic tracts. A hemiparesis and hemisensory defect of the contralateral side of the body to the lesion results from their involvement. Unilateral lesions may be caused by space occupying lesions such as neoplasms (deLahunta & Cummings, 1967) or abscesses. Ischaemia following vascular occlusions may also occur. Inflammation of both optic tracts may be caused by the distemper virus in dogs.

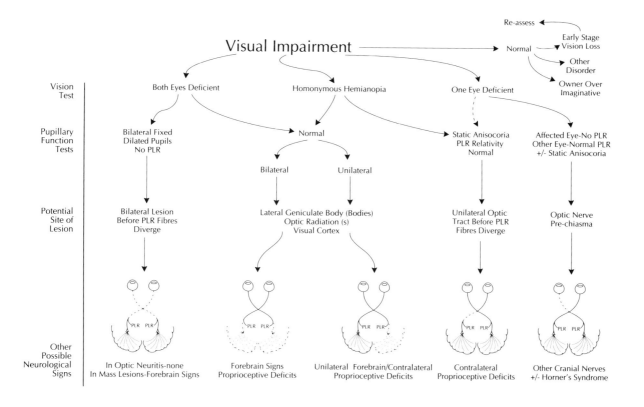

Figure 9.13
Flow diagram to help link the results of vision testing with those of pupillary light reflex testing.
(The broken lines on the visual pathway indicate the site of the lesion).

d. Lesions affecting the lateral geniculate nucleus, optic radiation or occipital cortex.

Homonymous hemianopia is present, as described for post chiasmal optic tract lesions (c). The pupillary light reflex (PLR) is normal. A patient with bilateral complete lesions will be blind with a normal PLR. The lateral geniculate nucleus and initial portion of the optic radiation are positioned just laterally to the internal capsule so lesions may also affect the sensory and motor components within this structure. The posterior part of the optic radiation branches away from the internal capsule toward the occipital cortex so lesions closer to the cortex may spare the internal capsule fibres.

Unilateral lesions may result from neoplasia, abscessation or trauma. Encephalitis and vascular occlusions are additional causes. Trauma resulting in cerebral swelling, or space occupying lesions such as hydrocephalus and neoplasia which result in brain herniation (pushing of posterior cerebrum under the tentorium towards the cerebellum), and encephalitis may all result in bilateral visual defects along with other severe neurological abnormalities.

SECTION II.   ANISOCORIA

Anisocoria is a difference in size of pupils. It may result from intraocular disease (e.g. glaucoma, uveitis, synechiae) or by interference with the nervous control of the pupils.

Anisocoria of a neurological origin may result from lesions of the PLR arc, or of the sympathetic nerve supply to the eye, or from cerebellar disease.

LESIONS WITHIN THE AFFERENT PATHWAY OF THE PUPILLARY LIGHT REFLEX

Afferent nerve fibres involved in the PLR diverge from fibres concerned with vision just before the lateral geniculate nucleus. Lesions affecting the fibres prior to that point also affect vision and are considered in Section 1.

The fibres concerned with pupillary response may be damaged as they pass between the optic tracts and the oculomotor nuclei. Lesions at these sites spare vision. The effect on the pupillary responses of lesions prior to the central decussation is the same as caused by lesions of the ipsilateral optic tract prior to the lateral geniculate nucleus.

LESIONS WITHIN THE EFFERENT PATHWAY FOR CONTROL OF PUPILLARY SIZE

(Parasympathetic control of pupil size — see figure 9.11). Lesions of the oculomotor nerve will affect the parasympathetic nerve supply to the pupillary sphincter muscle. Total lesions result in a dilated unresponsive pupil. The oculomotor supply to the extraocular muscles may also be affected, ptosis and a lateral and ventral strabismus result. Pharmacological testing may help to localise the site of the lesions within the PLR arc.

a.   Direct acting parasympathomimetic (e.g. *Pilocarpine* 1% drops). Topically administered *pilocarpine* can be used to differentiate between upper motor neurone (i.e. pretectal nucleus to oculomotor nucleus) and lower motor neurone (i.e. oculomotor nerve) lesions. Lower motor neurone lesions result in hypersensitivity to *pilocarpine*, the iris circular muscle fibres contracting more rapidly than normal. Upper motor neurone lesions do not result in this hypersensitivity.

b.   Indirect acting parasympathomimetics (e.g. 0.5.% *physostigmine* drops) cause no pupillary change with post ganglionic lesions. There is a rapid pupillary constriction when either preganglionic lesions or upper motor neurone lesions are present. (The ganglion referred to is the ciliary ganglion). The normal eye constricts within 40-60 minutes.

Feline dysautonomia may affect the parasympathetic control of the pupils resulting in fixed, dilated pupils.

SYMPATHETIC INNERVATION OF THE EYE

The sympathetic nervous system innervates the pupillary dilator muscles and interference with its supply to the iris results in a miotic (constricted) pupil. This occurs as part of Horner's syndrome.

The sympathetic nervous system supply to the eye is shown in Figure 9.14 (Barlow and Root, 1949).

Smooth muscle within the orbit, upper, lower and third eyelids is also innervated by the sympathetic nervous system. It keeps the eyeball protruded, the palpebral fissure widened and the third eyelid retracted.

The sympathetic innervation of the iris results in some dilation of the pupil which is increased by excitement, stress etc. Note that reduced tone in the pupillary constrictor muscle (parasympathetic supply) is responsible for pupillary dilation in reduced light.

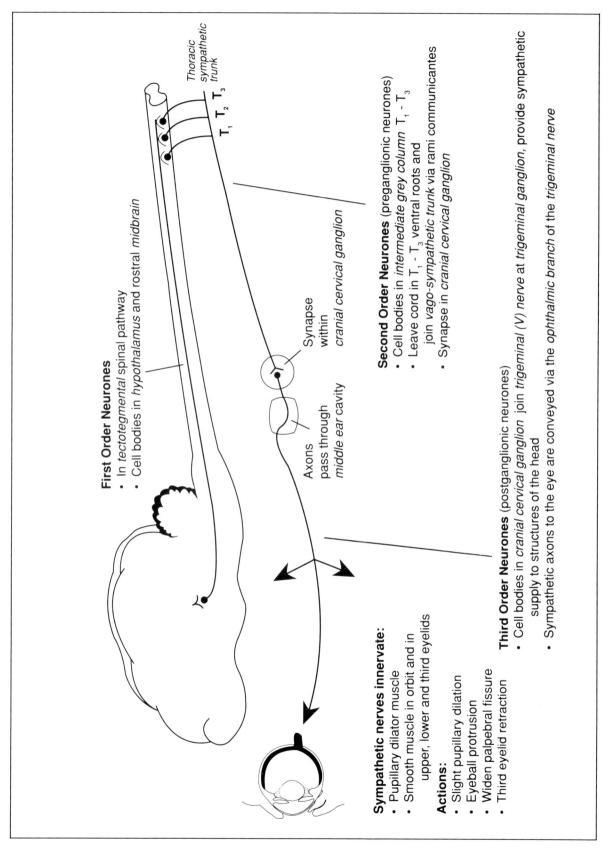

First Order Neurones
- In *tectotegmental* spinal pathway
- Cell bodies in *hypothalamus* and rostral *midbrain*

Second Order Neurones (preganglionic neurones)
- Cell bodies in *intermediate grey column* T_1 - T_3
- Leave cord in T_1 - T_3 ventral roots and join *vago-sympathetic trunk* via rami communicantes
- Synapse in *cranial cervical ganglion*

Third Order Neurones (postganglionic neurones)
- Cell bodies in *cranial cervical ganglion* join *trigeminal (V)* nerve at *trigeminal ganglion*, provide sympathetic supply to structures of the head
- Sympathetic axons to the eye are conveyed via the *ophthalmic branch* of the *trigeminal nerve*

Synapse within *cranial cervical ganglion*

Axons pass through *middle ear cavity*

Sympathetic nerves innervate:
- Pupillary dilator muscle
- Smooth muscle in orbit and in upper, lower and third eyelids

Actions:
- Slight pupillary dilation
- Eyeball protrusion
- Widen palpebral fissure
- Third eyelid retraction

Thoracic sympathetic trunk

T_1 T_2 T_3

Figure 9.14
Sympathetic nerve supply to eye and adnexa

153

Horner's syndrome — Interference with the sympathetic nerve supply to the head results in a combination of signs collectively referred to as Horner's Syndrome.

They are

> Miosis: the pupil on the affected side being smaller than the pupil on the unaffected side (anisocoria).

> Protrusion of the membrana nictitans: (third eyelid) due to lack of tone in smooth muscle retracting it and also secondary to the enophthalmia.

> Upper eyelid ptosis: (incomplete elevation) due to reduced tone in Muller's muscle; laxity of the lower eyelid may also be observed.

> Enophthalmia: resulting from a lack of tone in the orbital smooth muscle allowing the eye to sink back into the orbit.

These signs are shown by the patient illustrated in Figure 9.15. There may also be some reduction in intraocular pressure, and increased peripheral vasodilation resulting in a warmer pinna and a slight engorgement of conjunctival blood vessels.

Horner's syndrome may result from lesions of the sympathetic supply to the head at one of three anatomical levels, resulting in a first, second or third order Horner's syndrome. These levels and possible aetiologies of lesions are illustrated in Figure 9.16. Other clinical signs and pharmacological differentiation may aid localisation of the lesion.

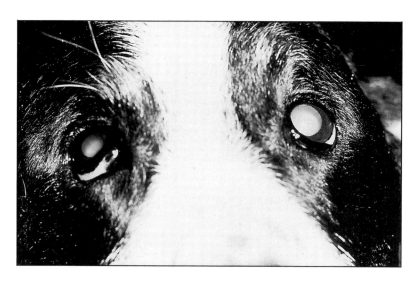

Figure 9.15
Dog with Horner's syndrome.
Note ptosis, third eyelid protrusion and miosis in dog's right eye.

Pharmacological differentiation (Bistner *et al*, 1970)

10% *phenylephrine* is administered topically to both eyes and the time taken to dilate the pupils is noted. The pupil of a normal eye and the eye with a first order Horner's syndrome will dilate in 60—90 minutes. If the Horner's syndrome is second order the pupil dilates in about 45 minutes and in the case of a third order lesion dilation occurs in about 20 minutes. The increased sensitivity to *phenylephrine* in second and third order Horner's syndrome is due to denervation hypersensitivity. In addition to dilating the pupil, other local signs of Horner's syndrome may be abolished by topical *phenylephrine*. Radiographs of the anterior thorax, cervico-thoracic spine and middle ear may help localise the lesion, though in many cases the aetiology remains obscure.

ANISOCORIA IN PATIENTS HAVING SUFFERED INTRACRANIAL TRAUMA

Intracranial trauma may result in abnormalities in pupil size. Unilateral or bilaterally miotic pupils may occur. Severe midbrain, or bilateral oculomotor nerve damage results in non responsive, dilated fixed pupils. Cerebellar disorders may result in dilated, slowly responsive pupils, accompanied by protrusion of the third eyelid and widening of the palpebral fissure. Other signs of cerebellar disease will also be present.

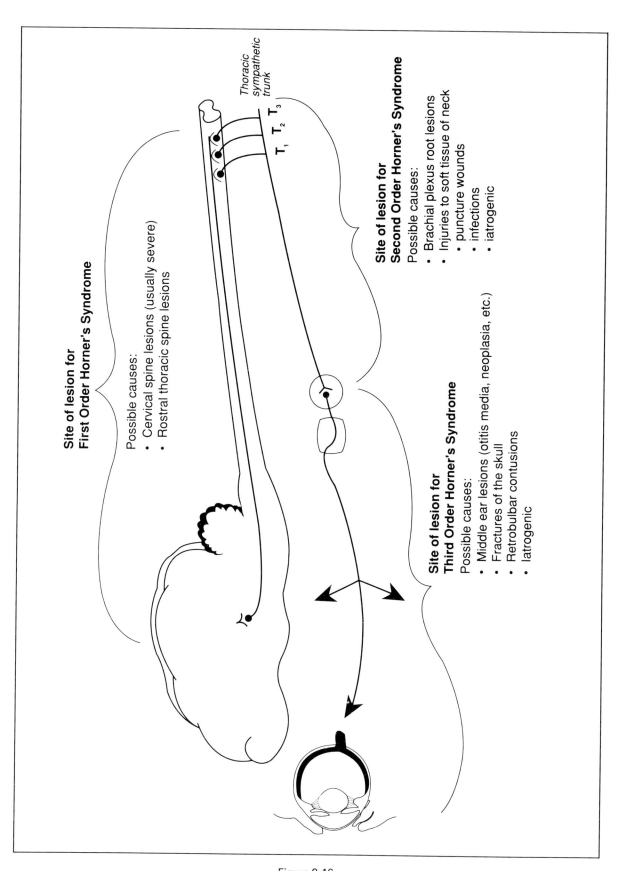

**Site of lesion for
First Order Horner's Syndrome**

Possible causes:
· Cervical spine lesions (usually severe)
· Rostral thoracic spine lesions

*Thoracic
sympathetic
trunk*

T₁ T₂ T₃

**Site of lesion for
Second Order Horner's Syndrome**

Possible causes:
· Brachial plexus root lesions
· Injuries to soft tissue of neck
  · puncture wounds
  · infections
  · iatrogenic

**Site of lesion for
Third Order Horner's Syndrome**

Possible causes:
· Middle ear lesions (otitis media, neoplasia, etc.)
· Fractures of the skull
· Retrobulbar contusions
· Iatrogenic

Figure 9.16.
Sites of lesions resulting in Horner's syndrome and possible aetiologies

SECTION III. EYE POSITION AND EYE MOVEMENTS

STRABISMUS/ABNORMALITIES OF EYE POSITION

Squints or strabismus are not uncommon. They may occur as a congenital abnormality or as a result of lesions of the extraocular muscles or their nerve supply. Congenital strabismus may be seen in any breed of dog or cat. A common example is the bilateral convergent strabismus (esotropia) of some Siamese cats.

Traumatic proptosis of the globe may cause tearing of the rectus muscles (usually the medial rectus muscle). If the globe is subsequently saved, a strabismus will result. A divergent strabismus or exotropia results from tearing of the medial rectus muscle. Retrobulbar swelling (due to infection or neoplasia) may cause strabismus in addition to exophthalmia.

A full knowledge of the actions and innervations of the extraocular muscles (Figure 9.17) is required to enable one to investigate the aetiology of a squint. Disorders of eye movement can be observed during the oculocephalic reflex (see Part 1). Surgery to correct squints in animals is possible but is seldom necessary.

Nerve supply to the extraocular muscles

Oculomotor nerve (III). This innervates dorsal, medial and ventral rectus muscles, the ventral oblique muscle and the levator palpebrae superioris. Parasympathetic fibres, which travel within the nerve, supply intraocular smooth muscle. Interference with the parasympathetic component of the oculomotor nerve results in a fixed, dilated, unresponsive pupil. When the general somatic efferent component of the nerve is affected there is a lateral and ventral strabismus (the 'down and out eye') and an upper lid ptosis (drooping).

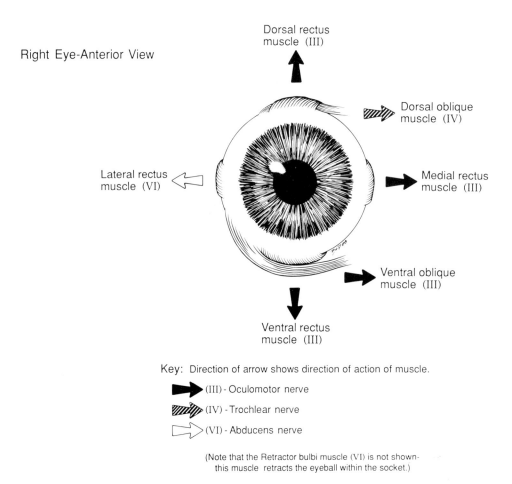

Key: Direction of arrow shows direction of action of muscle.

(III) - Oculomotor nerve

(IV) - Trochlear nerve

(VI) - Abducens nerve

(Note that the Retractor bulbi muscle (VI) is not shown-
this muscle retracts the eyeball within the socket.)

Figure 9.17
A diagram showing the extraocular muscles, their actions and innervation

Trochlear (IV) nerve. The trochlear nerve innervates the dorsal oblique muscle. Lesions result in rotation of the globe with the dorsal portion turned laterally. This is easier to detect in cats with their particular pupil shape.

Abducens (VI) nerve. This innervates the lateral rectus and retractor bulbi muscles. Lesions of the abducens nerve result in a medially diverted globe (esotropia) which cannot be abducted.

DISORDERS OF EYE MOVEMENTS (ABNORMAL NYSTAGMUS)

The coordination of eye movements is a complex mechanism with inputs from the vestibular systems, cerebellum and higher centres. Communication between the nuclei of the nerves to the extraocular muscles occurs via the medial longitudinal fasciculus and helps coordinate the extraocular muscles.

Vestibular influence on eye movements. The vestibular system is involved in controlling eye movements and position as well as maintaining the position of the trunk and limbs in reference to position or movement of the head. See Figure 9.18.

Normal nystagmus and the oculocephalic reflex. Nystagmus is an involuntary rhythmical eye movement with a slow and fast phase. Usually the slow phase is a slow movement of the eyes from their central position, the fast phase then rapidly recentres the eye's positions. The nystagmus produced by the oculocephalic reflex is due to the vestibular system and will occur in blind dogs (so long as the necessary vestibular system and pathways are normal).

Higher centres also influence the normal nystagmus induced by rotation, the autonomic 'pursuit' eye movements co-ordinated by the cerebral cortex allow fixation on a moving object in the surroundings or a stationary object if the head is moving . Nystagmus induced, for example, when looking out of a moving train's window, is a result of this system. It is called opticokinetic nystagmus and requires an intact central visual pathway.

Nystagmus is said to occur in the direction of the fast phase, that is, if the animal's head is rotated to the left nystagmus occurs to the left. In normal nystagmus the eyes move in unison. After the head has stopped moving the nystagmus stops; if it continues this is abnormal. However, if the animal is rotated rapidly and then stopped, there is normally a post rotatory nystagmus for a few moments. Dorsoventral as well as mediolateral nystagmus should be checked by the oculocephalic reflex.

Abnormalities of nystagmus. Abnormal nystagmus occurring when an animal's head is unrestrained is called 'spontaneous nystagmus'. Nystagmus occurring when an animal's head is held by the examiner in an abnormal position is called 'positional nystagmus'.

Peripheral vestibular disease results in spontaneous horizontal nystagmus. The direction of the nystagmus (i.e. the fast phase) is away from the side of the lesion. The nystagmus occurs in the same direction whatever position the head is put into. Other signs of vestibular disease such as head tilt, circling, loss of balance etc, may also be present.

Central vestibular disease may result in vertical or positional nystagmus (where the direction of nystagmus alters as the head's position is altered). Other neurological signs typical of vestibular disorders may be present. Cerebellar disorders may result in nystagmus, this being a form of intention tremor of the extraocular muscles.

A congenital nystagmus may sometimes be observed in puppies or kittens with no other detectable neurological abnormality. This is usually seen as continual fine oscillations of the globes. Congenital blindness may result in continuous, almost random eye movements described as 'searching nystagmus'. If the potential for vision is later restored, these movements will remain.

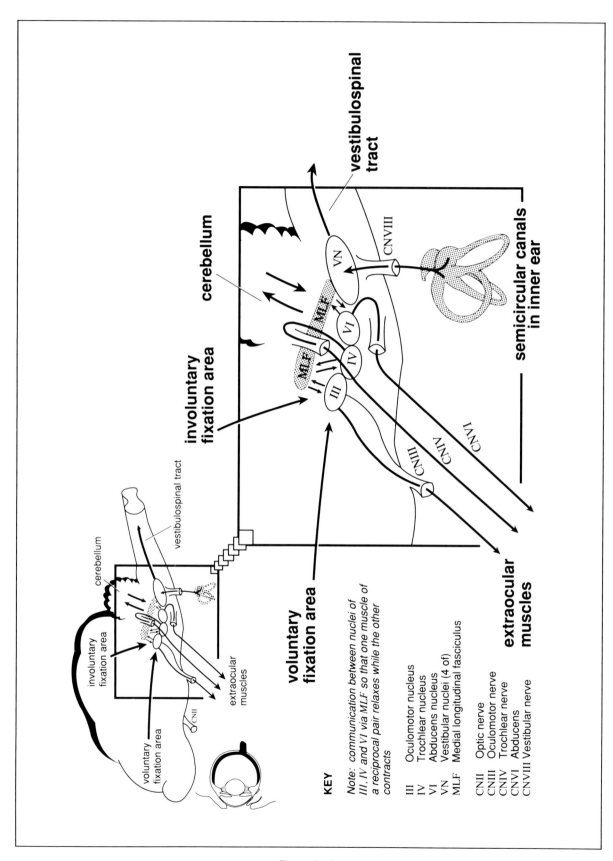

Figure 9.18
Diagram to show the pathway for vestibular influence of eye movements

158

SECTION IV.   DISORDERS OF BLINK

The normal blink is important for the well being of the eye. A deficiency of blink results in varying degrees of corneal disease. Lack of normal blink may result from lesions of the afferent (sensory) or efferent (motor) arms of the blink reflex.

ABNORMALITIES OF BLINK DUE TO SENSORY DEFICIT

Sensory Innervation of the Eye. Sensory innervation of the globe and adnexa is via the trigeminal (V) nerve. The ophthalmic branch of the trigeminal nerve supplies sensory innervation to the globe and middle portion of the upper eyelid. Branches of the maxillary branch of the trigeminal nerve supply the lateral parts of the upper eyelid, the lower eyelid and surrounding skin. The trigeminal nerve transmits sensory impulses to the trigeminal nucleus in the brain stem. After synapsing, these impulses cross to the contralateral thalamic nuclei and from there to the cerebral cortex for conscious perception. The corneal reflex is used to assess corneal sensation, the efferent arm of this reflex is via the facial (VII) nerve.

Denervation of sensory supply to the globe. A neurotrophic keratitis results from a sensory deficit of the cornea. Ulceration usually affects most of the cornea within the interpalpebral fissure. Note that the menace reflex will cause the animal to blink if the eye is still visual.

Infranuclear lesions (i.e. those occurring between the sensory nerve endings and cells of trigeminal nuclei) may result in total anaesthesia or partial anaesthesia. Hypalgesia of the three branches of the trigeminal nerve due to a supranuclear lesion is quite common. Often a supranuclear facial nerve palsy is present as well, due to the close proximity of thalamic nuclei (V) and the internal capsule(VII).

Lesions of the trigeminal nerve may result from neoplasia, infection or skull fractures. Attempts should be made to identify the site and cause of the lesion and to treat it if possible. A neurotrophic keratitis should be treated symptomatically, giving covering antibiosis and tear substitutes.

ABNORMALITIES OF BLINK DUE TO MOTOR DEFICITS

Motor innervation of eyelids. The facial nerve (VII) supplies the muscles of facial expression, and carries parasympathetic nerves innervating the lacrimal glands. It passes from the brain alongside the auditory nerve until it enters the facial canal which passes adjacent to the medial wall of the tympanic cavity. Fibres innervating the lacrimal gland pass via the major petrosal nerve and are given off just as the facial canal bends to become adjacent to the tympanic cavity. This close anatomical association between the facial nerve and the tympanic cavity is of clinical significance. The facial nerve emerges through the stylomastoid foramen and innervates the muscles of facial expression including the orbicularis oculi muscle which is responsible for blinking. The ability to blink may be checked by a number of reflexes such as the menace test and corneal reflex.

Lesions of the facial nerve. Facial nerve paralysis results in inability to blink. When the animal is stimulated to attempt to blink by the menace test or corneal reflex, the globe is retracted and the third eyelid flicks across the cornea, but the upper and lower lids are incapable of closing the palpebral fissure. The cornea will be unaffected in cases where the parasympathetic supply to the lacrimal gland is spared and the third eyelid can adequately distribute the tear film. The cause of the facial nerve lesion should be identified and treated if possible. Ocular treatment is not usually necessary unless lacrimal function is impaired, in which case tear substitutes should be used.

Hemifacial spasm. This is the result of increased motor activity of the facial nerve. It may, at first glance, be confused with facial nerve paralysis of the contralateral side. It has been reported in dogs with chronic otitis media (irritation of facial nerve) and following facial paralysis; central causes have also been suggested (Parker *et al,* 1973; Roberts and Vainisi, 1967).

SECTION V.   DISORDERS OF LACRIMATION

The afferent arm for the tearing reflex is via the trigeminal nerve. The efferent arm takes the following route; preganglionic axons leave the brain stem within the facial nerve and pass via the major petrosal nerve which leaves the facial nerve within the facial canal in the medial wall of the middle ear cavity. The major petrosal nerve passes through the pterygoid canal to end in the pterygopalatine ganglion. The preganglionic axons synapse with postganglionic cell bodies in the pterygopalatine ganglion, the post-ganglionic axons then pass to innervate the lacrimal glands.

Tear production may be measured by the Schirmer tear test. A specially shaped strip of filter paper is hooked between the lower lid and cornea and left in situ for one minute (Figure 9.19). The length of strip which is wet with tears after this time is measured. The normal reading is about 15—25 mm/minute.

Lesion of the afferent arm of the tearing reflex. Sensation conveyed from the cornea, conjunctiva and to a certain extent the nasal mucosa via the trigeminal nerve acts as the afferent arm of the reflex to increase tear production. Lesions of the trigeminal nerve have been discussed above.

Lesions of the efferent arm of the tearing reflex. Lesions of the parasympathetic supply to the lacrimal gland may be accompanied by facial nerve lesions. They result in much reduced tear production; the Schirmer tear test reading may be zero. This leads to corneal desiccation and possibly corneal perforation. Lesions may occur secondary to otitis media.

There are also non neurological causes of dry eye (keratoconjunctivitis sicca), such as gradual destruction of the secreting tissue of the gland (possibly immune mediated in West Highland white terriers) and drug toxicities. These should be differentiated from neurological causes.

The cause should be identified and treated, if possible. Topical tear substitutes and ointments can be used and oral parasympathomimetics such as *pilocarpine* may be of benefit particularly in neurogenic cases. A parotid duct transposition may be performed if medical treatment fails to control the condition.

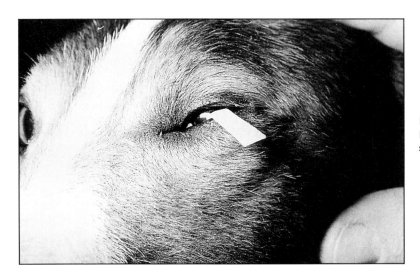

Figure 9.19
Photograph of a Schirmer tear test strip in use

All photographs for Chapter 9 (except 9.15) were taken by David Gunn.

REFERENCES

BARLOW, C. M. & ROOT, W. S. (1949). The ocular sympathetic path between the superior cervical ganglion and the orbit in the cat. *Journal of Comparative Neurology* **90**, 195.

BARNETT, K. C., KELLY, D. F. and SINGLETON, W. B. (1967). Retrobulbar and chiasmal meningioma in a dog. *Journal of Small Animal Practice* **8**, 391.

BEDFORD, P. G. C. (1982) The diagnosis of ocular disease in the dog and cat. *British Veterinary Journal* **138**, 93.

BISTNER, S., RUBIN, L., COX, T. A. and CONDON W. E., (1970). Pharmacological diagnosis of Horner's Syndrome in the dog. *Journal of the American Veterinary Medical Association* **157**, 1220.

BRAUND, K. G., VANDEVELDE, M., ALBERT, R. A., HIGGINS, R. J. (1977). Central (post retinal) visual impairment in the dog — a clinical pathological study. *Journal of Small Animal Practice* **18**, 395.

deLAHUNTA, A. and CUMMINGS, J. F. (1967). Neuro-ophthalmological lesions as a cause of visual deficit in dogs and horses. *Journal of the American Veterinary Medical Association* **150**, 994.

FISCHER, C. A. and JONES, G. T. (1972). Optic neuritis in dogs. *Journal of the American Veterinary Medical Association* **160**, 68.

PALMER, A. C., MALINOWSKI, W. and BARNETT, K. C. (1974). Clinical signs including papilloedema associated with brain tumours in twenty-one dogs. *Journal of Small Animal Practice* **15**, 359.

PARKER, A. J., CUSICK, P. K., PARK, R. D. and SMALL, E. (1973). Hemifacial spasms in a dog. *Veterinary Record* **93**, 514.

ROBERTS, S. R. and VAINISI, S. J. (1967). Hemifacial spasm in dogs. *Journal of the American Veterinary Medical Association* **150**, , 381.

RUBIN, L. R. (1974). *Atlas of Veterinary Ophthalmoscopy.* Lea and Febiger, Philadelphia, p. 218.

SKERRITT, G. C., OBWOLO, M. J. and SQUIRES, R. A. (1986). Bilateral blindness in a dog due to invasion of the optic chiasma by a glioma. *Journal of Small Animal Practice* **27**, 97.

WILLIAMS, J. O., GARLICK, E. C. and BEARD, D. C. (1961). Glioma of the optic nerve of a dog. *Journal of the American Veterinary Medical Association* **138**, 377.

FURTHER READING

deLAHUNTA, A. (1973) Small animal neuro-ophthalmology. *Veterinary Clinics of North America* **3**, (3) 491.

de LAHUNTA, A. (1983). *Veterinary Neuroanatomy and Clinical Neurology* 2nd ed. W. B. Saunders Co., Philadelphia, pp115-123 and 279-303.

KAY, W. J. (1981). Neuro-ophthalmology. *In Veterinary Ophthalmology.* **20**, pp 672-698. Ed. K. N. Gelatt, Lea and Febiger, Philadelphia.

SCAGLIOTTI, R. H. (1980). Current concepts in veterinary neuro-ophthalmology. *Veterinary Clinics of North America: Small Animal Practice* **10**, (2) 417.

SLATTER, D. H. and deLAHUNTA, A. (1981). Neurophthalmology. *Fundamentals of Veterinary Ophthalmology.* Ed. D. H. Slatter, W. B. Saunders Co., Philadelphia, pp571-661.

CHAPTER 10

NEUROLOGICAL DEFICITS IN MULTIPLE LIMBS

Simon J. Wheeler B.V.Sc., Ph.D., M.R.C.V.S.

The identification of neurological deficits affecting more than one limb should allow the clinician to localise the lesion to an area of the nervous system using the information given in Part I of this book. A careful clinical and neurological examination should be performed in all cases to avoid mis-diagnosing the problem because, in some cases, the true origin of the locomotor disturbance may not be in the nervous system. Some examples of conditions which mimic neurological presentations are given in Table 10.1.

Neurological deficits in multiple limbs usually indicate that a lesion is present cranial to the affected limbs or that there is multifocal disease. Use of the various ancillary aids described in Part I will allow a diagnosis to be reached. This chapter describes the aetiology, treatment and prognosis for conditions causing such signs. Generally, spinal diseases are dealt with in this chapter whilst other classes of disease, such as peripheral neuropathies and myopathies, are covered elsewhere in this book (Chapters 13 and 14).

Spinal diseases causing the types of clinical signs described here are frequently accompanied by pain or hyperaesthesia and these may be the only signs present at many stages of some diseases. It may be more accurate to consider these conditions as having the **potential** to cause the neurological deficits described in many circumstances. The presence of pain or an area of hyperaesthesia is extremely useful in the localisation of lesions whether or not neurological deficits are present and animals should be evaluated carefully in this regard.

In this chapter the differential diagnosis is considered from an initial 'base line' condition, which provides a starting point in evaluating a case. Features are described which will assist the examiner to reach the correct diagnosis in any particular case. The conditions which should be considered are somewhat different in juvenile animals than in adults, thus these groups are treated separately. Many conditions differ in the neurological picture they produce only by virtue of the anatomical site at which they occur. The considerations discussed in one section may well apply elsewhere in the chapter, depending on the site of the lesion. The chapter is arranged as follows:

DISORDERS AFFECTING ALL LIMBS

FOCAL DISORDERS — GENERALISED DISORDERS

JUVENILES — ADULTS — JUVENILES — ADULTS

DISORDERS AFFECTING THE HIND LIMBS

FOCAL DISORDERS — GENERALISED DISORDERS

JUVENILES — ADULTS — JUVENILES — ADULTS

Table 10.1
Conditions mimicking neurological presentations

A	**BILATERAL ORTHOPAEDIC CONDITIONS** Osteochondritis dissecans Anterior cruciate ligament rupture Tibial crest avulsion Limb / pelvic fractures
B	**GENERALISED ORTHOPAEDIC DISEASES** Panosteitis Polyarthritis Hypertrophic osteodystrophy
C	**SOFT TISSUE DISORDERS** Muscle contractures: — Infraspinatus Gracilis Quadriceps Achilles tendon rupture
D	**VASCULAR DISEASE**

Table 10.2
Some conditions causing neurological deficits in all limbs based on
presence of pain and time course of the condition

	ACUTE	SUBACUTE	CHRONIC
Pain only or predominant sign		Meningoencephalitis	Hypervitaminosis A
	Disc protrusion	Vertebral osteomyelitis	
		Disc protrusion	
	Fracture/dislocation	Atlanto-axial subluxation	
	Discospondylitis	Discospondylitis	Discospondylitis
			Granulomatous meningoencephalitis
		Cervical spondylopathy	
	Inflammatory disease	Inflammatory disease	Cervical spondylopathy
		Neoplasia	
			Neoplasia
			Cervical spinal stenosis
		Distemper myelitis	Storage diseases
		Toxoplasmosis	Feline infectious peritonitis
			Toxoplasmosis
	Ischaemic myelopathy	Central/peripheral neuropathies	Central/peripheral neuropathies
			Degenerative disorders
Neurological deficit predominant or only sign			

164

DISORDERS AFFECTING ALL LIMBS

The presentation of a dog or cat with neurological deficits in all limbs should alert the clinician to the possibility of either a focal lesion in the cervical spinal cord or brain, or a diffuse lesion affecting various parts of the central nervous system (CNS) and/or the peripheral nervous system (PNS). Some such disorders may well not affect all limbs, for example, only the forelimbs or the limbs on one side of the body may be involved. The general neurological status of the animal may be described as follows: —

Quadriparesis — muscular weakness in all limbs due to a lesion of the nervous system (NS).

Quadriplegia — total motor paralysis due to a NS lesion.

Ataxia — incoordinate gait due to interference with NS function.

Hemiparesis/hemiplegia — deficits on one side of the body.

FOCAL DISORDERS

The neurological examination may indicate a lesion cranial to C_6 although sometimes it may not be possible to further localise the lesion on the basis of the neurological signs alone. Concurrent cranial nerve signs and a change in the animal's attitude indicate the presence of a lesion within the brain and particular note should be made of vestibular signs or abnormalities of the eyes. Tremor or hypermetria may indicate a cerebellar lesion. However, the absence of any specific cranial signs does not completely eliminate the possibility of a cranial lesion being present.

The majority of cases in this category will have cervical cord lesions. Diagnosis will be aided by radiography and CSF analysis. Plain radiography will provide the diagnosis in the majority of cases but myelography may be necessary to identify some lesions not involving bone. CSF analysis may provide useful information in inflammatory, degenerative or neoplastic disorders.

The differential diagnosis for this category of cases is outlined in Table 10.2. Particular note should be taken of the breed and age of the animal and of the presence or absence of pain. Pain frequently is a feature of cervical cord lesions; in fact, neurological deficits in isolation are seen less commonly.

Base line diagnosis

Cervical disc extrusion is the 'base line' diagnosis for this category of cases. Certain specific breeds feature in all series of cases, particularly beagles, dachshunds, corgis and all types of spaniels. Thus it is typically the chondrodystrophic breeds which are involved. One exception to this is the Doberman which suffers from disc protrusions as part of the syndrome of **cervical spondylopathy**. Cervical disc extrusion occurs very rarely in dogs of less than 2 years old. The presentation of a young dog with neck pain and/or quadriparesis should alert the clinician to other possibilities which are discussed below.

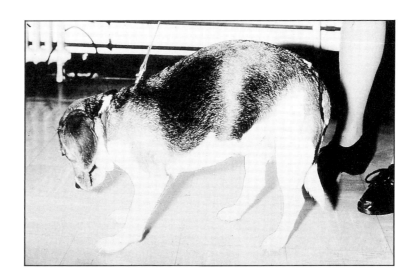

Figure 10.1
Beagle in typical posture of dog with severe neck pain due to cervical disc extrusion.

(Courtesy Professor L. C. Vaughan, Royal Veterinary College.)

Figure 10.1 shows a beagle in the posture typical of a dog with severe cervical pain, which frequently is the only sign in the early stages of the disease. Overt pain localised to the neck may not be evident in some dogs, rather there is generalised discomfort. However, it is usually possible to appreciate spasm of the neck muscles which helps to identify the origin of the pain in cases where this is not immediately apparent. The commonest neurological sign is paresis or lameness of one forelimb, though a full range of signs referable to a cervical cord lesion may be seen. Some acute cases, or those which are longstanding, may have profound deficits.

The diagnosis is based on the clinical signs and confirmed by radiography (Figure 10.2). The vast majority of cases involve one of the first four cervical discs with the $C_{2/3}$ disc the most commonly affected. Treatment by the use of anti-inflammatory drugs and cage rest may be successful. Despite medical treatment, many cases require surgical intervention at some stage. The majority of dogs will respond to cervical fenestration though some will require decompression via a ventral 'slot' (Denny, 1978; Wheeler, 1986, 1987). Ventral decompression should be performed if there are marked neurological deficits or myelographic evidence of a large amount of extruded disc material in the spinal canal. The prognosis is good, though some dogs may undergo a prolonged recovery following fenestration.

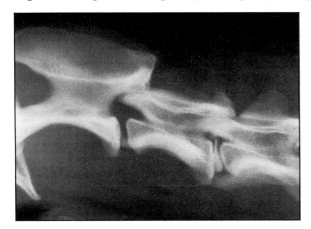

Figure 10.2 a.
Lateral radiograph, cervical spine
demonstrating $C_{3/4}$ disc extrusion.

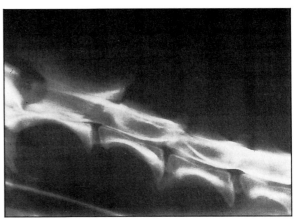

Figure 10.2 b.
Myelogram showing cord compression
due to disc extrusion.

FOCAL DISORDERS IN JUVENILES

Other conditions must be considered in young dogs with signs of a cervical lesion.

Inflammatory disorders

Inflammatory disorders often lead to one predominant clinical feature. However, careful evaluation of the case usually reveals a multifocal problem. This may be reflected in localised neurological signs but with hyperaesthesia present at a number of locations. Such a presentation is strongly suggestive of inflammatory CNS disease. Whilst inflammatory disorders are not strictly 'focal' in nature, the clinical signs are somewhat different from the generalised disorders described later in this chapter.

Meningitis and meningoencephalitis are frequent causes of neck pain though neurological signs may be restricted to dullness or depression. The clinical signs are often undulating in severity, particularly if short courses of treatment are administered. Various causative agents are involved but attempts at isolation of organisms often are unsuccessful (Braund, 1980) and in some cases a non-infectious inflammatory process may be occurring. The diagnosis is based on the clinical signs, normal radiological findings and evaluation of CSF, which usually reveals a pleocytosis with an increase in protein. In cases where the course of the disease is episodic the laboratory findings may prove normal between bouts. It may be possible to culture bacteria from the CSF in some instances. Treatment involves the administration of a suitable antibiotic for a prolonged period, often accompanied by corticosteroids in the early stages. **Feline infectious peritonitis** may lead to such signs in cats.

Canine distemper virus (CDV) infection leads to a wide range of clinical and neurological signs in dogs, the most common being myoclonus (Chapter 8). However, CDV infection can lead to other presentations and this possibility should always be considered in the type of case being considered here.

A routine vaccination programme does not preclude the possibility of CDV associated disease being present. Confirming the diagnosis may prove difficult, though the analysis of CSF for CDV neutralising antibody may be useful.

Toxoplasmosis is another condition which should be considered and again serological testing is required to confirm the diagnosis. Where Toxoplasmosis is diagnosed, treatment with *clindamycin* (100mg/kg BID parenterally) may effect a cure.

Other inflammatory processes such as **discospondylitis** occur in young dogs and may lead to pain or neurological dysfunction (see below).

Development disorders

Atlanto-axial subluxation is the other major condition to consider in young dogs with pain and/or neurological deficits. Small breeds are usually affected early in life but traumatic cases can occur in any type of dog at any age. The diagnosis is confirmed radiographically (Figure 10.3). Great care must be taken when manipulating dogs with this condition as hyperflexion of the neck can cause a precipitous worsening of the neurological status. A number of congenital defects underlie the condition including absence of the dens, separation or fracture of the dens or defects in the ligamentous structures (Geary *et al,* 1967). Treatment involves two principles; limiting spinal cord damage and stabilising the subluxated joint. Limitation of damage may best be achieved by medical treatment and immobilisation with a neck cast though surgical decompression may be indicated in some cases. Stabilisation of the joint is performed by one of a number of surgical procedures, some of which are hazardous. Wiring the dorsal arches of the vertebrae has been favoured by many surgeons though, currently, ventral stabilisation is the preferred technique (Denny, 1988).

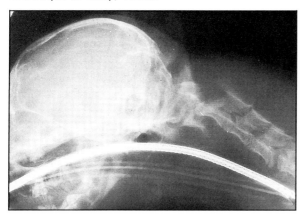
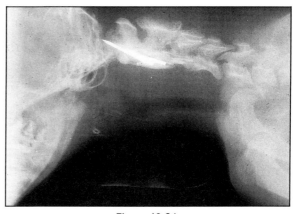

Figure 10.3 a	Figure 10.3 b
Lateral radiograph demonstrating abnormal alignment of $C_{1/2}$ due to atlanto-axial subluxation	Post operative radiograph following ventral fixation.

Other disorders predominantly affecting young animals include the following conditions. **Stenosis** of the spinal canal may occur, leading to progressive neurological deficits. The diagnosis is made from plain or contrast radiographs. Treatment by decompression and stabilisation is possible though clinical signs often cease to progress near one year of age. The basset hound is prone to a malalignment of the cervical vertebrae leading to similar signs. The various **lysosomal storage diseases** also should be considered; see Chapter 8.

FOCAL DISORDERS IN ADULTS

Traumatic lesions

Spinal fractures or luxations can occur in the cervical spine. Road accidents are the most common cause although falls and other traumatic incidents may also be involved. Careful radiographic examination will usually provide the diagnosis and should help in assessing whether surgical intervention is indicated. Decompression of the cord in this area is not performed frequently and surgery usually is restricted to fracture fixation (Figure 10.4). External fixation with neck casts is suitable in many instances. The course of action is influenced to a great degree by the neurological status, any deterioration being a definite indication for surgical intervention. Medical therapy aimed at limiting spinal cord damage and relieving pain should be considered, particularly in the early stages (See Chapter 6). Many cases of cervical fracture, even where there are profound neurological deficits, will recover eventually.

Vascular disorders

Ischaemic myelopathy due to fibrocartilaginous embolism also features an acute onset of signs, without the pain associated with fractures. The brachial plexus outflow segments are more often affected than the more cranial parts of the cord and these cases demonstrate lower motor neurone (LMN) deficits in a forelimb. Lesions usually originate unilaterally, leading to a marked asymmetry of signs with secondary changes in the cord leading to the rapid development of bilateral neurological deficits. The diagnosis is based on the clinical signs with the absence of pain and the asymmetry being important features. The absence of myelographic evidence of a space occupying lesion excludes the presence of tumours, disc extrusions etc., though the cord may be swollen in the very acute stages of ischaemic myelopathy. The course of the disease is usually a very rapid progression over a few hours and some owners report that the animal is in discomfort during the early stages. Treatment is with corticosteroids for the first few days accompanied by careful nursing and attention to bladder function. The prognosis is variable; LMN deficits rarely improve whereas upper motor neurone (UMN) losses often recover (Griffiths, 1973; Zaki and Prata, 1976).

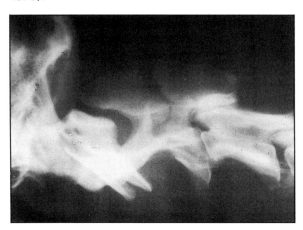

Figure 10.4 a
Fracture of C$_2$

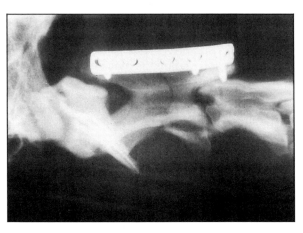

Figure 10.4 b
Repair by plating dorsal spinous process.
(Courtesy Mr. D. G. Clayton Jones, Royal Veterinary College).

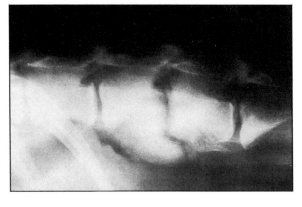

Figure 10.5
Lateral radiograph, lumbar spine of dog
with discospondylitis.

Inflammatory disorders

Other inflammatory brain and spinal cord diseases are seen. Acute inflammation of the central nervous system may occur, but more common is the chronic type of presentation seen in **granulomatous meningoencephalitis (GME)**. This disease is recognised uncommonly in the UK though it does occur, causing initially low grade, poorly localising neurological signs and hyperaesthesia in adult dogs (Braund, 1985). The pug is prone to a similar disorder which may be related to GME or canine distemper. Confirmation of the diagnosis is aided by CSF evaluation, and treatment with corticosteroids may induce a temporary remission. Despite treatment, the long term prognosis for these conditions is poor.

Discospondylitis in the cervical spine usually leads to a subacute onset of neck pain and neurological signs in animals of any age. The condition arises from infection of the intervertebral disc space with extension into the vertebral end plates, vertebral bodies and the spinal canal. The causative organism usually arrives by haematogenous spread though cases associated with foreign body migration or which follow disc surgery have been seen. Diagnosis is confirmed radiographically (Figure 10.5) and it is often possible to isolate the causative agent from blood or urine and thus determine the specific antibiotic sensitivity. Some very early cases may not show radiographic signs but nuclear imaging will reveal an area of increased vascularity at the site. Treatment with prolonged courses of antibiotics may be successful.

Specific therapy should be used wherever possible though in the absence of this information the cephalosporins or *cloxacillin* are most likely to effect a cure. Treatment should be maintained for six weeks (Kornegay, 1983). Surgical curettage of the affected disc may also be considered as the cervical spine is easy to approach and many dogs do respond rapidly to such treatment. **Vertebral osteomyelitis** occurs less commonly. The diagnosis is apparent on radiographs and management is similar to that for cases of discospondylitis.

Degenerative disorders

Cervical spondylopathy ('Wobbler's syndrome') is a significant cause of subacute or chronic neurological dysfunction in certain breeds of dog. Whilst the majority of the pathological changes which occur are degenerative in nature, there is a significant congenital component involved in the development of this disorder. Great Danes and other giant breeds are usually affected in the first two years of life whilst Dobermans generally present between 4 and 7 years old, though occasional individuals are affected at an earlier age. The clinical signs are variable with neck discomfort or pain being a frequent feature. Initially, neurological signs may be restricted to the hind limbs with ataxia, proprioceptive losses, paresis and hyperactive local reflexes. Closer examination often reveals abnormalities of the forelimbs with increased tone of the extensor muscles leading to a rather short foreleg action. In mildly affected animals the clinical signs may be more apparent at slower gaits. The severity of the clinical signs varies from a mild gait abnormality to virtual quadriplegia, and neck pain is often a feature (Denny *et al,* 1977; Mason, 1979; Seim and Withrow, 1982; Read *et al,* 1983). Many severely affected cases are long standing and some are exacerbated by a traumatic incident. Some Great Danes exercise fairly normally but find it impossible to stand still, developing muscle tremors and eventually lying down.

The differential diagnosis in these cases warrants careful consideration. In dogs showing only hind limb deficits the possibility of a thoracolumbar lesion should not be ignored. Similarly, non-neurological causes of gait abnormalities should not be overlooked, particularly in young Great Danes, where osteochondritis dissecans or generalised bone diseases are prevalent. Radiography and myelography are required to evaluate cases fully. Findings can be difficult to interpret as changes may be subtle and can also be identified in clinically normal dogs, especially if flexed views of the spine are taken. Bony abnormalities, evident on plain films, often are not consistent with the site of spinal cord compression subsequently revealed by myelography. Some of the radiographic findings are illustrated in Figure 10.6.

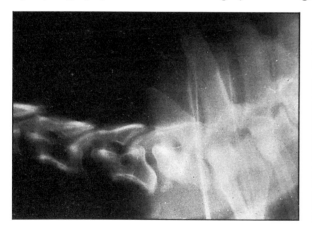
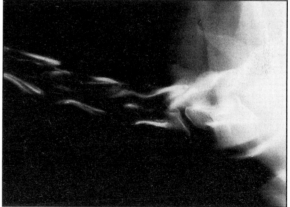
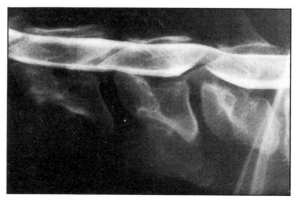

Figure 10.6 a (above left)
Figure 10.6 b (above right)
Figure 10.6 c (right)

Lateral radiographs demonstrating changes seen in spine in cervical spondylopathy.

a. vertebral body malposition or 'tilting' with abnormal shape of vertebral body and angulation of cranio-ventral aspect
b. stenosis of vertebral canal
c. disc protrusion causing compression of spinal cord as demonstrated myelographically.

The underlying lesion in this condition may be a primary bony abnormality, degenerative joint disease, secondary disc and ligament changes or often a combination of these. An assessment of these changes is required to determine the best treatment in an individual case. In acute cases, medical and surgical treatment may be necessary to limit spinal cord damage. Administration of anti-inflammatory drugs in the first instance may be accompanied by surgical decompression which is best accomplished via a ventral 'slot'. Decompression may also be beneficial in less acute cases where there is significant protrusion of disc material or ligamentous hypertrophy. Stabilisation by lag screw fixation has also proved useful in cases where vertebral malalignment is a major component. Some dogs may not be suitable candidates for surgery particularly where there is canal stenosis or osteoarthritis of the dorsal articular facets (Figure 10.7). There is considerable controversy concerning surgical treatment and the diversity of opinion reflects the guarded prognosis these cases carry, a fact which should always be remembered when embarking on treatment.

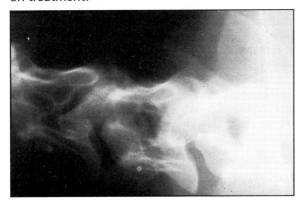 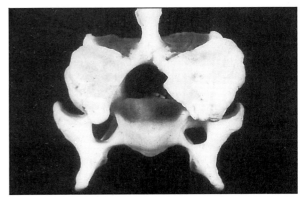

Osteoarthritis of the dorsal vertebral articulations of one year-old Great Dane.

Figure 10.7 a	Figure 10.7 b
Lateral radiograph of cervical spine	Specimen demonstrating impingement on spinal canal.

Neoplasia

Neoplasms are an important cause of spinal pain and neurological dysfunction in dogs and cats. Whilst the animals usually present with an insidious progression of signs of spinal cord compression, a relatively acute history does not preclude the possibility of a spinal tumour being present. Tumours can occur in any age of animal but they are more prevalent in older individuals. It should be remembered that some tumours of neural origin occur in young dogs and lymphoma is seen in young cats. Tumours are relatively infrequent in dogs but account for up to 50% of spinal cases in cats (Prata, 1977; Wright *et al*, 1979; Luttgen *et al*, 1980; Wright, 1985; Fingeroth *et al*, 1987; Wheeler, 1989b). Radiography is the most productive diagnostic aid in these cases and myelography is usually required to identify the lesion (Chapter 5). CSF analysis may also provide useful information.

Tumours are classified according to their location in the spinal canal. Extradural tumours are mainly primary bone tumours or, less commonly, metastatic in origin. In cats, lymphoma is the most common tumour type and is usually extradural. Tumours in this site are often painful with progressive neurological signs. If there is major bone destruction, vertebral collapse may occur leading to an acute onset of severe neurological deficits (Figure 10.8). Some extradural tumours can be removed surgically and lymphoma cases may be treated medically or by radiotherapy (Gorman, 1987).

Intradural/extramedullary tumours are usually either meningiomas or nerve sheath tumours (a broad classification which includes neurofibromas, neurofibrosarcomas etc.). A study of canine meningiomas showed a predilection for the cervical spine, with dogs showing general discomfort and progressive neurological signs (Fingeroth *et al*, 1987). Meningiomas may be removed surgically and carry a reasonable prognosis unless they involve the brachial or lumbosacral outflow segments. Nerve sheath tumours are more prevalent in the brachial plexus area and often may be palpated in the axilla. Surgical removal of tumours in this area is difficult and leaves a residual LMN deficit, and the rate of recurrence is high.

Intramedullary tumours are the least common type in dogs and are derived from the glial cells or are metastatic. Pain is not usually a feature of such masses, rather there is a gradual progression of neurological signs. Glial tumours may occur in younger dogs and generally they are not amenable to treatment. In summary, the prognosis for spinal tumours is guarded though recent advances in therapy have improved the outlook.

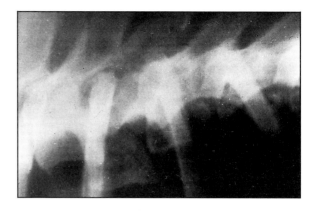

Figure 10.8
Lateral radiograph demonstrating thoracic vertebral body collapse following bone destruction due to osteosarcoma.

GENERALISED DISORDERS

JUVENILES

Many of the generalised **central/peripheral neuropathies** occur in young dogs (Chapter 14). Some of the conditions causing episodic weakness, such as the congenital form of **myasthenia gravis,** should also be considered (Chapter 13). **Juvenile ataxias** have been recognised in several breeds including smooth haired fox terriers, Jack Russell terriers and bull mastiffs and some may have a hereditary basis (Bjorck *et al,* 1957; Hartley and Palmer, 1973; Carmichael *et al,* 1983). In the terriers the nervous system changes are predominantly in the spinal cord. In the mastiffs there is cerebellar degeneration and closer inspection of these dogs also reveals visual deficits. Further cases of this condition, which is progressive, have now been recognised. Ataxia and generalised tremor is seen in cerebellar disorders (Chapter 8) and in hypomyelinating syndromes in some breeds e.g. springer spaniel, weimaraner. Some of these disorders show spontaneous improvement during the first year of life.

Hereditary spinal muscular atrophy has been reported in a number of breeds, including Swedish Laplands, Brittany spaniels and pointers. Individuals show gait abnormalities at an early age with muscular weakness and atrophy. The signs are progressive, eventually resulting in quadriplegia due to a loss of cell populations in the CNS (Griffiths, 1986).

ADULTS

In addition to the conditions described above, multifocal CNS diseases of any type may lead to neurological deficits in multiple limbs. Acquired **muscle diseases** are seen in adult dogs as are the various disorders affecting the neuromuscular junction, such as **myasthenia gravis** and **botulism** (Chapter 13). Other conditions causing neurological signs in all limbs include **Hypervitaminosis A** in cats (Chapter 16) and certain peripheral neuropathies such as **distal denervating disease** (Chapter 14).

DISORDERS AFFECTING THE HIND LIMBS

This group of presenting signs is relatively common and hence familiar to the clinician in small animal practice. The approach to these cases in terms of lesion localisation and assessment of severity has been covered in Part 1. The diagnosis will usually be assisted by radiographic examination and CSF evaluation, with other tests indicated if LMN deficits are present. The differential diagnosis of conditions causing these signs is given in Table 10.3. As with cervical lesions, pain is often a major feature of thoraco-lumbar or lumbar spinal disorders and in some of the conditions described, neurological dysfunction may not be evident at certain stages of the disease. Particular types or breeds of dogs are susceptible to some conditions (Appendix 1) but, whilst a knowledge of such predilections is useful, it should not be used as the only basis for diagnosis.

Base line diagnosis

Thoraco-lumbar (T/L) disc extrusion is the 'base-line' diagnosis for cases in this category. The intervertebral discs between T_{11} and L_2 account for the majority of extrusions in dogs. Various methods have been used to classify disc disease but it is useful to divide cases into three groups: —

Disc disease in the chondrodystrophic breeds

Acute disc extrusions in the non-chondrodystrophic breeds

Chronic disc disease in the non-chondrodystrophic breeds

Degenerative disc disease in the chondrodystrophic breeds is familiar to most clinicians and the clinical signs of disc protrusion or extrusion are well recognised. The condition may arise any time after one year of age but it is unusual for aged individuals to be affected and in such cases other differential diagnosis are more likely. Disc protrusion or extrusion mainly occurs following disc degeneration which is usually present at many sites in the spine. All the clinical signs associated with T/L spinal cord compression may be seen and the course of the disease may be acute or chronic. The diagnosis is based on the clinical signs and confirmed radiographically. Good quality, correctly positioned radiographs will provide the diagnosis in the majority of cases. Myelography is of benefit if decompressive surgery is envisaged. The radiographic signs are illustrated in Figure 10.9.

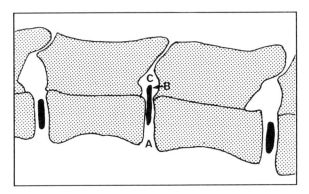

a.

Figure 10.9
Radiographic signs in thoracolumbar disc protrusion.(Modified from *British Veterinary Journal* **142**, 95 by permission).
a. Diagramatic representation;
Key:
A — Narrowing of intervertebral space
B — Extrusion of mineralised material into the spinal canal
C — Decreased size and opacification of intervertebral foramen

b and c. Lateral spinal radiographs

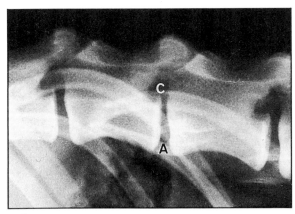

b.

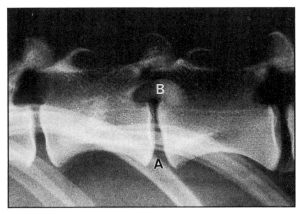

c.

d. Myelographic findings on lateral   e. ventro-dorsal projections

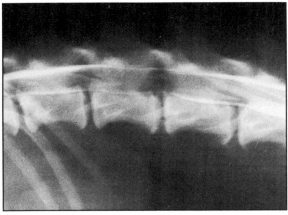

d.

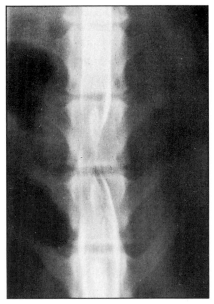

e.

172

Treatment may be conservative or surgical and good management is essential if a satisfactory outcome is to be achieved. The method of treatment selected is influenced to a significant degree by the surgical expertise available. Whilst the eventual outcome may be similar for many cases whichever method is employed, surgical intervention usually leads to a faster recovery and certainly dramatically reduces the incidence of recurrences (Davies and Sharp, 1983). The following protocol is suggested: —

Dogs with their first episode of pain, with or without paresis, may be treated conservatively, with strict cage confinement. Should this prove unsuccessful or if recurrence occurs, then fenestration should be performed (Denny, 1978).

Paraplegic dogs ideally require rapid surgical intervention, preferably hemilaminectomy, with fenestration alone an alternative (Wheeler, 1989a).

Dogs where deep pain sensation is absent carry a guarded prognosis and surgery, if contemplated, must be decompressive and be carried out within 48 hours of the onset of signs. Decompression within this time significantly improves the prognosis for these dogs.

If urinary retention and overflow is present the bladder must be carefully managed; see Chapter 12.

If conservative treatment is selected it must be undertaken with a positive attitude. Cage rest is the mainstay, preferably under veterinary supervision and corticosteroids should be administered only in the earliest stages. The patient must be kept rested for at least two weeks and under no circumstances may a return to activity be allowed as soon as pain subsides or limb function returns. The worst possible course of action in these cases is to treat dogs showing back pain with anti-inflammatory drugs and then immediately allow free activity. This frequently results in an initial improvement with consequent increase in activity but is often followed by a rapid, severe worsening of the condition with permanent loss of function.

Table 10.3
Some conditions causing hind limb neurological deficits
based on presence of pain and time course of the condition

	ACUTE	SUBACUTE	CHRONIC
Pain only or predominant sign	Disc protrusion Fracture/Dislocation	Meningoencephalitis Discospondylitis Disc protrusion	Hypervitaminosis A Lumbosacral spondylopathy
	Inflammatory diseases	Inflammatory diseases Neoplasia Progressive myelomalacia	Discospondylitis Neoplasia Toxoplasmosis Canine distemper Feline infectious peritonitis Syringomyelia Vertebral abnormalities
	Aortic embolisation		
Neurological deficit predominant or only sign	Ischaemic myelopathy	Myelitis Toxoplasmosis	Degenerative myelopathy Central/peripheral neuropathies

One unfortunate sequel to a small number of cases is the development of **progressive myelomalacia**. It occurs in approximately 2% of dogs which become paraplegic (Davies and Sharp, 1983) and an anterior and posterior progression of the spinal cord disease develops (Griffiths, 1972). This leads to a loss of local reflexes, respiratory depression, general lethargy (in marked contrast to most paralysed disc cases) and distress. Clinical signs are usually evident within a week of the paraplegic episode and death rapidly ensues. The importance of this syndrome is in its recognition which will allow euthanasia at an early stage. The signs may not be evident until after decompression has been carried out where an aggressive surgical policy is followed, though this possibility is not a contraindication to such treatment as the condition has a low prevalence.

Paraplegia due to **acute disc extrusions** may occur in medium sized or larger dogs of any age where there is no evidence of disc degeneration and no previous episodes of pain. There may be a history of trauma though this is not always true; some dogs are found to have suffered an extrusion overnight. There is usually a severe neurological deficit, most cases being paraplegic without deep pain sensation. Radiography confirms the diagnosis. Treatment is as for paraplegic cases described above with decompressive surgery reserved for those cases where there is myelographic evidence of a persistent compressive lesion. Often the spinal injury is a result of the dynamic effects of the disc extrusion with no persistent compression and here conservative treatment is indicated.

Chronic disc disease in the non-chondrodystrophic breeds affects middle aged or older dogs of the larger breeds. They usually present with a slow progression of hind limb ataxia and paresis, for which the differential diagnosis is degenerative myelopathy or neoplasia. Radiography and myelography confirm the diagnosis. The condition results from a Hansen Type II disc protrusion which causes a slowly progressive cord compression. Treatment with anti-inflammatory drugs may be successful. Surgical intervention is unlikely to lead to improvement due to the longstanding nature of the spinal cord disease and may at best only prevent further deterioration. On occasion affected dogs seem to be suffering from a degenerative myelopathy in addition to the disc protrusion which may account for the poor response to surgery in some cases.

Cats also suffer from disc protrusions though it is uncommon to see clinical signs associated with them. There are a small number of reported cases but other conditions, such as **neoplasia** or **aortic thrombo-embolism** are more prevalent causes of paraplegia in this species (Chapter 15).

JUVENILES

As in the cervical spine, the presentation of a young animal with signs of thoracolumbar spinal disease warrants special consideration. Disc disease very rarely occurs in dogs less than one year of age. Some of the **central/peripheral neuropathies** will initially show hind limb signs, for example, **progressive axonopathy** in boxers. **Congenital abnormalities** of the spine should be considered, particularly vertebral body defects or the various dorsal arch defects such as **spina bifida**. Other signs of the defect may give a clue to the diagnosis, such as the presence of a dermoid sinus or a palpable abnormality of the dorsal spines and radiography should identify the lesion.

ADULTS

(Some of the conditions described occur regardless of the age of the animal.)

Traumatic lesions

Trauma may lead to **fractures** or **dislocations** of the spinal column, with those occurring as far caudally as L_5 (L_6 in cats) involving the spinal cord itself and those more caudal involving the cauda equina. Spinal cord injury due to cord concussion following trauma can occur in the absence of bony damage. The neurological assessment of the case is of paramount importance as radiographs taken after the injury only show the changes present at the time of examination and do not always accurately reflect the degree of spinal cord damage. The possibility of damage to other body systems must be considered in animals which have been involved in a road accident.

The treatment of spinal injuries is a matter of some controversy and once again the available surgical expertise has some bearing on the decision. Surgery should be performed only if it is likely to improve the prognosis or make the animal more comfortable. Decompressive surgery is indicated if there is persistent cord compression by bone fragments or other foreign bodies and it does allow direct inspection of the spinal cord. The disadvantage of such surgery lies in the tendency of some procedures to increase instability and the absence of any benefit in relieving non-compressive cord injury. Spinal stabilisation should be carried out in selected cases particularly where there is instability at the fracture site, where the vertebral body is compressed or where the spinal canal has been explored surgically. Recent studies suggest that vertebral body plating is biomechanically the most efficient method of fixation in many fractures (Walker *et al,* 1986) although carefully applied external body casts also may be valuable. The use of bone screws or pins and methyl methacrylate cement is probably the most useful and readily performed method of internal fixation. Screws or pins are driven into the vertebral bodies and the protruding portions fixed in a mass of bone cement (Figure 10.10). The management of the spinal fracture case can be challenging and treatment must aim to relieve pain and preserve or enhance neurological function.

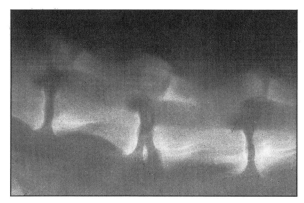 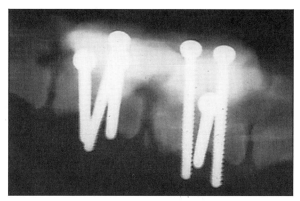

Figure 10.10
Radiographs demonstrating lumbar spinal fracture/luxation and subsequent repair
with bone screws and methyl methacrylate bone cement.

A number of the conditions described above are capable of causing a picture of acute paraplegia. **Ischaemic myelopathy** may occur in the thoracolumbar or, more frequently, the lumbosacral cord. A sudden onset of asymmetric signs in the absence of pain should indicate this possibility. **Aortic thrombo-embolism** in cats is a significant cause of such signs; see Chapter 15.

A more chronic picture of hind limb dysfunction is seen in a number of conditions. **Neoplasia** and **discospondylitis** are both possibilities, the features of which are described above. Also, both conditions occasionally can lead to a relatively acute presentation and always should be considered in such circumstances.

Degenerative disorders

Degenerative myelopathy is the most common cause of progressive hind limb dysfunction in older German shepherd dogs and is seen in some other breeds. Typically, there is a chronic progression of ataxia, paresis and proprioceptive loss. Crossing of the limbs and dragging of claws are frequent signs. Many cases are asymmetrical and sometimes there is patellar areflexia but visceral dysfunction is not a feature and pain sensation remains intact. The aetiology is unclear but degeneration is present in the dorsolateral funiculi of the white matter of the spinal cord and in the dorsal spinal roots. The diagnosis is based on the clinical signs and the elimination by myelography of the presence of any space occupying lesion. The course of the condition, whilst being progressive, is extremely variable and thus the time scale of the deterioration is difficult to predict. Medical treatment appears to have little effect on the outcome of cases (Griffiths and Duncan, 1975).

Lumbo-sacral spondylopathy is the term used to describe a number of pathological changes which occur at the lumbo-sacral (L/S) joint. Large breed dogs are most frequently affected, particularly those which work, such as police, shooting or trials dogs. Occasionally smaller dogs or, rarely, cats are involved.

The clinical signs referable to L/S lesions form a quite distinct clinical picture of low back pain which is relatively easily differentiated from the type of pain seen in thoracolumbar lesions. Affected dogs become less keen to exercise, are reluctant to jump and sometimes resist taking up a sitting position. Low grade pain or hyperaesthesia may be present over the L/S joint which may lead to signs of self mutilation. Lameness of one hind limb may be present and care must be taken to eliminate the more common orthopaedic causes of such signs. Severly affected cases may have great difficulty walking, be reluctant to stand or have marked paresis of the limbs. Signs of LMN deficits may also be present, particularly atrophy of the muscles of sciatic innervation and poor hock flexion. Signs of visceral dysfunction also may exist, particularly a dribbling urinary incontinence.

The aetiology of the syndrome is complex. There is often an underlying spinal stenosis, particularly in the German shepherd dog. Hansen type II disc protrusions compress the cauda equina, spondylosis deformans may impinge on the nerve roots and discospondylitis may be seen at this site (Tarvin and Prata, 1980; Denny, 1982). The diagnosis is based on the clinical signs and confirmed radiographically. Degenerative spinal disorders are a frequent finding at this site in middle aged, large dogs and the radiographic signs must be interpreted with care. Myelography and the use of flexed and extended views are particularly helpful (Lange, 1989). Some of the radiographic findings are demonstrated in Figure 10.11. Electrophysiological testing may be informative. Treatment of these cases is usually surgical as medical methods often provide only transient improvement at best. Most are treated by dorsal laminectomy and foramenotomy if the nerve roots are compressed (Denny, 1982). Many cases of discospondylitis respond to antibiotic therapy though some lesions at the L/S joint seem particularly intractable and curettage of the disc space may be achieved via a trans-abdominal approach. Generally the prognosis for these cases is favourable.

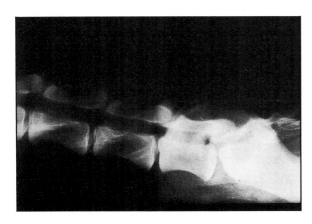 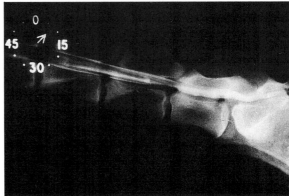

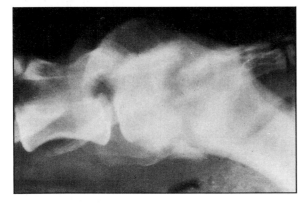

Figure 10.11 a (above left)
Figure 10.11 b (above)
Figure 10.11 c (left)
Radiographic signs in lumbosacral spondylopathy.

a. lateral radiograph demonstrating stenosis;
b. myelogram demonstrating displacement of cauda equina;
c. lumbosacral discospondylitis.

Other conditions which may cause the signs described have been covered earlier in this chapter. In addition, some of the disorders covered in Chapter 15 should be considered in cats. The majority of spinal diseases can be diagnosed by clinical examination and the use of regularly employed diagnostic aids, particularly radiography. Also, many are amenable to therapy and the application of appropriate treatment will enhance the prognosis.

REFERENCES

BJORCK, G., DYRENDAHL, S. and OLSEN, S. E. (1957). Hereditary ataxia in smooth haired fox terriers. *Veterinary Record,* **69**, 871.

BRAUND, K. G. (1980) Encephalitis and Meningitis. *Veterinary Clinics of North America,* **10 (1)**, 31.

BRAUND, K. G. (1985) Granulomatous meningoencephalitis. *Journal of the American Veterinary Medical Association,* **186,** 160.

CARMICHAEL, S., GRIFFITHS, I. R. and HARVEY, M. J. A. (1983). Familial cerebellar ataxia with hydrocephalus in bull mastiffs. *Veterinary Record,* **112,** 354.

DAVIES, J. V. and SHARP, N. J. H. (1983). A comparison of conservative treatment and fenestration for thoraco-lumbar disc disease in the dog. *Journal of Small Animal Practice,* **24,** 721.

DENNY, H. R. (1978). The surgical treatment of cervical disc protrusions in the dog; a review of 40 cases. *Journal of Small Animal Practice* **19,** 251.

DENNY, H. R. (1978). The lateral fenestration of canine thoracolumbar disc protrusions. *Journal of Small Animal Practice* **19,** 259.

DENNY, H. R., GIBBS, C. and GASKELL, C. J. (1977). Cervical spondylopathy in the dog; a review of 35 cases. *Journal of Small Animal Practice* **18,** 117.

DENNY, H. R., GIBBS, C. and HOLT, P. E. (1982). The diagnosis and treatment of cauda equina lesions in the dog. *Journal of Small Animal Practice* **23,** 425.

DENNY, H. R., GIBBS, C. and WATERMAN, A. (1988). Atlanto-axial subluxation in the dog; a review of 30 cases and an evaluation of treatment by lag screw fixation. *Journal of Small Animal Practice* **29,** 37.

FINGEROTH, J. M., PRATA, R. G. and PATNAIK, A. K. (1987). Spinal meningiomas in dogs. *Journal of the American Veterinary Medical Association,* **191,** 720.

GEARY, J. C., OLIVER, J. E. and HOERLEIN, B. F. (1967). Atlanto-axial subluxation in the canine. *Journal of Small Animal Practice,* **8,** 577.

GORMAN, N. T., Ed. (1986). *Oncology.* Churchill Livingstone, London.

GRIFFITHS, I. R. (1972). The extensive myelopathy of intervertebral disc protrusion in dogs ('the ascending syndrome'). *Journal of Small Animal Practice,* **13,** 425.

GRIFFITHS, I. R. (1986). Inherited neuropathies in dogs. *Veterinary Annual,* **26,** 28.

GRIFFITHS, I. R. (1973). Spinal cord infarction due to emboli arising from the intervertebral discs in the dog. *Journal of Comparative Pathology* **83,** 225.

GRIFFITHS, I. R. and DUNCAN, I. D. (1975). Chronic degenerative radiculomyelopathy in the dog. *Journal of Small Animal Practice* **16,** 461.

HARTLEY, W. J. and PALMER, A. C. (1973). Ataxia in Jack Russell terriers. *Acta Neuropathologica* **26,** 71.

KORNEGAY, J. N. (1983). Discospondylitis. In *Current Veterinary Therapy,* VIII, (Ed. R. W. Kirk) W. B. Saunders Co., Philadelphia.

LANG, J. (1989). Flexion-extension myelography of the canine cauda equina. *Veterinary Radiology* **29,** 242.

LUTTGEN, P. J., BRAUND, K. G., BRAUNER, W. R. and VANDEVELDE, M. (1980). A retrospective study of 29 spinal tumours in the dog and cat. *Journal of Small Animal Practice,* **21,** 213.

MASON, T. A. (1979). Cervical vertebral instability (Wobbler syndrome) in the dog. *Veterinary Record,* **104,** 142.

PRATA, R. G. (1977). Diagnosis of spinal cord tumours in the dog. *Veterinary Clinics of North America,* **7 (1),** 165.

PRATA, R. G. (1981). Neurosurgical treatment of thoraco-lumbar discs; the rationale and value of laminectomy with concomitant disc removal. *Journal of the American Animal Hospital Association,* **17,** 17.

READ, R. A., ROBINS, G. M. and CARLISLE, C. H. (1983). Caudal cervical spondylomyelopathy (Wobbler syndrome) in the dog: a review of 35 cases. *Journal of Small Animal Practice,* **24,** 605.

SEIM, H. B. and WITHROW, S. J. (1982). Pathophysiology and diagnosis of caudal cervical spondylomyelopathy with emphasis on the Doberman Pinscher. *Journal of the American Animal Hospital Association,* **18,** 117.

TARVIN, G. and PRATA, R. G. (1980). Lumbosacral stenosis in dogs. *Journal of the American Veterinary Medical Association* **177**, 154.

WALKER, M. C., SMITH, K. G. and NEWTON, C. D. (1986). Canine lumbar spinal internal fixation techniques. *Veterinary Surgery,* **15**, 191.

WHEELER, S. J. (1986). Surgical conditions of the canine spine. *British Veterinary Journal,* **142**, 95.

WHEELER, S. J. (1987). Cervical disc surgery. *In Practice,* **9 (3)**, 105.

WHEELER, S. J. (1989a). Thoracolumbar disc surgery. *In Practice,* **10 (6)**, 231.

WHEELER, S. J. (1989b). Spinal tumours in cats. *Veterinary Annual,* **29**, 270.

WRIGHT, J. A., BELL, D. A. and CLAYTON JONES, D. G. (1979). The clinical and radiological features associated with spinal tumours in 30 dogs. *Journal of Small Animal Practice,* **20**, 461.

ZAKI, F. A. and PRATA, R. G. (1976). Necrotising myelopathy secondary to embolisation of herniated intervertebral disc material in the dog. *Journal of the American Veterinary Association,* **169**, 222.

CHAPTER 11

NEUROLOGICAL DEFICITS IN ONE LIMB

Nicholas J. H. Sharp, B.Vet.Med., M.V.M., M.R.C.V.S., Dip.A.C.V.S.

In a number of conditions the major presenting sign may be a neurological deficit to one limb. If this is a deficit resulting in weakness of the limb, then the correct term is *monoparesis*. If the motor deficit is complete and the animal is unable to move the limb at all then the correct term is *monoplegia*.

The term *mononeuropathy* refers to a condition affecting one specific peripheral nerve. A severe mononeuropathy of the sciatic nerve will, of course, result in an obvious monoparesis of the affected hind limb. However, that limb is not totally paralysed or monoplegic as, by definition, the other peripheral nerves to that limb are functional and the animal can still move the limb.

FORELIMB

ANATOMY OF THE BRACHIAL PLEXUS

Detailed descriptions are available in standard veterinary anatomy and neurology texts. However, a working knowledge of the anatomy of this area does not require great detail, yet will considerably aid diagnosis. The brachial plexus is derived from cord segments C_6 to T_1 and less frequently C_5 and/or T_2 also make a contribution. We may remember the order in which the main peripheral nerve arise from the plexus as:

Suprascalpular	Musculocutaneous	Radial	Median/Ulnar
$C_{6(7)}$	$C_{7(6,8)}$	$C_7, C_8, T_1, (T_2)$	$C_8, T_1, (T_2)$

It can be seen that the nerve located on the most cranial part of the plexus is derived from the most cranial nerve root, and so on (see Figure 11.1).

The area of mixing of the contributing spinal nerves and the arising peripheral nerves is called the *common brachial plexus bundle.* To consider the main nerves of the plexus individually.

Suprascapular nerve — supplies motor fibres to the spinatus muscles on the lateral aspect of the scapula which provide lateral support to the shoulder joint.

Musculocutaneous nerve — supplies motor fibres to the muscles that flex the elbow (e.g., biceps brachii). It supplies sensation to the medial forearm ending at the first digit (dew claw). It also sends a sensory anastomotic branch to the median nerve.

Radial nerve — is the most important nerve of the forelimb. It innervates the extensor muscles of the triceps group which fix the elbow, the muscles that extend the carpus, and the digital extensor muscles. It is sensory to the whole cranial aspect of the forearm and foot except the fifth digit.

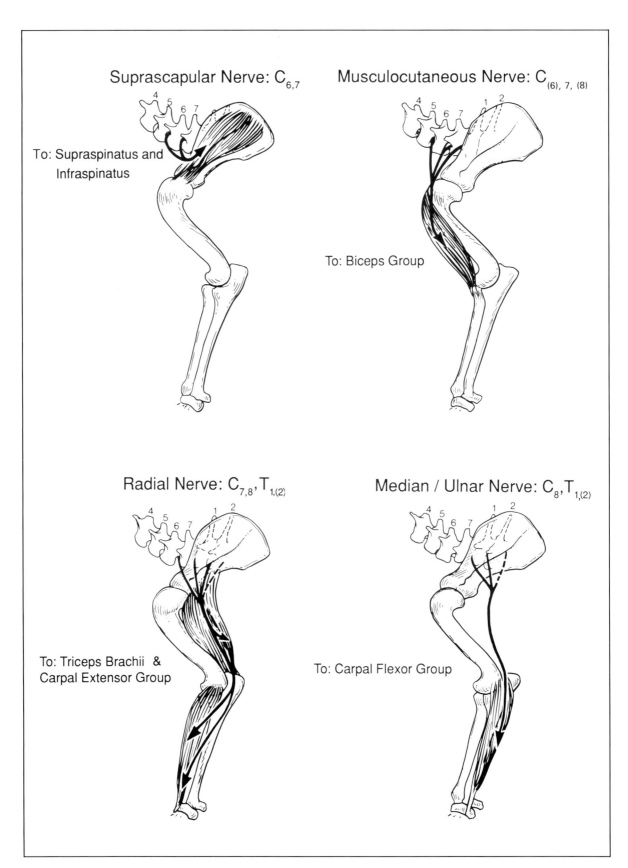

Figure 11.1
Main peripheral nerves arising from the brachial plexus

Median/Ulnar nerve — together innervate the muscles that flex the carpus and digits. The ulnar nerve supplies sensation to the caudal aspect of the forearm and foot. Sensation to the caudal aspects of the first, second and part of the third digit is shared with the median nerve.

Again, the tendancy for the most cranially located nerve to innervate the most cranial muscle mass, etc., can be seen.

The other peripheral nerves arising from the brachial plexus, such as the axillary and subscapular, are obviously important, but need not be considered clinically in the evaluation of plexal dysfunction.

Two other important components to the anatomy of the brachial plexus are the lateral thoracic and sympathetic nerves. Both arise from the caudal portion of the plexus and the relevance of this will become apparent in the section on neurological examination.

Lateral thoracic nerve — arises from C_8 and T_1 cord segments and innervates the cutaneous trunci muscle. It is responsible for the motor portion of the panniculus reflex on the ipsilateral side of the body.

Sympathetic nerves — provide the sympathetic supply to the head and neck, leaving the spinal cord through the rami communicantes of T_1 and T_2 spinal nerves. These enter the stellate ganglion near the first rib and then send fibres to pass along the sympathetic portion of the vagosympathetic trunk. They therefore supply the smooth muscles of the iris and third eyelid, causing mydriasis and retraction respectively.

NEUROLOGICAL EXAMINATION

Assessment of lower motor neurone disease of the forelimb is best considered under the four following syndromes:

> Dysfunction of the cranial brachial plexus
> Dysfunction of the caudal brachial plexus
> Dysfunction of the complete brachial plexus
> Dysfunction of the radial nerve alone

Cranial brachial plexus

Dysfunction in this location results in denervation over the suprascapular and musculocutaneous peripheral nerve fields. It is usually caused by an avulsion of the roots of the cranial brachial plexus or, by a tumour occupying the C_6 or C_7 nerve roots or the cranial portion of the common plexus bundle.

Clinically the animal will have weak shoulder extension and this joint may be easily subluxated both laterally or medially. More readily assessed will be poor or absent elbow flexion, evaluated either by attempting a forelimb placing response or by asking the dog to 'shake hands'. Occasional weakness may be detected over the radial nerve field. Sensation in the limb distal to the elbow joint is intact except, perhaps, for a small area on the medial antebrachium.

Caudal brachial plexus

Dysfunction here results in denervation over the radial, median and ulnar peripheral nerve fields. It is usually caused by an avulsion of the roots of the caudal brachial plexus, or by a tumour occupying the $C_{7,8}$ or T_1 nerve roots or the caudal portion of the common plexus bundle.

Clinically the animal will show a marked forelimb proprioceptive deficit, 'dropped' elbow and carpus and an inability to bear weight on the limb, which will knuckle over onto the dorsum of the foot.

Sensation to the limb distal to the elbow may be absent except for a small area on the medial aspect of the forearm. The panniculus reflex may also be absent and the animal may demonstrate a partial Horner's syndrome.

Complete brachial plexus

Dysfunction of the entire plexus causes a combination of the previous two syndromes with resultant paralysis over all peripheral nerve fields. A large neoplasm or complete avulsion of all nerve roots to the brachial plexus are the main causes of this syndrome.

The animal is unable to flex the elbow joint or bear any weight on the limb. Analgesia, if present, is usually complete distal to the elbow joint and also extends for a variable distance proximal to this level. A loss of the ipsilateral panniculus reflex and/or a partial Horner's syndrome will usually be seen.

Radial Nerve

Inability to fix the elbow and carpal joints, a 'dropped' elbow and knuckled over foot will result from this injury along with selective sensory denervation to the cranial forearm. Horner's syndrome and loss of the panniculus reflex **do not** occur. If the lesion is distal to the triceps muscle innervation, then elbow extension will be preserved.

Two very important components of the neurological examination in forelimb monoparesis/plegia are:

Panniculus reflex — this reflex is best considered as two identical reflexes, one for each side of the body. The sensory component of the reflex has a dermatomal input over one side of the trunk. The motor component arises from the ipsilateral cord segments C_8 and T_1 (lateral thoracic nucleus) and innervates the ipsilateral cutaneous trunci muscle via the lateral thoracic nerve. A spinal cord lesion or avulsion of the nerve roots at C_8 and T_1 on one side will therefore abolish the ipsilateral panniculus reflex. Provided that the contralateral C_8 and T_1 cord segments are intact, a strong consensual response will be obtained on stimulation of the flank on the original side. This is because ascending sensory stimuli can cross over to the contralateral spinal cord below the level of the lesion (Chapter 3).

Horner's Syndrome — Complete Horner's syndrome comprises miosis, enophthalmus, ptosis and prolapse of the third eyelid and can therefore be easily recognised. Lesions solely affecting T_1 and T_2 nerve roots nearly always result in a partial Horner's syndrome where only the miotic pupil occurs. This can easily be missed, particularly in animals with a dark iris, unless assessed from a distance of two feet or so from the animal's face using a bright ophthalmoscope. The reflection from the tapetal fundus, as seen from car headlights at night, will clearly delineate the pupillary apertures and allow camparison of the two diameters. Even mild yet significant unilateral miosis can be detected in this manner (Chapter 9).

LESION LOCALISATION

The degree of involvement of the ipsilateral hindlimb or the contralateral limbs should be assessed to differentiate UMN from LMN disease (see Chapter 3.).

The animal should be assessed for evidence of Horner's syndrome, panniculus loss or involvement of more than one peripheral nerve in order to differentiate a lesion affecting the plexus from one involving only the peripheral nerve(s).

From the neurological examination it should be possible to categorise the deficit and thus localise the lesion to one of the following areas:

A. $C_1 - C_5$ spinal cord — UMN signs, other limb(s) involved

B. $C_6 - T_2$ spinal cord — LMN signs, other limb(s) involved

C. $C_6 - T_2$ nerve roots/the brachial plexus — unilateral LMN signs,
   $\pm$ Horner's syndrome or panniculus loss

D. Radial nerve — unilateral LMN signs, no Horner's syndrome or panniculus loss

A. UMN: C_{1-5} cord segments

Lesions at this level are unlikely to cause unilateral forelimb signs without involvement of the ipsilateral hindlimb, and frequently deficits are also apparent on the contralateral side of the body.

Occasionally, intervertebral disease at $C_{2,3}$, $C_{3,4}$, or $C_{4,5}$ can cause predominantly a monoparesis of one forelimb. This may also be the presenting feature of infarcts or spinal cord tumours in this region and has been recorded in a dog with a fracture of C_2 vertebral body.

B. LMN: $C_6 - T_2$ cord segments

Cord compression in this region associated with cervical vertebral instability, disc protrusion, neoplasia or discospondylitis may cause monoparesis, but is again likely to also cause deficits in other limbs. A myelogram may be necessary to rule out a lesion at this location.

C. $C_6 - T_2$ nerve roots of brachial plexus

Conditions at this level are usually either tumour, avulsion or inflammatory in basis.

NEOPLASIA OF THE BRACHIAL PLEXUS AND ASSOCIATED NERVE ROOTS

Tumours in this region may be referred to under the general term nerve sheath tumour (NST) but have also been described as Schwannomas, neurofibromas, neurolemmomas, neuromas and neurofibromas. In man, the Schwann cell has been confirmed to be the predominant neoplastic cell in all tumour types. In the dog, it is unclear whether the Schwann cell, the perineurial fibroblast, or both, are responsible for the malignant cell line. The terms malignant Schwannoma or neurofibrosarcoma are the most applicable for use in animals. Regardless of the term, these tumours are nearly always malignant in behaviour. (Figure 11.2).

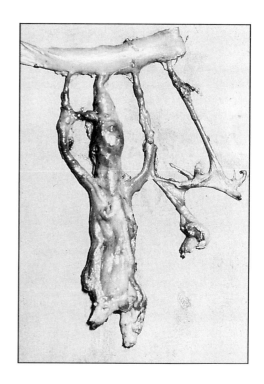

Figure 11.2
Typical appearance of a brachial plexus nerve sheath tumour in a dog
(Courtesy of Dr. S. J. Wheeler).

A proportion of tumours in this region can be of non neural origin and simply invade part of the plexus. These tend to be larger than primary neural tumours and so may be more easily detected, but by their nature carry a worse prognosis. Examples would include osteo- and chondrosarcomas (Griffiths and Carmichael, 1981).

Forty-five tumours affecting the brachial plexus have been described in the small animal literature to date, forty two in the dog and three in the cat. (The feline tumours will be considered separately.) Twenty of the forty two dogs (48%) showed gross, and/or clinical or radiographical evidence of spinal cord compression or invasion. In at least four of these cases the tumour appeared to arise primarily in a dorsal nerve root and therefore be situated predominantly or completely within the spinal canal. The rest appeared to arise peripherally and only invade the spinal cord as a terminal event. This situation is the reverse of that occurring in the lumbosacral plexus where the majority of tumours appear to arise within the spinal canal (Bradley et al, 1982).

The mean age at presentation for the forty two dogs was 7.4 years, with a median of 7 years and a range of 2.5 — 13 years. Approximately three quarters of the dogs were of medium or large breed. All initially demonstrated a foreleg lameness or paresis, which in some dogs progressed to involve one or more of the remaining limbs. Classically each dog had shown a chronic intractable forelimb lameness for 6 — 8 months prior to presentation (Wheeler et al, 1986).

Clinical Features

It can be seen from Table 11.1, that marked muscle atrophy of the involved limb is the most useful diagnostic feature together with the history of chronic lameness or paresis of one forelimb. The spinatus muscle group over the scapula seems to be the most frequently involved and the neurogenic nature of the atrophy is confirmed by electromyography to be due to denervation. Most animals show evidence of a lower motor neuron deficit but one quarter of recorded cases only showed lameness and demonstrated no neurological deficit in the affected limb.

Other useful features are the presence of a palpable mass in the axilla in the conscious or anaesthetised animal. This may be small, firm and cord-like in the case of a mass within the nerve bundle, or large in tumours of non-neural origin which involve nerve by direct infiltration or compression of the plexus. In some animals, no mass is palpable but hyperaesthesia is usually evident on palpation of the axilla. This can cause a marked aggressive response or even a detectable reaction in the anaesthetised animal. In some dogs this hyperaesthesia is hard to localise clinically and may suggest a cervical or thoracolumbar lesion.

Ipsilateral loss of the panniculus response and partial or complete Horner's syndrome may also be present. Complete Horner's syndrome would suggest invasion of the stellate ganglion in addition to T_1 and T_2 nerve roots.

Table 11.1
Clinical features of brachial plexus tumours

Feature	Percentage
Limb muscle atrophy	88
Axillary mass	69
Axillary hyperaesthesia	60
Panniculus loss	54
Horner's syndrome	29

Radiography

Plain radiography was unrewarding in most cases documented although oblique views of the spine may reveal enlargement of an affected intervertebral foramen. Myelography revealed a higher incidence of spinal cord involvement than was apparent from the neurological examination. In one series, only half of the affected dogs with positive myelographic findings showed hindleg neurological defects. This would suggest that myelography be performed in all cases if the full extent of the tumour is to be appreciated.

The classic appearance of a nerve root tumour that has extended to an intradural location is of an intradural extramedullary lesion, see Chapter 5. Chest metastasis is rare but thoracic radiographs should always be taken.

Treatment

In dogs with spinal cord involvement, a dorsal laminectomy is recommended to both confirm the diagnosis and to determine if removal is possible. Nerve sheath tumours are usually slow growing and sometimes even large lesions may only cause compression yet not have invaded the spinal cord. In such cases removal is worthwhile and may result in long term remission (Alexander et al, 1974; Braund et al, 1979). If the peripheral extent of the mass within the associated spinal nerve is not visible at laminectomy, successful removal of the intradural mass should be followed by exploration of the spinal nerves and brachial plexus, usually via a separate approach.

Two surgical approaches to the canine brachial plexus have been described. The craniomedial approach through the axilla gives very good exposure of the common brachial plexus bundle and more peripheral portions of the musculocutaneous, radial, median and ulnar nerves (Knecht and Green, 1977). The craniolateral approach gives very good exposure to the more proximal portion of the common plexus bundle and the ventral branches of the spinal nerves $C_6 - T_1$ (Sharp, 1988). It also allows the more proximal portions of these spinal nerves to be exposed. In that most tumours involve both the spinal nerves and plexus, a craniolateral approach is preferred initially. It only requires transection of the thin omotransversius muscle and if exposure to the more distal plexus is required, this approach can easily be combined with the craniomedial dissection. (Figure 11.3).

The craniolateral approach is undertaken with the dog placed in lateral recumbency and a curved skin incision is made over the cranial border of the scapula. The proximal communicating branch of the cephalic vein should be divided between ligatures. The omotransversius muscle is transected over the cranial border of the scapula. The dissection is then continued ventrally through the deep fascia, along the dorsolateral border of the cleidobrachialis muscle. The omotransversius muscle is retracted cranially, the cleidobrachialis muscle is retracted cranioventrally and the scapula is elevated to provide craniodorsal exposure of the axilla. The brachial plexus is exposed by careful separation from the surrounding loose subscapular fat and fascia. The ventral branches of the seventh and eighth cervical and the first thoracic nerves can be exposed by section of the superficial and deep portions of the scalenus muscle, just cranial to the first rib. Care must be taken at this stage to avoid damage to the vessels and nerves of the thoracic inlet. Following exploration, fascicular nerve biopsy can be performed (Braund et al, 1979) or the procedure continued as a forequarter amputation (Harvey, 1974).

Careful exploration and gentle palpation of the plexus should cause no long term problems and is preferable to delaying surgery until therapy is impossible. Normal peripheral nervous tissue is white and feels soft when gently palpated. Nerve sheath tumours are often discoloured off white or grey, but the most useful criterion is that they are much firmer than normal nerve tissue, which is usually apparent even if the affected nerve trunk is not yet enlarged.

Grossly involved tissue is normally non functional so may be biopsied with little ill effect. Less obvious cases should undergo careful fascicular biopsy. Following exploration and biopsy, the neurological deficit may be more pronounced (Chapter 4).

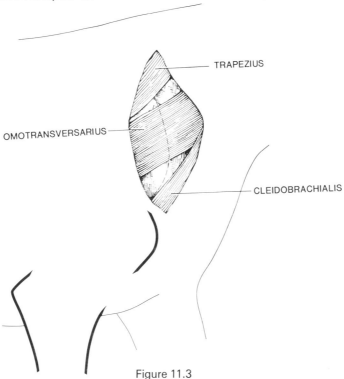

Figure 11.3
Craniolateral approach to the canine brachial plexus, showing sites of skin incision and section of the omotransversarius muscle at the cranial border of the scapula
(From *Veterinary Surgery* **17**, 18, reproduced by permission).

It is preferable at the time of diagnosis of plexal neoplasia to amputate the forequarter and remove spinal nerves $C_6 - T_1$ as far proximal as is feasible. This is suggested because these neoplasms have very diffuse and ill-defined borders and are very prone to recurrence. To give the dog the best chance of long term remission or cure, a radical approach is the best course of action. Local resection of the neoplastic portions of the plexus will usually leave the animal with a severe neurological deficit and also has a strong tendency towards early recurrence. The suitability of the candidate for forequarter amputation should be considered with respect to arthritis in the hindlimbs or contralateral forelimb. The procedure of dorsal laminectomy followed by forequarter amputation has been performed successfully to date in two large breed dogs, with the animals requiring approximately one week of adjustment in each case. If doubt remains regarding the diagnosis at initial exploration, amputation should await histopathological confirmation of the diagnosis. Amputation should not be performed if the proximal extent of the tumour cannot be defined.

Prognosis

It has been suggested that nerve sheath tumours are usually benign. Although evidence of chest metastases were documented in only one of twenty-two cases (4.6%) and local or distant metastasis in eight of twenty-eight cases (29%) coming to post mortem, these tumours are very locally invasive in nature. They are difficult to remove completely, particularly as the exact extent of the neoplasm may be very difficult to discern on gross examination of the nerves. This is supported by the high number of cases destroyed due to the extensive nature of the mass at exploration and by the high recurrence rate following attempted removal. Six of eight cases recorded in the literature where treatment was attempted have had early recurrence of disease, with only two dogs possibly disease free at two and ten months respectively and an additional one destroyed at 14 months due to recurrence (Troy et al, 1979; Bradley et al, 1982).

Therefore a high index of suspicion should be observed in a middle aged or older dog with chronic intractable forelimb lameness and poorly localisable pain, particularly if any neurological deficit is present. Rapid institution of diagnostic procedures such as electromyography and myelography will be needed for diagnosis with early exploratory surgery to be employed as a further diagnostic tool. Once confirmed, amputation with removal of all involved spinal nerves at as proximal a level as possible offers the best long term prognosis. Nerve sheath tumours do not appear to be particularly radiosensitive. The prognosis for non neural tumours is generally poor as most are sarcomas with high invasive and metastatic potential.

Feline brachial plexus tumours

Only three such cases have been recorded, one due to a chondrosarcoma, one lymphosarcoma, and one due to reticulosis (Shell and Sponenberg, 1987). These carry an even worse prognosis than in the dog due to their high potential for involvement of other body regions, which occurred in each of these three cats. The clinical features were similar to those in the dog although two of three cases showed Horner's syndrome. Two cats were two years of age and one was five.

BRACHIAL PLEXUS NEURITIS

This condition in man, although uncommon, is well recognised, but only two cases have been documented in the dog (Alexander et al, 1974). Although both dogs showed bilateral involvement, 71% of 136 human cases in one series were unilateral. The aetiology is not known but in man some cases follow administration of vaccines, sera or other foreign proteins and the neuropathy is preceded by malaise, vomiting and urticaria. One dog demonstrated these signs and the cause was confirmed to be a horse meat diet; in the second the cause was not found and there was no preceding illness. Weakness and atrophy predominantly affects the shoulder muscles but all limb muscles may be involved. The prognosis is good in man but full recovery usually takes months or even years. One dog could not walk and was destroyed, the second remained ambulatory but showed only minimal improvement over four months. Other cases have been seen in the dog and have shown considerable variation in severity. (Figure 11.4).

VASCULAR LESIONS

A unilateral partial ischaemia to one forelimb has been described in a dog following a road traffic accident (McCoy and Trotter, 1977). Immediately following the accident, the dog could use the leg but paralysis developed within a further eight hours. The triceps muscles were firm and swollen and the pulse at the brachial artery was absent. Necrosis and thrombosis of the intrathoracic subclavian artery were diagnosed and surgically corrected. Limb use returned but was compromised by ischaemic contracture of the triceps muscle causing severe fixation of the elbow joint.

AVULSION OF THE NERVE ROOTS OF THE BRACHIAL PLEXUS

This is by far the most common forelimb nerve injury encountered in small animals (Griffiths *et al*, 1974). It is frequently referred to simply as brachial plexus avulsion. Avulsion of the nerve roots is a preferable term because the injury is nearly always immediately at the origin of the nerve roots from the spinal cord and not at a more peripheral portion of the plexus such as the common plexus bundle. The reason for the predisposition of the more proximal site is because as the traction injury is transmitted up the limb it affects firstly the peripheral nerves, then the common plexus bundle, then the ventral branches of the spinal nerves and finally the dorsal and ventral nerve roots which attach to the spinal cord. The nerve roots are the weakest of these structures as they lack a well defined perineurium, which is one of the three main connective tissue components of peripheral nervous tissue. Therefore, the traction injury, if severe enough, causes rupture at the site where the roots originate from the spinal cord. Furthermore, the ventral roots appear more susceptible to rupture than the dorsal roots (Griffiths, 1974).

The traction injury is the result of severe trauma. In dogs and cats this usually occurs during a road traffic accident (RTA) or occasionally when an animal is hung by the foot in a fence. In man, most cases are the result of an automobile injury but mild dysfunction can result from such unusual causes as rucksack paralysis and pallbearer's palsy!

As the presence of a root avulsion is usually devastating in terms of the resulting paralysis, the complication of any co-existing orthopaedics repairs, prolonged nursing care and the poor overall prognosis; every RTA should be screened for the existence of this injury. This is much easier than it would seem and will be covered below.

Although the clinical signs are variable, nearly all cases can be divided into one of the categories described earlier in the chapter.

Caudal plexal deficits — This results from injury to C_7 or $C_8 - T_2$ nerve roots and accounted for roughly one third of the cases documented in one series (Griffiths, 1977). It probably results from a cranial traction on the limb. The salient features are an inability to bear weight on the limb which is usually carried in a flexed position, because innervation to the biceps brachii and brachialis muscles is preserved. The animal may show loss of the ipsilateral panniculus reflex and/or a partial Horner's syndrome. Analgesia is usually only present distal to the elbow joint.

Cranial plexal deficit — Injury to C_6 and C_7 nerve roots alone is uncommon and results only in loss of shoulder movement and elbow flexion. This probably results from a caudal traction on the limb. The animal usually is able to bear weight on the limb almost normally. Panniculus reflex loss is not seen nor is Horner's syndrome present. Shoulder muscle atrophy will frequently be evident. Analgesia, if present, may affect the medial aspect of the antebrachium and the skin overlying the dorsocranial border of the scapula. Hemiplegia of the diaphragm (phrenic nerve, C_5) may also be demonstrable using fluoroscopy.

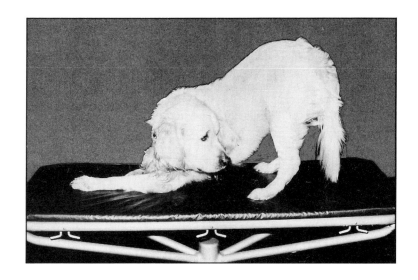

Figure 11.4
Dog with chronic bilateral
brachial plexus neuritis and
associated forelimb weakness
(Courtesy Dr. S. J. Wheeler).

Complete plexal deficit — This is the most common presentation and results from damage to nerve roots $C_6 - T_2$. It probably results from severe traction or possibly abduction of the limb. The animal is unable to bear weight on the limb or flex the elbow joint but may still be able to protract the limb by using the brachiocephalicus muscle. Ipsilateral loss of the panniculus reflex and Horner's syndrome may be seen. Analgesia is usually present both proximal and distal to the elbow joint.

Diagnosis — It would seem prudent to screen all animals that cannot obviously use their forelimb(s) following trauma for a possible avulsion injury. This can be performed very quickly by checking for evidence of anisocoria (see Chapter 9), checking the panniculus reflex on both sides of the flank and by ensuring that the animal can flex his limb in response to a painful stimulus applied to the nailbed of the fifth or preferably the fourth digit.

Further diagnostic procedures should include electrophysiological techniques if possible. Electromyographic examination performed 5—7 days after injury will confirm denervation of various muscles groups and help differentiate a pure radial nerve injury. To further quantitate the deficit, nerve conduction velocities and the amplitude of evoked muscle action potentials are useful, particularly if they can be repeated one or two months later to determine if any recovery has taken place. In particular, an inability to electrically excite the radial nerve is a poor prognostic sign. Myelography is of little value in this condition.

Prognosis — This is generally very poor for a useful recovery of function, particularly following complete avulsion. Occasional animals have been encountered with an apparent complete avulsion but which then make a full recovery within one week. Presumably, in such cases, the injury is purely neurapraxic and there is no loss of continuity of the nerve roots. In cases with caudal avulsion and preservation of some ability to bear weight on the limb, the prognosis is better. The presence of normal deep pain sensation over the limb suggests sparing of the dorsal roots which may correlate with a less severe injury to the ventral roots. In general, if no recovery has taken place within one month, useful function is unlikely to be regained subsequently. The prognosis is often quite favourable with cranial plexal avulsions because the animal can still bear weight on the limb, and the lack of analgesia to the distal limb renders excoriation of the digits unlikely.

Pathology — The lesion occurs predominantly inside the dura mata, at the junction of the spinal cord and the nerve roots. Usually there will be a complete loss of continuity in the most severely affected roots while adjacent roots may be only incompletely avulsed. In severe cases, the torn roots often end up attached as a fibrous mass to the first rib (Griffiths, 1974).

Management — This condition is, unfortunately, not amenable to any form of therapy directed at the lesion itself. The final outcome depends on the original degree of damage sustained. In animals that show no improvement over one month or in which excoriation of the digits or carpus occurs, amputation is often the best solution.

Tendon relocation is one surgical option to lessen the effects of the denervation. Two approaches are available, directed at allowing extension of the elbow and carpus respectively. The tendon of the biceps brachii muscle can be re-attached to the olecranon in an attempt to take over the function of the triceps muscle. Similarly, a carpal flexor muscle can be used to take on the role of a carpal extensor (Bennett and Vaughan, 1976). Although these techniques can work well, it is essential that the muscle to be relocated has normal function in order to take on its new role. Even a subclinical denervation in that muscle may result in a lack of adaptation and subsequent failure of the procedure. It should be remembered that the radial nerve originates from $C_7 - T_2$ nerve roots which also give rise to both the median and ulnar nerves. As the median and ulnar nerves innervate the carpal flexor muscles, these too may be partially denervated.

Carpal arthrodesis is an alternative to prevent the carpus from collapsing. One disadvantage with this procedure can be that the digits remain paralysed and so weight bearing on the digital pads is uneven and may result in excessive wear. In addition, the limb will usually remain analgesic and so cannot benefit from the normal protective reflexes.

Proper client education is essential in avulsion injuries to stress the fact that surgery is only an attempt to salvage function from a paralysed limb and that if it does not work, amputation may still prove necessary.

Complications following traumatic injuries to the brachial plexus — Long term disuse of a limb can have several severe sequelae such as contracture of joints due to muscle fibrosis or abrasion of the foot. The abrasion may become so severe as to erode portions of the digits, set up an osteomyelitis in the phalangeal bones and introduce infection into tendon sheaths, which will then further exacerbate the contractures. Trophic ulcers are the result of ulceration of denervated pads (Read, 1986). The denervated skin is less resistant to the pressure of weight bearing, has poor vascular tone, may contact the ground at an unusual angle, and cannot be protected by normal reflexes. Trophic ulcers may also occur following carpal or hock arthrodesis for the same reasons and can therefore invalidate these corrective procedures. These ulcers can be very difficult to deal with although surgical techniques are described which involve transfer of normally innervated skin into the affected area.

During the waiting period, while any reversible component to the nerve injury is recovering, strict attention to hygiene, prompt attention to wounds, protection of the foot, if possible by a leather or wire mesh boot, and physical therapy to keep joints and muscles mobile, are all crucial. This calls for a large time commitment on the part of the owner, and compliance from the animal. Therefore, strict owner and case selection is crucial. In some instances, as a long term salvage procedure, limb amputation is often the most practical course of action with severe injuries. If the animal can carry the limb in flexion, then the major complication of abrasions can be avoided. Animals with major orthopaedic injuries or severe arthritis in another limb are poor candidates for amputation and euthanasia may then be a consideration.

Paraesthesias can be an unfortunate complication during the management of any neuropathic patient. They may have a delayed onset as a result of nerve entrapment or reinnervation, and have been described in up to 15 per cent of animals with neurological deficits resulting from pelvic fractures. Similar figures are not available for brachial plexus lesions. The resultant self mutilation usually resolves over a variable period of time, usually within two to three months. Needless to say, it considerably complicates case management. It should raise the possibility of nerve exploration and neurolysis if the lesion is in an accessible area.

RADIAL NERVE

This nerve is occasionally subject to injury in small animals although well documented cases are rare (Wheeler *et al*, 1986). Fractures of the humerus or first rib are said to be responsible for the damage although many such cases in the past were unrecognised nerve root avulsion injuries, which had also sustained incidental fractures at the time of trauma. Nine per cent of humeral fractures in man have associated radial nerve palsy; similar figures are not available for dogs and cats although the incidence does not appear to be nearly as common.

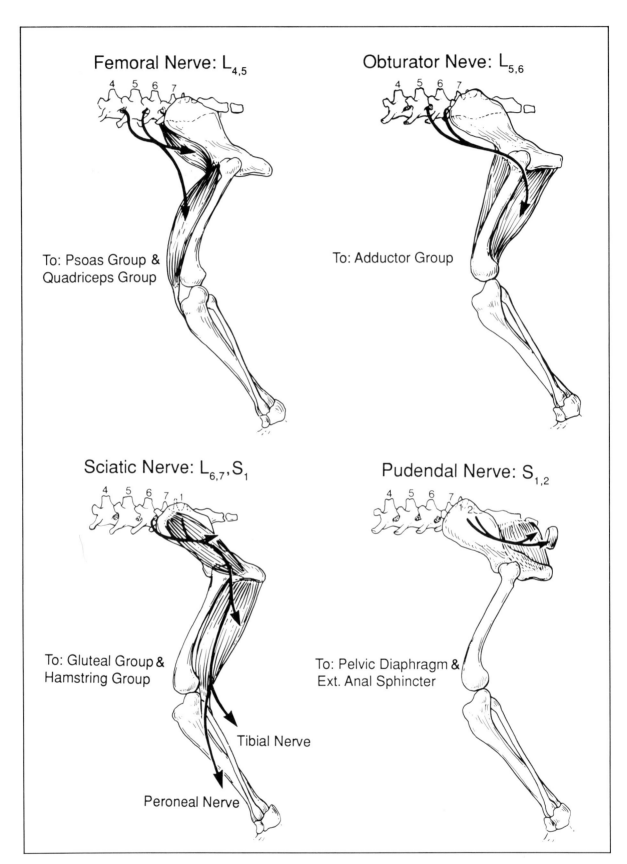

Figure 11.5
Main peripheral nerves arising from the lumbosacral plexus

190

HINDLIMB

ANATOMY OF THE LUMBOSACRAL PLEXUS

The lumbosacral plexus is derived largely from cord segments $L_4 - S_2$. If we remember the order (from cranial to caudal) in which the four main peripheral nerves to the hindlimb and pelvic region arise:-

$$\text{Femoral} \quad - \quad \text{Obturator} \quad - \quad \text{Sciatic} \quad - \quad \text{Pudendal}$$

it is logical that their approximate derivation from the plexus is as follows (see Figure 11.5):-

$$\text{Femoral} \quad - \quad \text{Obturator} \quad - \quad \text{Sciatic} \quad - \quad \text{Pudendal}$$
$$L_{4,5} \qquad\qquad L_{5,6} \qquad\qquad L_{6,7}, S_1 \qquad S_{1,2,(3)}$$

This is a reasonable estimation as there is some degree of variation from animal to animal and, in addition, each cord segment also contributes to more than one peripheral nerve.

Due to the disparity in lengths of the spinal cord and vertebral column, the last three lumbar segments reside over the 4th lumbar vertebrum and the three sacral segments lie over the 5th lumbar vertebrum (Figure 11.6). In the cat and sometimes in small breeds of dogs, the three sacral segments may reside over the $L_{5/6}$ disc or even the L_6 vertebral body. To consider each peripheral nerve individually (and see Figure 11.5):-

Femoral Nerve — arises from the most cranial portion of the plexus and innervates the most cranial muscle mass in the hindlimb — the quadriceps group (Figure 11.5). This group of muscles extend the stifle joint and together with the psoas muscle group, which is also innervated by the femoral nerve, flex the hip joint. The saphenous branch of the femoral nerve supplies sensation to the medial aspect of the limb, usually as far as the medial aspect of the second digit but occasionally only as far as the first digit.

Obturator Nerve — is a purely motor nerve and supplies the adductor group, comprising the Adductor magnus, Pectineus and Gracilis muscles (Figure 11.5).

CORD SEGMENTS

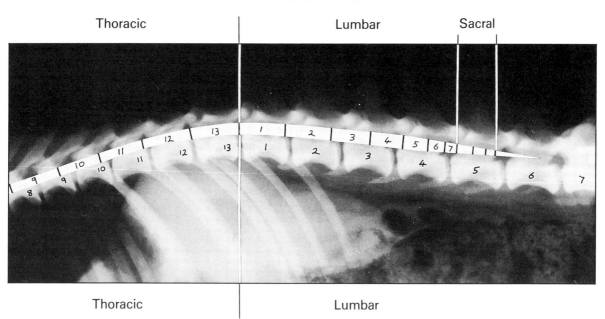

Figure 11.6
Diagram to show the relative positions of spinal cord segments and vertebral bodies
(From Wheeler, S. J. (1985) The approach to spinal disease in dogs *British Veterinary Journal* **141**, 222, reproduced by permission).

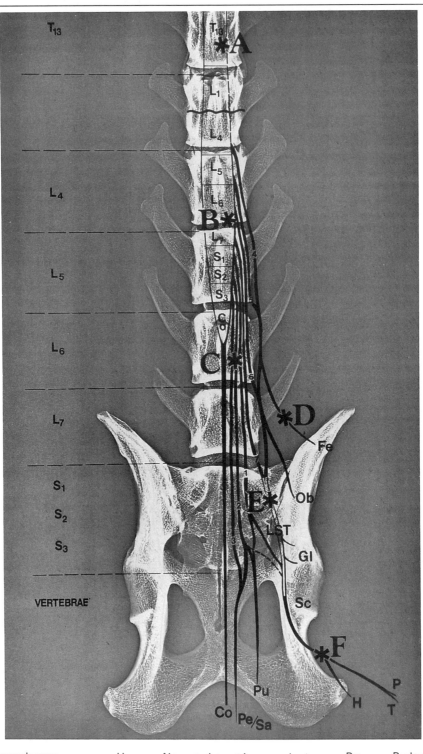

Fe — Femoral nerve	H — Nerve to hamstring muscles		Pu — Pudendal nerve
Ob — Obturator nerve	T — Tibial nerve	Sc	Pe — Pelvic nerves
Gl — Gluteal nerves	P — Peroneal nerve		Sa — Sacral nerves
LST — Lumbosacral trunk	Sc — Sciatic nerve		Co — Coccygeal nerves

Figure 11.7
Diagram to show the six possible sites of injury that may result in hindlimb monoparesis/monoplegia.
(see Table 11.2).

Sciatic Nerve — The intrapelvic portion of the sciatic nerve is termed the lumbosacral trunk (Figure 11.7). The cranial and caudal gluteal nerves arise from this trunk, before it exits the pelvis at the greater sciatic notch to become the sciatic nerve. The sciatic nerve then innervates the most caudally situated muscle group on the thigh — the hamstring group. These muscles serve to flex the stifle joint and, together with the gluteal group which is innervated by the gluteal nerves, to extend the hip joint (Figure 11.5).

At the level of the stifle joint the sciatic nerve then divides into peroneal and tibial branches.

The peroneal nerve is the cranial branch which innervates the skin and the muscle groups on the craniolateral surface of the tibia and foot. It therefore activates the hock flexor muscle group and the digital extensors.

The tibial nerve branches caudally and innervates the skin and the muscle groups on the caudal aspect of the tibia and foot. It therefore activates the hock extensors and the digital flexors.

Pudendal Nerve — is the most caudally derived of the major branches of the lumbosacral trunk and does not innervate any major limb muscles. It is motor to the muscles of the pelvic diaphragm and the external anal sphincter (Figure 11.5). It is also sensory to the skin of the anus, perineum and genitalia.

The pelvic and sacral nerves arise independently from the caudal plexus (S_{1-3}) and supply autonomic innervation to the pelvic viscera. They are largely responsible for control of urinary and faecal continence. The most caudal portion of the cauda equina is made by the coccygeal nerves to the tail.

NEUROLOGICAL EXAMINATION

The two aims of the neurological examination in a case of hindlimb monoparesis/plegia are to localise the lesion and to assess its severity. The aims in localising the lesion are threefold:- firstly by defining the deficit as either UMN or LMN; secondly by defining the LMN disorder into one or more of the following types of deficit:-

Femoral	(F)
Sciatic	(Sc)
Sacral	(Sa)
Coccygeal	(Co)

Finally, to localise the lesion according to the following classification scheme:-

A: T3 – L3 SPINAL CORD

B: L4 – S$_2$ SPINAL CORD

C: L4 – COCCYGEAL NERVE ROOTS

D: FEMORAL NERVE

E: L6 – S1 SPINAL NERVES AND LUMBOSACRAL TRUNK

F: SCIATIC NERVE

LESION LOCALISATION

To define the deficit as UMN or LMN:

For differentiating the features of UMN and LMN disease, the reader is directed to Chapter 3. In essence UMN lesions result in an increase, or no alteration, in spinal reflexes to the affected limb; whereas LMN lesions will result in subtle or profound reflex losses. The most sensitive indicator of mild lower motor neuron disease is usually a weakness in carpal or hock flexion. This should be compared with the normal limb or that of a control animal. In addition, marked muscle atrophy will usually develop in the affected limb.

To define the LMN deficit

Lesions affecting the lumbosacral plexus can be divided into four relatively distinct LMN deficits, which may be present either alone or in combination. The obturator nerve is rarely damaged in isolation and lesions are not recognised as a distinct clinical entity in small animals, although they may be present subclinically. The four types of deficit are:

Femoral nerve: Lesions may be due to damage to L_4 or L_5 cord segments, nerve roots and/or spinal nerves or the femoral nerve itself. Of the four types of neurological deficit, the femoral nerve deficit is the least commonly encountered because the nerve and its spinal nerves of origin are very well protected within the sublumbar musculature. Occasional trauma or neoplasia in this area can affect these structures. Deficits more commonly result from damage to the spinal cord segments or nerve roots which lie within the spinal canal. This type of lesion is therefore also likely to cause contralateral limb signs.

Femoral nerve deficits cause severe gait dysfunction due mainly to an inability to fix and therefore bear weight through the stifle joint. Hip flexion is also markedly reduced and analgesia/hypalgesia may occur over the medial aspect of the thigh, crus, metatarsus and second digit. The patellar reflex will usually be reduced or absent.

Sciatic Nerve: Lesions result from damage to $L_6 - S_1$ cord segments, their nerve roots and/or spinal nerves, the intrapelvic lumbosacral trunk or the sciatic nerve itself (see Figure 11.7).

Complete lesions of the sciatic nerve result in an inability to extend the hip joint, flex the stifle joint and to both flex or extend the hock joint. The digits are also paralysed. Even with such profound deficits the animal can still fix the stifle joint (via the femoral nerve) and can often bear some weight on the leg. The foot usually knuckles and the hock collapses. Analgesia may be present over the whole limb distal to the stifle, except on the medial aspect (supplied by the saphenous branch of the femoral nerve).

Pure tibial nerve deficits are rare. The main features will be loss of hock extension so that the animal walks in a plantigrade manner. Analgesia, if present, will occur on the caudal aspect of the limb distal to the stifle.

Peroneal nerve deficits are much more commonly seen than tibial deficits. In man, random injuries to the main trunk of the sciatic nerve in the thigh cause peroneal deficits up to six times more often than tibial deficits. The tibial and peroneal branches of the sciatic nerve are well defined and can be easily separated up to the level of the greater sciatic notch of the pelvis. The fascicles within the tibial division are small and are surrounded by a higher proportion of connective tissue compared with the large fascicles of the peroneal division which have less protecting connective tissue. Therefore a bullet or bite wound to the sciatic nerve in the caudal thigh will frequently present with a deficit predominantly reflecting the peroneal nerve. The same is also true for an injury to the intrapelvic structures contributing to the sciatic nerve, although for reasons that are less well defined. In addition it has been suggested that the peroneal division lies slightly ventral to the tibial and so is more susceptible to injury from a protruding intramedullary pin at the level of the greater trochanter.

To detect a sciatic neuropathy is relatively easy if the animal is able to walk and so demonstrate conscious proprioceptive deficits in the limb and paresis of the appropriate muscle groups. Similarly, analgesia of the distal limb with sparing of the medial aspect usually leaves little doubt as to the presence of a deficit to the sciatic nerve. However, to diagnose a moderate sciatic neuropathy in a dog with severe pelvic fractures is both very important and often much more difficult. The conscious response to a painful stimulus, caused preferably by using haemostats on the nailbed, is assessed and compared to the other hindlimb and to one or both forelimbs. Most neurologically intact animals with pelvic fractures are well able to respond consciously to such stimulus even if they are somewhat reluctant to move the limb. If hypalgesia is suspected, the animal's response to a similar stimulus on the medial aspect of the second digit and medial metatarsus should be normal provided that the femoral pathways are intact.

The second useful diagnostic feature is an inability of the animal with sciatic motor deficits to actively flex the hock joint. The withdrawal reflex is mediated through the sciatic nerve, except for some hip flexion (psoas muscle) and weak stifle flexion (sartorius muscle) which are made possible by the femoral nerve. Hock flexion is, however, mediated solely by the peroneal division of the sciatic nerve. This is evaluated by applying a painful stimulus to the digits while also gently extending the hock. If in doubt, the opposite limb should be evaluated or a control dog assessed. If analgesia or hypalgesia over the sciatic field is suspected, then the sensory field of the femoral nerve should be stimulated. Most neurologically intact animals with pelvic fractures are well able to firmly flex the hock joint against moderate resistance, particularly if this does not involve movement of the whole limb. The most sensitive means of detecting reflex contraction of the hock flexor muscles is by the use of an EMG needle to detect motor unit potentials (see page 203).

Therefore, an inability to flex the hock joint and particularly hypo/analgesia over the sciatic field should arouse a high index of suspicion for sciatic nerve damage. Early recognition may have a considerable bearing on the overall case management. For prognosis, see the section on assessing the severity of a lesion.

Sacral deficit: This is a general term used for deficits of the sacral cord segments, nerve roots, and/or spinal nerves or the pudendal, pelvic and/or sacral nerves. These structures together innervate the external anal sphincter muscle and the muscles of the pelvic diaphragm, supply sensation to the perineal region and are in large part responsible for urinary and faecal continence (see Chapter 12). The anal reflex and control of urination are good indicators of the integrity of this region. The anal reflex is mainly mediated through S_1 nerves and cord segments, while urinary and faecal continence are mainly mediated through S_2 nerves and cord segments.

Coccygeal nerve: Lesions result from injury to the coccygeal cord segments or nerves and produce motor and/or sensory disturbance to the tail.

In any animal with a suspected neurological problem the clinician must not omit to conduct a thorough assessment of the musculoskeletal system so that, for example, a cruciate ligament rupture is not missed. Similarly, any dog presenting with an orthopaedic lesion following trauma must have an assessment of its neurological status. Over ten per cent of dogs and cats with pelvic fractures or fracture/dislocations have associated neurological deficits.

Localising the lesion by area:
Having defined the deficit by neurological examination, the clinician should now be able to localise the lesion to one or more of the areas described in Table 11.2 and illustrated in Figure 11.7.

Table 11.2
Classification Scheme for Lesion Localisation. (The areas correspond to Figure 11.7)

AREA	DEFICIT
A: $T_3 - L_3$ SPINAL CORD	UMN
B: $L_4 - S_2$ SPINAL CORD	LMN, F, Sc, Sa, or Co
C: $L_4 -$ COCCYGEAL NERVE ROOTS	LMN, F, Sc, Sa, or Co
D: FEMORAL NERVE	LMN, F
E: $L_6 - S_1$ SPINAL NERVES AND LUMBOSACRAL TRUNK	LMN, Sc, (Sa)
F: SCIATIC NERVE	LMN, Sc

LMN	=	Lower motor neurone type deficit
UMN	=	Upper motor neurone type deficit
F	=	Femoral deficit
Sc	=	Sciatic deficit
Sa	=	Sacral deficit
Co	=	Coccygeal deficit

A. UMN LESIONS AFFECTING CORD SEGMENTS $T_3 - L_3$. Because it is difficult to selectively damage one half of the spinal cord and yet cause no damage to the contralateral half, lesions at this level nearly always show bilateral hindlimb deficits. Occasionally, an animal may present with almost completely unilateral signs in the limb ipsilateral to the cord lesion. Careful sequential neurological examination or evaluation of the initial signs of the disease will, in most cases, provide evidence of contralateral limb dysfunction. In UMN lesions, the spinal reflexes should be normal or hyperactive.

The following conditions may cause such a deficit:-

Infarct (Ischaemic myelopathy):- After resolution of early oedematous change in the contralateral spinal cord, a unilateral infarct will often leave the animal with a resulting neurological deficit in the ipsilateral hindlimb. Pain sensation is usually preserved to the affected limb, due to cross over of nociceptive fibres in the spinal cord distal to the infarction. Lesions in the $T_3 - L_3$ area usually have a better prognosis than those occurring in the lumbosacral enlargement, where the crucial lower motor neurones (ventral horn cells) themselves are located.

Neoplasia:- A gradual progression of the neurological deficit and frequently also the presence of spinal hyperaesthesia are the main presenting signs. Bone lysis on plain radiography or myelographic demonstration of the lesion should confirm the diagnosis.

Intervertebral disc disease:- Due to the wide range of possible presenting signs in this condition, cases with almost complete lateralisation can be encountered. The likely breed incidence, focal thoracolumbar hyperaesthesia, and the radiographic demonstration of an extradural lesion should confirm the diagnosis.

B. LMN LESIONS AFFECTING CORD SEGMENTS $L_4 - S_2$

As shown in Figure 11.6, these six spinal cord segments overlie the three vertebral bodies L_3, L_4, and L_5. Caudal to $L_{5/6}$ disc space lie the coccygeal segments and the nerve roots of the cauda equina. Even if predominantly unilateral, lesions affecting cord segments $L_4 - S_2$ are likely to result in bilaterally diminished patellar or withdrawal reflexes and frequently also sacral deficits such as urinary and faecal incontinence. In addition, sensory loss to the affected hindlimb(s) and to the perineum may be present. Damage to this region of the cord usually has a very bleak prognosis because the loss of large numbers of ventral horn cells cannot be replaced.

The most common conditions are:-

Infarct

Neoplasia

Intervertebral disc — Roughly 10 per cent of disc protrusions occur between discs $L_{3/4}$ and $L_{5/6}$ inclusive. Again, due to the wide variation in presenting signs with disc disease, marked lateralisation of signs is sometimes seen.

Degenerative myelopathy — Early signs in this condition are often markedly lateralised. The involvement of dorsal nerve roots is clinically associated with depression of the patellar reflex in up to 70% of cases, which may cause the clinician to localise the lesion to this area of the spinal cord.

C. LESIONS OF NERVE ROOTS L_4 — COCCYGEAL

Lesions occurring at this level of the nervous system will obviously cause clinical signs very similar to those at B, as can be seen from Table 11.2. Survey radiographs and myelography, epidurography and, in some cases CSF analysis, should aid in differentiating between lesions in these two regions.

Fracture of L_6 and L_7 vertebral bodies — Only nerve roots (and not spinal cord) overlie the L_6 and L_7 region of the spinal canal. Nerve roots are more able to displace than spinal cord in the face of an overriding fracture and surprisingly little deficit may result even with severe displacement of fragments. Fractures at this level can have a marked variation in clinical signs. Signs may be lateralised and occasionally appear as a monoparesis/plegia. Of L_7 vertebral body fractures reported in the dog, almost half presented with minimal clinical signs consisting only of pain and reluctance to walk. These dogs returned to normal within six weeks or so without surgical intervention. Dogs with more severe clinical signs showed sciatic deficits, in most cases combined with urinary and faecal incontinence (Slocum and Rudy, 1975). Following either surgical or conservative therapy, a proportion of cases may be left with permanent deficits, usually referable to either the peroneal nerve or as a disturbance of continence.

Fracture/luxations of the sacrococcygeal area — Animals with fractures or luxations in the sacrococcygeal area often present with weakness or lameness in the hindlegs and some may show marked lateralisation of signs. Hindlimb dysfunction occurs with this injury due to an associated traction injury to the more proximal nerve roots of the cauda equina. This produces a neurapraxic injury, often combined with axonal damage and demyelination. This usually improves clinically within one week of the injury. The severity of the sacral and coccygeal deficits varies and this can be used as a guide to prognosis. In a review of over fifty cats with this injury, all those showing only coccygeal deficits recovered. Seventy five per cent of cats, which in addition demonstrated urinary retention, recovered. Cats showing these deficits together with decreased anal tone or perineal sensation had only a 60% recovery rate. Cats with coccygeal deficits, urinary retention, decreased anal tone and perineal sensation combined with a lack of urethral sphincter tone (as assessed by ease of bladder expression) had the worst prognosis, with only 50% recovering. The most important information from this series was that all cats that did not recover the ability to urinate normally within one month of the injury remained incontinent. Although tail amputation has been advocated to prevent further traction on the cauda equina, it did not affect the overall recovery rate in this series (Smeak and Olmstead, 1985). It may be of benefit, however, in preventing soiling of, or accidental trauma to, the tail.

Neoplasia of nerve roots $L_4 - S_2$ — Tumours arising from the lumbosacral roots or spinal nerves have been described with much less frequency than tumours in the brachial plexus region. Signs of contralateral limb dysfunction appear early as most lumbosacral tumours are located intradurally, whereas intradural invasion usually is a delayed event with tumours of the brachial plexus.

Lumbosacral spondylopathy — Lumbosacral malarticulation/malformation and lumbosacral stenosis are other terms used to describe this condition. The pathogenesis appears to be a combination of bony narrowing of the lumbosacral canal due to either congenital or acquired stenosis and/or subluxation, combined with soft tissue compression caused by hypertrophied ligamentous structures and in some cases also by Type II disc protrusions. Clinical signs vary and although weakness is usually bilateral, a unilateral sciatic type neuropathy is not unusual, with weak hock flexion being recorded as the main neurological deficit in one series (Denny *et al*, 1982). In addition, some dogs show associated anal hyporeflexia and faecal or urinary incontinence. The most common feature, however, is pain in the lumbosacral area. Plain radiography demonstrates lumbosacral spondylosis in most cases, but this is a very non specific sign. EMG is useful in confirming neurological deficits referable to the lumbosacral plexus, and epidurography, transosseous venography or CT scan may help to confirm the diagnosis. Myelography frequently provides useful information in the evaluation of the lumbosacral joint (Wheeler and Davies, 1985, Lang 1989). The response to conservative management is usually poor. Dorsal laminectomy provided good to excellent results in ten of 13 dogs in one series (Oliver *et al*, 1978), but was not helpful in another (Denny *et al*, 1982).

A similar condition has been seen in smaller or toy breed dogs and has been referred to as lumbosacral stenosis. Clinical signs were as described above and unilateral deficits seemed to predominate. Exacerbation of signs with exercise was reported to be a feature in these animals. This was thought to be due to an increase in nerve root compression at the level of the spinal foramen, caused by dilation of the spinal arteries and veins on exercise. All dogs in this series responded to surgical decompression (Tarvin and Prata, 1980).

Intervertebral disc protrusion — Lesions at L_7/S_1 are now being recognised more frequently, particularly in large breed dogs, either alone or as a part of the lumbosacral spondylopathy/cauda equina syndrome. Hindlimb lameness was most often unilateral in the seven dogs with this condition recorded by Denny *et al*, (1982).

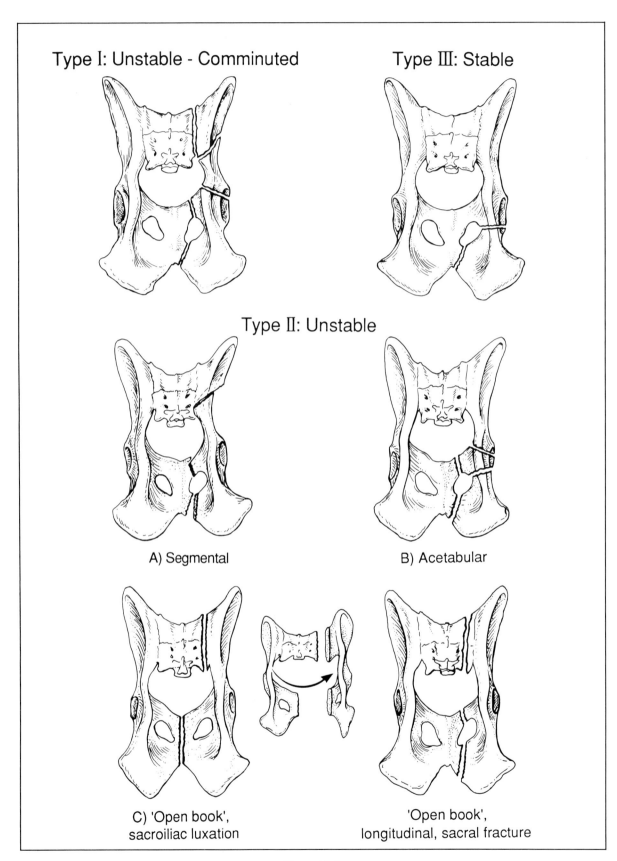

Type I: Unstable - Comminuted

Type III: Stable

Type II: Unstable

A) Segmental

B) Acetabular

C) 'Open book',
sacroiliac luxation

'Open book',
longitudinal, sacral fracture

Figure 11.8
Diagrams to show the three main types of pelvic fracture

Inflammation of the cauda equina — This may result from meningitis due to distemper, toxoplasmosis, or FIP and can also be a feature of Coonhound paralysis. Signs may be unilateral or bilateral. A polyradiculoneuritis of unknown aetiology analagous to cauda equina neuritis in horses has been described in two dogs, one of which had unilateral onset of signs (Griffiths *et al*, 1983).

Discospondylitis — Dogs with lumbosacral discospondylosis may show pain and lameness of one hindlimb together with muscle atrophy and EMG evidence of denervation in one or both hindlimbs.

Aortic emboli — Although not a primary neural lesion, the resultant ischaemia causes a peripheral neuropathy to be superimposed on the more obvious ischaemic myopathy. Although the clinical signs and pulse deficit may be less marked in one hindlimb, paraparesis/plegia is nearly always seen with this condition.

D. INJURY TO THE MAIN TRUNK OF THE FEMORAL NERVE

Injuries to this structure are rare. They may occur following prolonged caudal limb extension over the edge of a table, such as during perineal hernia surgery. Masses in the region of the psoas muscles may also cause femoral nerve deficits.

E. INJURIES TO THE VENTRAL BRANCHES OF L_6, L_7 AND S_1 SPINAL NERVES OR THE LUMBOSACRAL TRUNK

This area is perhaps the most important location for serious nerve injury to occur in the whole of the lumbosacral plexus, mainly because of the close proximity of these structures to the pelvis. Of 474 fractures or luxations occurring in dogs and cats, 26% involved the pelvis (Kolata and Johnston, 1975). In a retrospective survey of pelvic fractures or luxations occurring over a 4.5 year period, 35 dogs and cats reflecting 11% of the total number of animals seen, had associated neurological deficits (Jacobsen and Schrader, 1987).

Pelvic fractures can be classified as: — (Figure 11.8)

Type I   Comminuted

Type II   a. Segmental with two major fracture lines, one on either side of the acetabulum

b. Fractures through the acetabulum

c. 'Open book' involving the pubic symphysis area together with either a sacroiliac luxation or a longitudinal sacral fracture. The isolated hemipelvis is free to rotate, or open like a book (see inset).

Type III   Stable

Type I and II fractures have the highest incidence of associated neural and soft tissue injuries. In 1972, a post mortem survey was conducted of 42 human cadavers with pelvic fractures that were of the 'open book' type (Type IIc). Forty-seven per cent of these had evidence of gross or histopathological damage to nerves of the lumbosacral plexus. The most frequently damaged structures were the lumbosacral trunk and superficial (= cranial) gluteal nerve, both of which lie in intimate association with the sacroiliac joint (Huittinen, 1972). In the same year 68 clinical patients were also evaluated following pelvic fractures of the 'open book' type and 46% of these had associated neurological deficits, many of which were permanent (Huittenen and Slatis, 1973).

In a prospective survey over one year, ten of 25 (40%) Type II pelvic fractures in dogs and cats had concomitant neurological deficits. Five of these were 'open book' (Type 11c) fractures involving the sacroiliac joint or sacral wing, and five were segmented iliac shaft (Type IIa) fractures. (Sharp, 1982).

Of another 34 canine pelvic fractures with documented neurological deficits, 41% of these occurred in association with sacroiliac luxations. Segmental iliac shaft fractures accounted for a further 53% of the 34 cases (Jacobsen and Schrader, 1987).

In general therefore, the following three types of pelvic fracture in the dog and cat have a very high incidence of sciatic type neurological deficits:-

a.   sacroiliac luxations

b.   longitudinal sacral fractures (sacral wing)

c.   ilial shaft fractures

The damage usually occurs either to the lumbrosacral trunk or the ventral branch of S_1 spinal nerve, both of which are very close to these fracture sites and are only poorly protected by surrounding soft tissue. The resultant injury causes a neurological deficit which is clinically indistinguishable from an injury to the sciatic nerve itself. In addition, cases may also show mild sacral signs such as anal hyporeflexia, presumably due to damage to the S_1 ventral spinal nerve. These animals are nearly always continent due to sparing of the S_2 spinal nerve (See page 191). The exception to this statement is that fractures of the sacral wing which extend through the sacral foraminae may damage S_2 and S_3 as well as S_1 spinal nerves and therefore usually result in sacral signs including incontinence or analgesia to the perineal area. Denervation of the tail however, is not seen with these pelvic injuries.

Diagnosis in such cases rests on the presence of a unilateral sciatic type neurological deficit and the radiographic confirmation of one of the three pelvic fracture types ipsilateral to the deficit. Unless there are two separate neurological lesions, the resultant deficit will always be unilateral.

Confirmation of an injury at this location of the lumbosacral plexus is obtained by EMG mapping of muscle denervation. As the lesion involves the L_6 spinal nerve and the lumbosacral trunk prior to the origin of the gluteal nerves and often also the obturator nerves, denervation will occur in muscles supplied both by the obturator nerve (adductor, pectineus, gracilis) and the gluteal nerves (gluteal muscle group). These features serve to distinguish a lesion at this level from a lesion of the main trunk of the sciatic nerve (see Figure 11.8 and F below).

Many animals suffer severe pelvic fractures including bilateral sacroiliac luxations or ilial shaft fractures, but never show clinical neurological deficits. Thus it is obviously futile to predict that a neurological deficit will occur in a given case. However, the presence of such fractures should give the clinician a high index of suspicion and certainly indicate the need for a thorough neurological examination. If a sciatic type deficit is diagnosed, it is highly likely to be related to damage occurring at the level of the fracture or luxation.

That a severe neurological deficit severely complicates the management of a dog with pelvic fractures is beyond doubt, particularly if there are also associated long bone fractures of either hindleg. Early recognition, or at least, suspicion, of neurological complications allows proper client communication and education. In particular, the prolonged nursing and increased recovery period additional to that required for the pelvic fracture itself, must be discussed.

General orthopaedic recommendations as to whether to perform internal fixation of the pelvic fracture/luxation should be followed. Candidates for surgery include animals in severe pain, those that are unable to stand and those where other orthopaedic injuries complicate case management. Surgery may allow visualisation of the injured intrapelvic nerves. Anastomosis of damaged nerve is not feasible due to the widespread nature of the lesion occurring in a traction injury of this type, but occasionally decompression of entrapped nerve is possible. Conversely, recognition of a severed nerve trunk can justify limb amputation.

Stabilisation of pelvic fractures might be expected to reduce repeated trauma to the already damaged nerve trunks. This is not necessarily supported by the results of one survey. The results were good or excellent in 11 of 13 dogs that underwent surgery, recovery occurring after 2 – 16 weeks of rehabilitation. However, 10 of 12 dogs that did not have surgery had similar results over 2 – 12 week periods. This would suggest that the bulk of the nerve damage occurs at the time of the original injury and does not seem to be exacerbated by an unstable fracture. Overall, 81% of the 34 dogs and cats had excellent or good recovery of neurological deficits following pelvic fractures (Jacobsen and Schrader, 1987).

In another series, 7 of 11 cases with sciatic paralysis associated with ilial shaft fracture recovered within 6 months and an eighth within 12 months. Three of four cases with sacral wing fractures or sacroiliac luxation also recovered within 6 months. These authors recorded some animals with a predominantly peroneal distribution to their weakness that learn to compensate for their disability by flipping the paw to prevent knuckling of the digits (Gilmore, 1984). An extreme example of this was seen in a five year old Border Collie that sustained an ilial shaft fracture and had an associated severe sciatic neuropathy causing total analgesia and almost complete denervation of muscles over the peroneal distribution. The dog dragged the foot, causing excoriation of the dorsum of the paw. This eventually healed by 3 months post injury. Re-examination at 5 months post injury revealed no recovery of the peroneal nerve deficit, although a considerable regeneration of the tibial nerve was demonstrated by electrophysiology. The dog was, however, able to run without dragging the digits and had resumed work as a cattle dog (Sharp, 1982).

It is also possible to cause iatrogenic damage to this area of the plexus during repair of pelvic or sacral fractures. Furthermore, the callus associated with a healing iliac shaft fracture can compress nerves at this site. These are two further reasons why preoperative identification of potential neurological deficits is important.

F. INJURY TO THE MAIN TRUNK OF THE SCIATIC NERVE

The sciatic nerve is vulnerable to injury after it leaves the pelvis, although this occurs less frequently than injuries to the more proximal structures discussed under E above.

A wide number of causes of sciatic nerve damage have been documented as shown in Table 11.3. The most important are either complications resulting from intramedullary pinning (Fanton et al, 1983) or from ischial and acetabular fractures (Chambers and Hardie, 1986). Clinically, these injuries are usually indistinguishable from those occurring to the intrapelvic portions of the sciatic nerve covered under area E. However, in the absence of an orthopaedic injury to the spine, sacrum, sacroiliac joint or iliac shaft, damage to the more proximal structures is unlikely. Without one of the previously mentioned orthopaedic injuries to explain the neurological deficit, the presence of an acetabular or ischial fracture has a high degree of correlation with an injury to the main trunk of the sciatic nerve in this region.

Conscious proprioceptive deficits, selective muscle atrophy, reduced hock flexion and/or reduced sensation over the sciatic or peroneal field will be seen. Radiography is of value to identify any recent or old orthopaedic injuries. Sacral deficits do not occur in association with pure sciatic nerve lesions unless another lesion is also present. The main means of differentiating sciatic nerve lesions from more proximal lesions is the absence of denervation in muscles supplied by the gluteal nerves (gluteal muscle group), obturator nerve (adductor group) and sacral nerves (sacrococcygeus muscle group) on electromyographic examination of a sciatic nerve injury.

Intramedullary pinning and sciatic neuropathy — An incidence of 14.5% of sciatic neuropathies was seen in 83 femoral fracture repairs. Interestingly, this appeared to be independent of the experience of the surgeon. The incidence was higher in cats than in dogs. All pins had been placed in a retrograde fashion. The onset of signs was immediate in three animals and delayed for 1 – 50 days (mean 16 days) in eleven. All cases showed pain over the greater trochanter area and all showed deficits referable to the sciatic field alone. Surgical exploration confirmed trauma from pin insertion as the cause in three cases and from cicatrix formation around the exposed pin in eleven. All animals improved following external neurolysis/pin removal or shortening and no animals were left with permanent neurological deficits (Fanton et al, 1983). Although excessive pin length was thought likely to be a contributory cause of the nerve damage, this was not proven. Sciatic nerve damage from this cause can be minimised by keeping the femur in adduction and the hip in a ventral position during pin placement. External rotation of the hip during pin replacement should be avoided.

Table 11.3.   Causes of injury to the sciatic nerve

Intramedullary pinning of the femur	Bites and lacerations
Ischial fractures	Femoral neck fracture
Acetabular fractures	Femoral shaft fracture
Anterodorsal hip luxation	Intramuscular injection
Surgery of the hip area	Rabies vaccination
Perineal hernia surgery	

Acetabular or ischial fractures — These injuries are occasionally associated with sciatic neuropathies. In one series of seven cases of sciatic neuropathy due to ischial or acetabular fractures, four of the cases were caused by the fracture itself and in the other three the sciatic nerve became entrapped by progressive fibrosis at the fracture site. Cranial displacement of the ischiatic tuberosity caused compression at the greater trochanter in five of the dogs. Diagnosis in each case was confirmed by an EMG pattern of denervation typical for damage to the main trunk of the sciatic nerve at this level with sparing of the gluteal muscles. In some cases, denervation was also absent in the hamstring muscle group, presumably because the branch to these muscles had left the sciatic nerve above the site of compression (Figure 11.7). Surgical exploration was performed on a delayed basis in each case and all lesions were demonstrated between the sacrotuberous ligament and the third trochanter. Limb amputation was performed in one dog and external neurolysis in the other six. The superficial gluteal muscle was used to protect the nerve in two dogs and a nerve cuff was utilised in one. All dogs had satisfactory return to function (Chambers and Hardie, 1986).

Perineal hernia repair — The sciatic nerve lies very close to the sacrotuberous ligament and can easily be damaged by attempts to pass a suture around this ligament. If this structure must be used in hernia repair, then the suture should be carefully passed through the ligament and not around it.

Post vaccinal rabies — An important, though fortunately very uncommon LMN disorder can follow rabies vaccination using live virus derived from chick embryo. Clinical signs appear 7 – 21 days post vaccination and begin in the pelvic limb following vaccination in the ipsilateral thigh. LMN signs are seen initially as the virus travels in the peripheral nerves to reach the spinal cord and generalisation can occur later. At present there is no evidence to suggest that the virus reverts to field virulence and recovery has been documented in dogs within one or two months. Appropriate notification of public health authorities should be made.

Distal lesions — Injuries to the tibial division of the sciatic nerve are rare. The clinical features have been described on page 194. The peroneal nerve is more vulnerable than the tibial division due to its more superficial location at the head of the fibula. Pressure from an orthopaedic cast, surgery of the stifle joint, particularly cruciate repair, or an injury in this area, can result in the clinical features described above. However, the majority of cases suffering peroneal type deficits have, in reality, sustained injury to the main trunk of the sciatic nerve or its origins.

ASSESSING THE SEVERITY OF A LESION

The diameter of a nerve fibre has a direct bearing on the susceptibility of that fibre to compression. Large myelinated fibres (mainly those supplying proprioceptive function) are the most sensitive type of nerve fibre to injury. The slightly smaller myelinated fibres controlling motor function are usually next affected. Small unmyelinated fibres supplying nociception (deep pain sensation) are the most resistant to compression. This applies equally well in both the peripheral and central nervous systems.

Thus, with increasing compression of, for example, the sciatic nerve, proprioceptive function will be compromised initially, then motor function, and finally deep pain sensation over the sciatic field will be lost.

This gradation of functional loss gives the clinician an indication of the severity of a given lesion. In general, the presence of intact deep pain sensation to a limb implies a better prognosis than if the limb is analgesic.

Nerve injuries can also be classified according to the functional integrity of the nerve. Compression, oedema and perhaps also local demyelination, can result in a complete block of impulse conduction in the nerve without loss of anatomical continuity. This is termed a neurapraxic type of injury. Recovery will usually occur within one to two weeks when the compression and oedema resolve. Local remyelination may take a little longer to reverse but neurapraxia is the mildest type of injury. If the injury is more severe, axons may degenerate distal to the lesion although their axon sheaths remain intact. This is termed axonotmesis. Recovery will now depend on regrowth of the axons from the site of injury, which normally occurs no faster than 1 mm per day. The most severe type of injury is termed neurotmesis and is when there is loss, not only of axonal continuity, but also of continuity of the whole nerve trunk. Recovery will then depend on axonal regrowth successfully crossing the resultant neuroma to reach the axon cylinders on the distal side of the lesion. This often proves to be impossible, or at best regeneration is only partial.

Two electrophysiological techniques may be of value in assessing the severity of a lesion. These are:

a. Motor and sensory nerve conduction studies and the recorded amplitudes of muscle evoked action potentials (see Chapter 4).

b. Immediately following an injury to the sciatic nerve, EMG can be used to determine if any voluntary motor function remains in the muscles innervated by the nerve. This should be established by attempting to induce a withdrawal reflex by stimulating the femoral sensory nerve field (first digit). Simultaneous EMG recording from the gastrocnemius muscles will record motor unit potentials if any reflex motor function remains.

SURGERY FOR LESIONS OF THE LUMBOSACRAL PLEXUS

This comprises two categories:-

Exploration of the sciatic nerve

Muscle relocation following peroneal nerve paralysis.

Exploration of the sciatic nerve

This nerve is easily located under the biceps femoris muscle during a standard approach to the proximal and midshaft portion of the femur.

More proximal exposure is obtained by extending this approach into a caudolateral approach to the hip joint where the incision through the fascia lata is continued caudal to the greater trochanter. The origin of the biceps femoris muscle on the sacrotuberous ligament is freed, taking care at this point to protect the caudal gluteal vessels.

A tenotomy of the superficial gluteal muscle allows maximum exposure of the sciatic nerve. If more exposure is required at this point, a middle gluteal tenotomy can be performed. However, the more muscle mass that is cut, the more adhesions that will form at this level, which may subsequently risk entrapment of the nerve.

Exposure of the lumbosacral trunk area can be obtained by a ventrolateral approach to the ilial shaft, if necessary combined with an ilial osteotomy.

Following exposure of the nerve, any fibrous scar or callus should be carefully dissected free. To then protect the sciatic nerve from subsequent adhesions, the superficial gluteal muscle can be passed under the nerve to keep it in a more superficial position. A silicone nerve cuff can also be used to protect the nerve. It should be laid around the damaged area and should not be too tight. A cross sectional area of two to three times that of the nerve itself is recommended. Therefore for a nerve of 6mm diameter, a cuff of between 8 and 10 mm diameter is ideal. The cuff should be anchored with fine epineurial sutures of (6/0) polypropylene or nylon.

Muscle relocation

Two techniques have been described to overcome peroneal nerve paralysis. The first attaches the tendon of the long digital flexor muscle, which is innervated by the tibial division of the sciatic nerve, to that of the long digital extensor muscle (Bennett and Vaughan, 1976). If the tibial division of the sciatic nerve is functional as determined by minimal muscle atrophy, and preferably also on the basis of nerve conduction studies, then this technique may be of value.

However, many animals with severe peroneal nerve dysfunction also suffer some degree of clinical or subclinical tibial nerve dysfunction which may prevent the long digital flexor from functioning adequately in its new role. In such cases a more elaborate alternative is required. The origin of the long digital extensor can be attached to the freed insertion of the vastus lateralis muscle. Unfortunately, as this new muscle apparatus crosses two joints, it may not work without concommitant arthrodesis of the hock joint (Lesser and Soliman, 1980). Complications associated with injuries to the lumbosacral plexus are similar to those encountered in the forelimb or described above.

REFERENCES

ALEXANDER, J. W., deLAHUNTA, A. and SCOTT, D. W. (1974). A case of brachial plexus neuropathy in a dog. *Journal of the American Animal Hospital Association* **10**, 515.

BENNETT, D., and VAUGHAN, L. C. (1976). The use of muscle relocation techniques in the treatment of peripheral nerve injuries in dogs and cats. *Journal of Small Animal Practice* **17**, 99.

BRADLEY, R. L., WITHROW, S. J. and SYNDER, S. P. (1982). Nerve sheath tumours in the dog. *Journal of the American Animal Hospital Association* **18**, 915.

BRAUND, K. G., WALKER, T. L. and VANDEVELDE, M (1979). Fascicular nerve biopsy in the dog. *American Journal of Veterinary Research* **40**, 1025.

CHAMBERS, J. N. and HARDIE, E. M. (1986). Localisation and management of sciatic nerve injury due to ischial or acetabular fracture. *Journal of the American Animal Hospital Association* **22**, 539.

DENNY, H. R., GIBBS, C. and HOLT, P. E. (1982). The diagnosis and treatment of cauda equina lesions in the dog. *Journal of Small Animal Practice* **23**, 425.

FANTON, J. W., BLASS, C. F. and WITHROW, S. J. (1983). Sciatic nerve injury as a complication of intramedullary pin fixation of femoral fractures. *Journal of American Animal Hospital Association* **19**, 687.

GILMORE, D. R. (1984). Sciatic nerve injury in twenty-nine dogs. *Journal of the American Animal Hospital Association* **20**, 403.

GRIFFITHS, I. R. (1974). Avulsion of the brachial plexus — 1. Neuropathology of the spinal cord and peripheral nerves. *Journal of Small Animal Practice* **15**, 165.

GRIFFITHS, I. R. (1977). Avulsions of the brachial plexus. In: *Current Veterinary Therapy VI* (ed. R. W. Kirk) W. B. Saunders Co., Philadelphia.

GRIFFITHS, I. R. and CARMICHAEL, S. (1981). Tumours involving the brachial plexus in seven dogs. *Veterinary Record* **108**, 435.

GRIFFITHS, I. R., CARMICHAEL, S. and SHARP, N. J. H. (1983). Polyradiculoneuritis in two dogs presenting as neuritis of the cauda equina. *Veterinary Record* **112**, 360.

GRIFFITHS, I. R., DUNCAN, I. D. and LAWSON, D. D. (1974). Avulsion of the brachial plexus — 2. Clinical Aspects. *Journal of Small Animal Practice* **15**, 177.

HARVEY, C. E. (1974). Forequarter amputation in the dog and cat. *Journal of the American Animal Hospital Association* **10**, 25.

HUITENNEN, V. M. (1972). Lumbosacral nerve injury in fracture of the pelvis. A postmortem radiographic and pathoanatomic study. *Acta Chir. Scandinavian,* Supplement 429.

HUITTENEN, V. M. and SLATIS, P. (1972). Nerve injury in double vertical pelvic fractures. *Acta Chir. Scandinavia* **138**, 571.

JACOBSEN, A. and SCHRADER, S. C. (1987). Peripheral nerve injury associated with fracture or fracture dislocation of the pelvis in dogs and cats: 34 cases. (1978 – 1982). *Journal of the American Veterinary Medical Association* **190**, 569.

KNECHT, C. D. and GREENE, J. A. (1977). Surgical approach to the brachial plexus in Small animals. *Journal of the American Animal Hospital Association* **13**, 592.

KOLATA, R. J. and JOHNSTON, D. E. (1975). Motor vehicle accidents in urban dogs: a study of 600 cases. *Journal of the American Veterinary Medical Association* **167**, 938.

LANG, J. (1989) Flexian-extension myelography of the canine cauda equina. *Veterinary Radiology* **29**, 242.

LESSER, A. S. and SOLIMAN, S. S. (1980). Experimental evaluation of tendon transfer for the treatment of sciatic nerve paralysis in the dog. *Veterinary Surgery* **9**, 72.

McCOY, D. M. and TROTTER, E. J. (1977). Brachial paralysis subsequent to traumatic partial occlusion of the right subclavian artery. *Journal of the American Animal Hospital Association* **13**, 625.

OLIVER, J. E., SELCER, R. R. and SIMPSON, S (1978). Cauda equina compression from lumbosacral malarticulation and malformation in the dog. *Journal of the American Veterinary Medical Association* **173**, 207.

READ, R. A. (1986). Probable trophic pad ulceration following traumatic denervation. *Veterinary Surgery* **15**, 40.

SHARP, N. J. H. (1982). *Traumatic hindlimb neuropathies,* MVM Thesis, Glasgow University.

SHARP, N. J. H. (1986). Craniolateral approach to the canine brachial plexus. *Veterinary Surgery* **17**, 18.

SHELL, L. and SPONDENBERG, P. (1987). Chondrosarcoma in a cat presenting with forelimb monoparesis. *Compendium of Continuing Education* **9**, 391.

SLOCUM, B. and RUDY, R. L. (1975). Fractures of the seventh lumbar vertebra in the dog. *Journal of the American Animal Hospital Association* **11**, 167.

SMEAK, D. D. and OLMSTEAD (1985). Fracture/luxations of the sacrococcygeal area in the cat. A retrospective study of 51 cases. *Veterinary Surgery* **14**, 319.

TARVIN, G. and PRATA, R. G. (1980). Lumbosacral stenosis in dogs. *Journal of the American Veterinary Medical Association* **177**, 154.

TROY, G. C., HUROV, L. I. and KING, G. K. (1979). Successful surgical removal of a cervical subdural neurofibrosarcoma. *Journal of the American Animal Hospital Association* **15**, 477.

WHEELER, S. J. and DAVIES, J. V. (1985) Iohexol myelography in the dog and cat: a series of one hundred cases, and a comparison with metrzamide and iopamidol. *Journal of Small Animal Practice* **26**, 247.

WHEELER, S. J., CLAYTON JONES, D. G. and WRIGHT, J. A. (1986). Diagnosis of brachial plexus disorders in dogs: a review of 22 cases. *Journal of Small Animal Practice* **27**, 147.

VISCERAL AND BLADDER DYSFUNCTION

DYSAUTONOMIA

Nicholas J. H. Sharp B.Vet.Med., M.V.M., M.R.C.V.S., Dip. A.C.V.S.

VISCERAL AND BLADDER DYSFUNCTION

INTRODUCTION

This section discusses neurogenic abnormalities affecting the bladder, colon and rectum. More detailed reviews exist, particularly of the physiology and of the effect of neural damage on micturition. It is not the aim of this chapter to duplicate these reviews, but to provide a simplified overview. This would seem justified because several aspects of the physiological control of the bladder still remain controversial and poorly understood.

ANATOMY

The anatomy of the lumbosacral plexus has been described in Chapter 11. From this structure three main sources of innervation to the pelvic viscera are derived:

Pelvic nerves arising from sacral cord segments $S_1 - S_3$ and supplying parasympathetic innervation to the bladder, rectum and genital smooth muscle.

Hypogastric nerves arising from $L_1 - L_{4/5}$ cord segments and supplying sympathetic innervation to the bladder, rectum and genital smooth muscle.

Pudendal nerves arising from sacral cord segments $S_1 - S_3$ and supplying somatic innervation to external anal and urogenital skeletal muscle.

Sensory fibres from this area reach the CNS via:

Pudendal nerves for sensation from the perineum and genitalia, **pelvic** and **hypogastric nerves** for visceral sensation. Note that visceral sensation can enter the spinal cord at either the sacral or the lumbar level.

The three most important target organs in the lower urinary tract are:

Detrusor smooth muscle that empties the bladder. This is either encouraged to:
— relax by sympathetic stimulation (ß effect) or
— contract by parasympathetic stimulation

Urethral smooth muscle that is caused to contract by sympathetic stimulation (α effect)

Urethral striated muscle that contracts via pudendal nerve stimulation.

Autonomic control of smooth muscle, for example the detrusor, occurs by diffusion of transmitter from terminal nerves to adjacent muscle cells. This causes a wave of depolarisation within the detrusor, the spread of which is facilitated across selected cells joined by tight junctions. If the bladder wall is overstretched, these tight junctions are damaged and the detrusor becomes ineffective. If the stretch is not reversed within 1—2 weeks, fibrosis may occur that will permanently disturb detrusor function.

PHYSIOLOGY OF MICTURITION

The course of events leading to micturition are as follows:-

Initially as the bladder passively fills with urine, there is only a very gradual increase in intravesicular pressure, largely due to the effect of adrenergic (sympathetic) stimulation that causes the detrusor muscle to relax (Figure 12.1).

As the bladder fills to a greater degree, tension in the detrusor muscle increases more rapidly until a threshold level is reached.

Sensory fibres in the bladder wall respond to this increase in tension, and at threshold level they activate parasympathetic neurons in the sacral spinal cord. This information is then relayed to the brain stem (pons).

Reflex efferent stimulation from the brain stem to the sacral cord causes sustained firing of parasympathetic neurons and results in sustained detrusor contraction.

Sensory stimulation of bladder wall stretch receptors not only stimulates parasympathetic nerves, but also reflexly inhibits both sympathetic and pudendal nerves resulting in sphincter relaxation.

Higher control via the brain stem is important to co-ordinate detrusor contraction with sphincter relaxation. Therefore the bladder empties against a low sphincter pressure.

When the bladder is empty, sensory nerves in the bladder stop discharging and urethral receptors also perceive that urine flow has stopped.

Parasympathetic stimulation then stops and the activity of sympathetic and pudendal nerves increases; thus the bladder relaxes to allow refilling to occur once more, and the sphincter closes.

The cerebral cortex can initiate the micturition reflex as it does during territorial marking, or it can inhibit micturition as in house training.

'Micturition fibres' running in the spinal cord are usually more resistant to the effects of compression than are proprioceptive or motor fibres. Therefore, most dogs become ataxic, paretic or paraplegic before losing full control of urination, though some fine tuning of the micturition reflexes may be lost at an earlier stage. This explains why paraplegic animals with good control of urination are sometimes encountered.

Full control of urinary continence is lost before the appearance of analgesia caudal to a spinal cord lesion, as micturition fibres are damaged before those carrying deep pain sensation.

Prognosis for recovery from spinal cord lesions deteriorates as the animal passes from paraplegia alone to paraplegia with incontinence. A much worse prognosis is usually suggested for those animals which are paraplegic, incontinent and which also lack deep pain sensation.

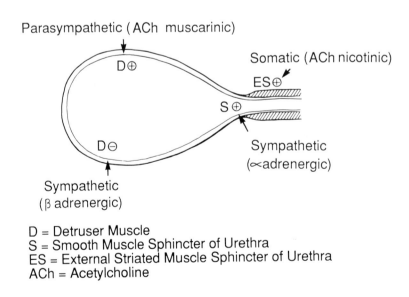

D = Detruser Muscle
S = Smooth Muscle Sphincter of Urethra
ES = External Striated Muscle Sphincter of Urethra
ACh = Acetylcholine

Figure 12.1
Diagram to show the innervation of the bladder and proximal urethra

EXAMINATION OF THE INCONTINENT PATIENT

Careful questioning of the owner and observation of the animal can help answer the following questions. This information is particularly important to obtain in a paraplegic animal, or one with sacral or pelvic fractures.

Even if recumbant or paraplegic, does the animal show any cerebral recognition of the need to urinate — such as showing discomfort, vocalising or attempting to get outside before urinating?

Does the animal attempt to retain urine and not just leak passively? This demonstration of house training may be seen in a continent recumbant or confined paraplegic animal which remains dry, but then eventually is forced to urinate on itself or its bedding. This differs from a continuous leakage of urine, an important feature which relates to sphincter incompetence or to passive overflow of urine following retention due to a UMN lesion (see below).

Does the animal have any other neurological deficits or could there be a non-neurogenic cause of abnormal micturition, for example bladder neoplasia or calculi? This topic has been thoroughly reviewed (Holt, 1983).

Some owners will think that an animal is continent because every time they pick it up, it urinates! The chances are that if this voiding occurs immediately (and often over them), then simply the increase in abdominal pressure or the tactile stimulation of lifting has caused voiding, and the animal is truly incontinent. If, however, the animal waits until it is outside, or at least attempts to wait, this may be a sign of partial or returning cerebral control.

If the animal does pass a flow of urine, is it a good volume in a steady flow? In other words, is the detrusor functioning properly?

This information can be obtained without touching the animal and is a very important facet of any assessment of a neurological case. The ability to void and the degree of overflow have, therefore, already yielded information regarding the animal's degree of cerebral control, detrusor function, and sphincter integrity. From the clinical examination, one can now determine:

If the animal does appear to urinate voluntarily, palpation of the bladder at the end of urination will identify the presence of any residual urine. The latter can be quantified by catheterisation and should be less than 0.2—0.4 ml/kg in dogs and less than 2 mls total in cats.

Manual expression of the bladder on a separate occasion gives subjective information on whether sphincter tone is normal, increased or decreased

A careful neurologic examination will define if an UMN or a LMN lesion is present, and in particular whether the anal reflex and perineal sensation are present, and if the tail is innervated.

Ancillary diagnostic aids include clinical pathology tests such as a complete blood count, serum creatinine, urinalysis and culture. These may identify systemic illness, sepsis or renal disease. Plain and contrast radiography may also be of value to identify associated orthopaedic injuries or genitourinary tract abnormalities (Holt, 1983).

The dynamics of the micturition reflex can be quantified using more sophisticated techniques explained in Chapter 4. This information (i.e. presence of a detrusor reflex, sphincter tone) can often be qualitatively obtained by the preceding careful historical and physical examination. In essence, a cystometrogram (CMG) measures the rise in intravesicular pressure as a volume of fluid is steadily instilled into the bladder. Eventually threshold should be reached and a detrusor reflex initiated. Measurement of these events can identify specific lesions or quantify the degree of damage.

Urethral pressure profilometry (UPP) records the change in pressure at the tip of a urinary catheter which is slowly withdrawn from the bladder lumen and along the length of the urethra. Any marked increase or decrease in sphincter tone is recorded.

Combining EMG recording from the anus with a CMG can also record electrical events of the micturition reflex. This is because the striated muscle of the external anal sphincter normally contracts synchronously with the external urethral sphincter. This may prove of value in identifying reflex dysnergia (see later) or poorly co-ordinated micturition responses.

TYPES OF MICTURITION ABNORMALITY

There is some disagreement as to the use of the term upper motor neurone (UMN) with respect to bladder lesions. This is because attempts to produce a bladder that will empty itself without higher control in dogs (LMN or reflex bladder) have failed. However, other authorities believe the state of a reflex bladder does exist and, clinically, dogs often appear to develop reflexive emptying. Two factors suggest that some degree of reflexive emptying of the bladder should occur:

The spinal reflex arcs to the bladder are intact in spinal cord lesions proximal to the sacral segments.

Isolated bladder smooth muscle will reflexly contract at a certain tension.

For simplicity, therefore, the terms UMN and lower motor neurone (LMN) will be employed. The micturition abnormality can be classified according to whether the detrusor or sphincter function is absent, depressed, normal or increased (see Table 12.1)

Table 12.1. Classification of Urinary Abnormalities

Category	Ability to void urine	Voluntary control	Residual urine	Anal reflex	Difficulty of manual expression
I Cerebral	+	±	+	+	+
II UMN, Sphincter normal	−	−	+ (+ +)	+	+ (+ +)
III UMN, Sphincter hyperactive	±	∓	+ +	+	+ +
IV LMN, Detrusor absent Sphincter absent	−	−	+	− (±)	− (± / +)
V LMN, Detrusor absent Sphincter absent	+	∓	+	+ (± / −)	±
VI LMN, Sphincter normal	−	−	+ +	+	+
+ = normal − = absent or none ± = decreased + + = increased					

I. UMN Lesion — cerebral cortex:

> Detrusor — normal
> Sphincter — normal

For example, dogs with brain tumours will often show a loss of house training due to lack of cortical control of the micturition reflex.

II. UMN Lesion — Brain stem to L7:

> Detrusor — absent (later normal)
> Sphincter — normal (or later hyperactive)

An example of this abnormality would be following a massive intervertebral disc protrusion at T_{13}/L_1.

Following severe cervical, thoracic or lumbar spinal cord damage or transection in animals, a phenomenon called spinal shock temporarily abolishes the portion of the micturition reflex that should take place in the sacral spinal cord. Spinal shock in man temporarily affects all spinal reflexes. In animals only the micturition reflexes appear susceptible, whereas the anal, pedal and patellar reflexes are not affected. Often, animals in this situation also lack deep pain sensation due to the severity of the lesion.

Initially the bladder fills until vesicular pressure exceeds the sphincter pressure and causes urine to dribble out (often termed urinary retention with overflow — UR + O). This is because no detrusor reflex is activated. Raising the intra-abdominal pressure (eg. by the animal coughing or when it is picked up) will also often cause an overflow of urine. The animal is, of course, incontinent and unaware of bladder filling at this stage.

If the spinal cord lesion is reversible, recovery of continence may occur in sequence with recovery of the other spinal cord functions. If the lesion is irreversible, a reflex or 'automatic' bladder may result. This usually occurs within three or four weeks of the original spinal cord injury as the micturition reflexes at the spinal level recover and start to function, but now without higher control. Therefore:

— Sustained detrusor function and complete emptying do not now occur. The detrusor and sphincter actions may be poorly coordinated. Lack of higher control on the pudendal reflexes may cause hypertonicity of the external sphincter (just as may occur to the patellar reflex in a UMN lesion). This sphincter disturbance further counteracts proper emptying.

With an automatic or reflex bladder, the results are:

— Emptying occurs without the animal's knowledge.

— Complete emptying may not occur, so residual volume is high.

— The sphincter may not relax properly so high vesicular pressures may develop, favouring a reflux of urine up one or both ureters, with a resultant risk of pyelonephritis.

High sphincter tone, if present, may make manual evacuation difficult or even dangerous. To overcome this, adrenergic blockers or skeletal muscle relaxants may be of value.

Because the lesion is UMN, the anal reflex will be intact with this type of lesion. This should differentiate it from a LMN lesion.

III. UMN Brain stem to L7:

Detrusor — normal
Sphincter — hyperactive

An example of this type of abnormality is a mild intervertebral disc protrusion at T_{13}/L_1.

This situation may occur in animals which do not have the complete loss of urinary control described in section II above. It can be seen in some paraparetic or paraplegic animals that are aware of the need to urinate and are able to void voluntarily. Such animals should always have intact deep pain sensation.

During voiding, the sphincter appears to be inappropriately activated, thus causing the stream of urine to spurt or stop abruptly. This situation, sometimes termed reflex dyssynergia, has been seen in dogs with intervertebral disc disease which are showing only mild to moderate paresis. The mechanism has not been documented by urodynamic investigations and could possibly be caused more by severe back pain inhibiting the dog from voiding or, conversely, causing bladder emptying due to sudden spasms of pain.

To overcome the higher sphincter tone, α adrenergic blockers or skeletal muscle relaxants may again prove helpful.

IV. LMN Sacral cord or cauda equina:

Detrusor — absent
Sphincter — absent

An example of a condition causing this deficit is a sacral fracture. Essentially, the sacral cord segments or nerve roots are damaged and if severe enough the animal will be incontinent and unaware of the need to urinate. There is no detrusor reflex. The bladder will fill and overflow easily due to the absent sphincter tone. In some situations, probably due to complete lack of bladder wall tone, the bladder may still distend considerably.

Manual expression can be performed with ease. Less severely damaged animals will retain sphincter tone as assessed by a resistance to this procedure, and have a more favourable prognosis than animals lacking sphincter tone. In certain individuals, this tone may paradoxically be somewhat excessive and require pharmacological blockade. Alpha adrenergic blockers are usually ineffective. *Dantrolene* or *diazepam*, which are skeletal muscle relaxants, have been reported to be helpful, presumably by acting on the external urethral sphincter. This suggests that the excessive urethral tone is mediated via an intact pudendal nerve supply.

The anal reflex is usually absent. Animals that retain an anal reflex and/or perineal sensation as further evidence of remaining pudendal function, usually have a more favourable prognosis. For more information regarding prognosis see Chapter 11.

V. LMN Pudendal or sympathetic nerves:

Detrusor — present

Sphincter — absent

This is thought to be the site of the lesion in hormonally responsive incontinence, seen usually in neutered animals. The sphincter is usually only intermittently incompetent and subject to leakage only under emotional stress or high abdominal or intravesicular pressures. The animal is otherwise continent and the residual volume is normal. Manual expression is relatively easy and the anal reflex may be depressed or absent in some cases.

Oestrogen or testosterone therapy may be employed, or an adenergic drug may be of value.

FeLV-associated urinary incontinence in cats falls into this category. The lesion in this instance is thought to involve the pelvic ganglia, it is unfortunately not normally responsive to hormone supplementation (see below).

VI. LMN failure of detrusor neuromuscular and muscular function:

Detrusor — absent

Sphincter — normal

This is either due to functional urethral obstruction, for example a calculus, or to some idiopathic cause. The result is bladder over-distension. This may cause the tight junctions of the detrusor smooth muscle to be damaged. The animal is unable to empty its bladder and is incontinent with overflow. It is, however, aware of bladder filling as sensory function remains, and so makes attempts to void. Voiding does not occur, although manual expression can usually be achieved. The anal reflex is usually intact.

An indwelling catheter for several days, together with *bethanecol*, are suggested as therapy. After catheter removal, an adrenergic blocker may aid voiding.

SPECIFIC CONDITIONS ASSOCIATED WITH URINARY INCONTINENCE

Urinary incontinence in FeLV-positive cats — has been described in a series of nine of eleven incontinent cats. The other two, although not FeLV tested, had also shown fecundity problems highly suggestive of FeLV infection (Barsanti & Downey, 1984). Six of these cats also showed anisocoria and atonic pupils, a sign that has previously been associated with FeLV infection. Other problems in some of the cats included abortion, neonatal kitten death, anorexia and weight loss, intermittent hypersalivation and vomiting, third eyelid prolapse and anaemia. The incontinence was intermittent in nature, usually consisting of dribbling while recumbent, asleep or when excited. Urination was otherwise normal. Although this appears similar to hormonally responsive incontinence (see below), half of the female cats in the series were entire and the neutered males did not respond to testosterone. A hormonal aetiology also does not account for the anisocoria. The lesion is likely to be affecting the pelvic ganglia. This could be related to the ciliary ganglion lesion that has been suggested to account for the anisocoria (Barsanti & Downey, 1984).

Post mortem findings provided no explanation to the aetiology. In contrast to feline dysautonomia (FD), widespread signs of autonomic dysfunction were not recorded and the dysuria usually noted in FD is one of bladder atony. This was not a feature of the FeLV associated condition.

Feline dysautonomia (FD) — is covered more fully later in this chapter. The incidence of dysuria varies from 17−39 per cent and affected cats are usually FeLV negative. The urinary dysfunction is due to lack of motor innervation to the bladder and urethra from the parasympathetic, sympathetic and in some cases also the somatic (pudendal) centres. This resembles the incontinence seen in category IV above (such as with a sacral fracture) except that the visceral and somatic afferent nerves are much less severely affected in FD than following trauma. Therefore, most incontinent cats with FD are aware of bladder filling and make repeated attempts to void by abdominal muscle contraction. Due to an absent detrusor reflex, the residual volume is high and lack of sphincter function renders manual expression easy in most cases. Combinations of *bethanecol* and *phenoxybenzamine* may aid affected animals, but the most useful treatment is frequent, careful manual expression of the bladder to avoid damage to the tight junctions, combined with nursing care to prevent urine scalding.

TREATMENT OF INCONTINENCE

Overdistension of the bladder can lead to permanent damage by disrupting the tight junctions of the detrusor muscle and causing subsequent fibrosis. It is imperative that this is **never** allowed to occur. Incontinent animals with elevated residual volumes are also prone to severe and even potentially life-threatening urinary tract infections. The aim should be to completely empty the bladder at least **three and preferably four** times daily. With manual evacuation, it is prudent to check the efficiency of expression by catheterisation at the end of the procedure. If expression stimulates voiding, which then results in complete emptying, this may identify a return of urinary voluntary control by the patient. However, manual expression may further damage a bladder where the detrusor has already been excessively stretched, and may be difficult or dangerous where sphincter pressure is high. Although some cases with raised sphincter pressure may be manageable with pharmacologic blockade and manual expression, catheterisation is usually preferable.

Intermittent aseptic catheterisation is the method of choice in most instances where manual expression is not possible, or is undesirable. If an indwelling catheter is used, it should only be used for one or two days and be connected to a closed system made from an old sterile IV set and empty IV drip bag. This technique is preferable, at least initially, in the management of females with detrusor damage caused by previous overdistension. The risk of ascending infection is outweighed by the atraumatic decompression provided by the indwelling catheter. In males, intermittent catheterisation is preferable. An indwelling catheter is very likely to introduce infection if maintained for more than one or two days. Use of antibiotics in such a case would only select for a resistant strain of bacteria and would not eliminate the infection. Careful manual evacuation should be continued after removal of the catheter in females, or if preferred, intermittent aseptic catheterisation can be substituted.

The presence of infection should be monitored by regular urinalysis and, where indicated, urine culture. Antibiotic therapy, if necessary, should be used for an adequate duration (14 days) in order to completely eliminate the infection. Antibiotic prophylaxis is not warranted and under no circumstances should it replace proper nursing care. Rigid attention to nursing in order to prevent urine scalding by the use of proper bedding materials, regular bathing, drying and application of emollients and/or petroleum jelly, should be performed three or four times daily.

PHARMACOLOGICAL MANIPULATION OF MICTURITION REFLEXES

The types of drugs commonly employed are shown in Table 12.2. As can be seen in Figure 12.1. the main neural control of the bladder is mediated by:

— ß adrenergic sympathetic relaxation of the detrusor muscle.

— Acetylcholine-induced (muscarinic) parasympathetic stimulation of the detrusor muscle.

— α adrenergic sympathetic stimulation of the smooth muscle internal urethral sphincter.

— Acetylcholine-induced (nicotinic) somatic stimulation of the striated muscle external urethral sphincter.

DRUG TREATMENT OF NEUROGENIC INCONTINENCE

α **blocking agent — Phenoxybenzamine —** This will block the α adrenergic sympathetic stimulation of urethral smooth muscle, and therefore help reduce sphincter tone. The suggested dose is 0.5 mg/kg b.i.d or t.i.d. Potential side effects include hypotension.

Table 12.2
Drug Treatment of Urinary Abnormalities (for explanation of categories see Table 12.1)

Category	Drug	Action	Comment
I			Dependent on type of abnormality displayed
II	α blocker/MR	Sphincter (S) or (ES) −	Used only if sphincter tone is increased
III	α blocker/MR	Sphincter (S) or (ES) −	
IV	MR	Sphincter (ES) −	Blockade of (S) alone usually is disappointing.
V	Hormonal therapy or α agonist	Sphincter (S) + +	
VI	Parasympathetic stimulant	Detrusor + +	

(S)	=	smooth muscle sphincter	+ + =	to stimulate
(ES)	=	skeletal muscle or external sphincter	MR =	skeletal muscle relaxant
−	=	to inhibit		

Skeletal muscle relaxant — Dantrolene — This relaxes the striated muscle external urethral sphincter and so helps to reduce overall sphincter tone. The suggested dose in dogs is 1 — 5 mg t.i.d. The starting dose in cats is suggested at 0.5 mg/kg b.i.d. gradually increasing to 2mg/kg b.i.d. This drug can cause hepatic enzyme elevation in humans. Other drugs that may have value are *diazepam* (2 — 10 mg t.i.d.), *methocarbamol* or *acepromazine*. Overdose of these may result in weakness or tranquillisation.

Hormonal therapy Diethylstilboestroel — Oestrogens act by facilitating α adrenergic receptor function, and so increase sphincter tone. This may prove of value in some bitches, although side effects of signs of oestrus or bone marrow suppression should be monitored. The suggested dose is 0.1 — 1mg for 3 — 5 days, then 1mg/week.

Oestrodiol cypionate — Is a more powerful oestrogen than *diethylstilboestroel* with a higher potential risk of oestrogenic side effects. The suggested dose is 0.1 — 1mg parenterally at intervals of weeks to months depending on response.

Testosterone — As *depotestosterone cypinate* this should be used at 2.2mg/kg parenterally at intervals of weeks or months depending on response. It should be used with care where perianal adenomas or prostatic disease are present.

α Stimulation — Phenylpropanolamine — This drug acts to increase tone in the urethral smooth muscle. The suggested dose is 12.5 — 50mg t.i.d. Potential side effects are urinary retention, anorexia and systemic sympathetic stimulation.

Parasympathetic stimulation — Bethanecol — This is the most effective drug to selectively stimulate the detrusor muscle. The suggested dose is 2.5 — 10mg t.i.d. subcutaneously or 2 — 15mg t.i.d. orally. General stimulation of the parasympathetic nervous system can occur with overdose. This can be countered with *atropine*.

NEURAL DISTURBANCES OF DEFAECATION

The innervation of the colon and rectum is derived from the sympathetic and parasympathetic nervous system in a similar manner to that of the bladder. However, the intrinsic neurons in the myenteric plexus of the gastrointestinal tract also play an important role in maintaining motility. The colon and rectum therefore appear to be less dependent on higher control in order to empty themselves. Even long term denervation at either the sacral level or higher often causes suprisingly few associated problems. Presumably, this is due to the fact that periodic incomplete emptying and elevated residual volume are not as deleterious as they are in the denervated bladder.

MEGACOLON — is defined as an enlarged colon where there is abnormal retention of contents. It is divided into two categories, congenital and acquired.

Congenital Megacolon — has not been documented to date in dogs or cats. It is described in humans, horses and mice. It results when a portion of foetal colon is not innervated by ganglion cells during their migration from the neural crests (Hirshchsprung's disease) (Hultgren, 1982). The affected colon remains permanently contracted, causing obstruction to the normal passage of faeces and dilation of the proximal portions of colon.

Acquired Megacolon — occurs most often in cats where prolonged distension of the colon or rectum results from obstruction. This could be due to an inflammatory or neoplastic stricture, pelvic canal narrowing following a pelvic fracture, or possibly when loss of neurones results from an active colonic inflammation (such as an Chagas disease in humans). The cause in cats, however, often seems to be idiopathic.

FELINE DYSAUTONOMIA — constipation is a common feature in this disorder and presumably relates to the general reduction in autonomic tone and to the loss of intrinsic gut neurones. Dehydration may be an important contributory factor.

DAMAGE TO THE SPINAL CORD OR CAUDA EQUINA — Animals with lesions at the thoracic or lumbar area tend to develop reflex emptying, often in response to tactile stimulation of the pelvic or perineal area. Although this 'reflex' is less obvious in animals with sacrococcygeal fractures, most cats reported with this injury can be managed by dietary means alone.

Treatment

The colon and the rectum appear able to spontaneously empty after denervation, nevertheless it is important to monitor defaecation and to prevent any excessive dilation.

To ensure adequate fluid balance, canned foods together with a stool softener such as Isogel (Allen & Hanbury) or bran, are used to give a bulky yet soft stool. Liquid paraffin may aid lubrication of dry faeces while enemas may relieve any periodic blockage. If blockage is severe, gentle manual evacuation under general anaesthesia may be required and in exceptional cases, a colotomy may prove necessary. Periodic manual evacuation is much less satisfactory than prevention of the problem. In recurrent constipation, reassessment of the diet should be made.

Hirschsprung's disease should respond to resection of the aganglionic section of the bowel. In acquired megacolon, removal of the obstruction, e.g. correction of prostatomegaly or reduction of a pelvic fracture, should improve the situation. Cats with idiopathic megacolon (where no cause can be identified) often respond well to subtotal colectomy. In feline dysautonomia, constipation can usually be managed by dietary therapy together with Danthron (Riker Laboratories) if necessary. This is a combined laxative and parasympathomimetic and is the best drug for use in stimulating defaecation. The only dose recommended is for cats with feline dysautonomia where 2 to 5 ml of a 5mg/ml solution are given daily.

DYSAUTONOMIA

GENERAL INTRODUCTION

Dysautonomias are important disorders in man but are usually encountered as complications of more widespread conditions such as amyloidosis, diabetes mellitus and the polyneuropathy of Landry-Guillian-Barré disease. Similar associations with these conditions or their counterparts in dogs or cats have not as yet been recorded.

The localised dysautonomia of Horner's syndrome is well recognised in animals. The aganglionic segment of bowel known as Hirschsprung's disease has been documented in man, the horse and mouse, but not in the dog or cat. Similar localised sympathetic disturbance is seen following brachial plexus avulsion or dorsolateral cervical disc explosions where vasomotor tone to a limb or limbs is lost, resulting in profound vasodilation and up to a 10°C increase in limb(s) temperature. After several weeks the limb is likely to become subnormal in temperature due to vascular pooling which becomes the predominant effect.

FELINE DYSAUTONOMIA

Key and Gaskell in 1982 were the first to draw attention to this fascinating clinical entity. In retrospect it appears that the first cases were seen simultaneously in both Scotland and England in late 1981. It is thought that the condition had not occurred prior to that time, at least in its current form, but this can not be proven. Disease incidence reached almost epidemic proportions in the summer and autumn of 1982 and again in 1983, with an apparent decline in the intervening period. Since 1984 the condition has been termed feline dysautonomia. At present it appears to be less common than in previous years and there is evidence to suggest that its clinical severity has also lessened (Baxter and Gruffydd Jones, 1987).

The pathophysiology and underlying pathological changes appear almost identical to the few sporadic cases of canine dysautonomia and to grass sickness of horses. This equine dysautonomia is widely recognised in the United Kingdom and to a lesser extent in other European countries.

Although the vast majority of confirmed cases have been reported from the United Kingdom, feline dysautonomia has been recognised in Norway and Sweden. Isolated cases have also been documented from the United States of America and the United Arab Emirates. There is no sex or breed distribution. Animals less than three years of age appear to be more susceptible but a wide age range from 6 weeks to 11 years has been recorded (Waltham Symposium, 1987).

Epidemiology

There have been several instances of siblings in the same household being affected. However, in households with several unrelated cats, cases tend to be isolated. Three of five kittens in one litter were affected and six of seven in another with the dams and other kittens remaining in good health. Direct contagion is not supported by epidemiological studies and no common environmental or managemental factor has been identified.

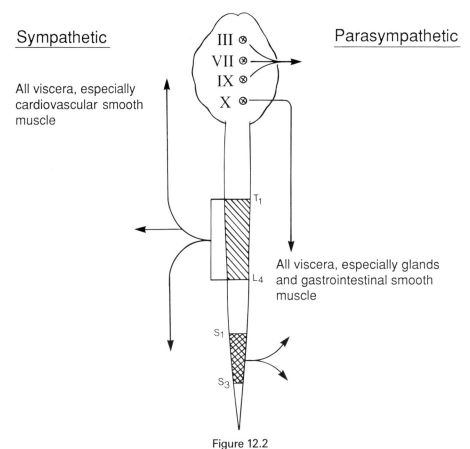

Figure 12.2
Diagram to show the origins and distributions of the sympathetic and parasympathetic divisions of the autonomic nervous system

Aetiopathogenesis

This remains unknown although a toxic or viral agent cannot be ruled out. Whatever the causal factor, it appears to have a primary effect on the pathways for protein biosynthesis in affected neurones. There is no evidence that a particular neurotransmitter is selectively inhibited and, furthermore, pharmocological studies have demonstrated that the receptors in tissues denervated by this condition are still functional (Waltham Symposium, 1987).

The autonomic nervous system provides motor innervation to visceral smooth muscle, cardiac muscle and glands (Figure 12.2). Its counterpart is the somatic nervous system which is motor to skeletal muscle. Clinical signs reflect dysfunction of both the sympathetic (e.g. third eyelid prolaspse, bradycardia) and parasympathetic (lack of ocular, nasal and oral secretions) divisions of the autonomic nervous system. Non-autonomic deficits referable to the somatic nervous system are also seen to a lesser extent (e.g. anal areflexia, hindlimb proprioceptive deficits).

Clinical Features

Onset of disease varies in rapidity from a few hours to several weeks. Some cats show prodromal signs of either mild upper respiratory or gastrointestinal irritation, or possibly autonomic hyperactivity manifest by serous oculonasal discharge and/or diarrhoea.

As can be seen from Figure 12.3, dilated pupils, oesophageal dysfunction, dry nose, reduced lacrimal secretions, prolapse of the third eyelid, regurgitation and constipation were seen in over 75 per cent of the 86 cases documented prior to 1984 (Rochlitz, 1984; Sharp *et al*, 1984). The clinical severity now seems to have lessened, with each of these features being seen in less than 60% of more recently affected cats. The one clinical feature that appears to have increased in frequency is dysuria (Baxter and Grufydd Jones, 1987).

Some cats with feline dysautonomia have been noted to go into a state of collapse lasting for 10−20 seconds. This was found to occur following sudden movement, such as being lifted from a basket onto the examination table. This is very likely to be a manifestation of orthostatic hypotension, which is the most common feature of dysautonomia in man. It occurs due to a lack of sympathetic vascular tone and subsequent failure to accommodate to sudden changes in body position. The result is a transient but profound fall in blood pressure and 'fainting'. The low resting blood pressure seen in affected cats, and lack of hypertensive response following the administration of an indirect acting sympathomimetic agent *(tyramine)* support this explanation (Waltham Symposium, 1987).

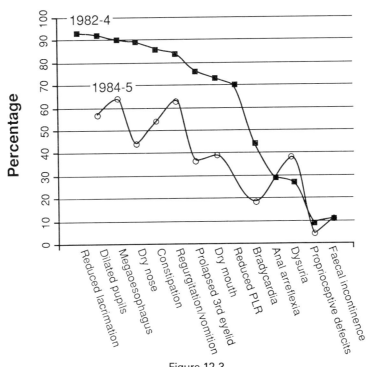

Figure 12.3
Graph to show the percentage incidence of clinical signs recorded for feline dysautonomia in 1982-4, as compared to 1984-5.

Diagnosis

Initially, diagnosis was based on the unusual combination of clinical features seen in this condition. However, in less severely affected cats, such as those encountered more recently, an objective means of diagnosis may be required.

One possible system is proposed in Table 12.3. A scoring system for the various clinical signs that are commonly associated with feline dysautonomia has been developed. The clinical features have been divided into two groups: group A consists of features that are either objective or frequently encountered in feline dysautonomia, but are otherwise uncommon in the cat; features in group B are less frequently encountered in the condition or more liable to be associated with other disorders. In combination, however, the features in group B would be very suggestive of feline dysautonomia. Using this system, the criteria necessary for a positive clinical diagnosis of feline dysautonomia are a total score of nine or more (grades 3 or 4). In the absence of another lesion to explain the clinical signs, such as a compressive lesion of the cauda equina (features 6, 7, 10 and 11), a score of five to eight (grade 2) gives a probable diagnosis on clinical grounds. A score of between one and four gives an inconclusive diagnosis on clinical grounds. Furthermore, this system allows the severity of the disease in individual cases to be characterised according to their overall grade from Grade 1 (mild) to Grade 4 (severe). Definitive diagnosis for feline dysautonomia at present requires histopathological confirmation of the pathognomonic lesions seen in autonomic ganglia.

Table 12.3
Grading System for Feline Dysautonomia

		Score
Group A — Clinical Features		
1.	Dry, crusty nose	2
2.	Reduced tear secretion (< 5mm/min) using Schirmer tear strip	2
3.	Mydriasis or reduced pupillary light response	2
4.	Bradycardia <120 beats/min	2
5.	Regurgitation with oesophageal dysfunction on contrast radiography	2
Group B — Clinical Features		
6.	Constipation	1
7.	Proprioceptive deficits	1
8.	Dry oral mucosae	1
9.	Prolapsed membrana nictitans	1
10.	Dysuria or bladder atony	1
11.	Anal arreflexia	1
	Maximum	16

Score	Clinical Grade	Clinical Diagnosis
1 — 4	1	Inconclusive
5 — 8	2	Probable
9 — 12	3	Positive
13 — 16	4	Positive

In equivocal cases the most objective criteria are contrast radiography of the oesophagus and the presence of reduced lacrimal secretions. The latter is assessed using the Schirmer tear strip which is left in the lacrimal sac for 60 seconds and the column of tear staining above the notch is measured in millimetres. Normal values are between 10 and 20 millimetres per minute. A reading below 5 millimetres is considered diagnostic. Oesophageal dilation affects primarily the intrathoracic portion of the oesophagus as can be demonstrated by plain radiography and/or by contrast studies. In some cats dysfunction is mild and restricted to retention of a small pool or bolus of contrast agent beyond five minutes following its oral administration. In other animals, contrast may be retained for over 24 hours and dysfunction of the cervical oesophagus may also be seen. Aspiration pneumonia may also be detected on thoracic radiography. A number of cats show evidence of delayed gastric emptying on barium contrast study. Small intestinal transit time is variable and may either be increased, normal or decreased. Distention of the urinary bladder or subjective evidence of constipation may also be demonstrated on abdominal radiography.

218

Further evaluation by pharmacological testing may be utilised in certain instances. *Atropine* will fail to produce a reflex tachycardia if the heart lacks sympathetic tone. However, mildly affected cats are likely to have partial autonomic drive to the heart rendering results sometimes equivocal. *Atropine* will also exacerbate any parasympathetic dysfunction such as dry mucous membranes or gastrointestinal paralysis, which may be undesirable.

The phenomenon of denervation hypersensitivity can also aid diagnosis (Canton & Sharp, 1988). Any target organ will become supersensitive to its physiological transmitter substance if it is deprived of that transmitter due to partial or complete denervation. Two ocular pharmacological tests based on the presence of denervation hypersensitivity have been utilised. In feline dysautonomia, ciliary smooth muscle frequently becomes supersensitive to acetylcholine due to the parasympathetic denervation. A 0.1% solution of *pilocarpine*, which mimics acetylcholine's muscarinic action, is applied to the cornea. The ciliary muscle should respond by causing miosis within 10 or 15 minutes. This concentration will have no effect in a normally innervated eye. Abrasion of the cornea (even by use of a Schirmer tear strip in the previous few days) may in some instances allow increased uptake of *pilocarpine* so that normally innervated ciliary muscle will respond. However, this response is not usually as rapid in onset, profound or sustained as in a denervated eye. For comparison the technique should be employed at the same time in a control cat. An occasional side effect of this drug is marked chemosis (oedema of the conjunctiva) which can be very distressing to the cat and owner, but usually reverses within 24 hours and responds well to topical corticosteriod and/or local anaesthetic. The events in denervation sensitivity of the ciliary muscle are directly analogous to the response of skeletal muscle to denervation.

The other ocular structure that can be evaluated by using this phenomenon is the prolapsed third eyelid. Unless denervated, this will not normally retract in response to a 1:10,000 solution of *epinephrine*. If too strong a solution is used it will cause some change to the position of the third eyelid of a normal cat, which should again be used as a control. Even the dilute solution should be used with care in a clinical case of feline dysautonomia. If an excess of drug is administered, it may be absorbed and in theory the hypersensitivity could be manifest in the cardiac nerves with possibly fatal results.

Differential diagnosis

A cat with cauda equina lesions, shock and dehydration due to either sacral fracture following a road traffic accident, or a cat with neurological disease due to FIP, might demonstrate some of the features of feline dysautonomia. These may include urinary retention, faecal incontinence, constipation, anal areflexia, proprioceptive hindlimb deficits and possibly prolapsed third eyelids. However, such a cat should not show any features in Group A (Table 12.3) and further evaluation should define the true cause of the clinical signs.

Feline leukaemia virus associated tonic pupils, which may be accompanied by a urinary incontinence, appears to be a distinct clinical entity and can be differentiated on several counts. There is no specific association of feline dysautonomia with FeLV. The FeLV-associated urinary incontinence is mild and consists of leakage during sleep with otherwise normal bladder emptying, whereas in feline dysautonomia there is usually marked bladder atony. Finally, the pupils in feline dysautonomia are fixed while in FeLV associated anisocoria they usually undergo a rapid spontaneous change in diameter over a short period of time.

Treatment

In the initial stages some severely affected cats will be hypoglycaemic and hypovolaemic with electrolyte disturbances which must be corrected by intravenous fluid therapy. *Metaclopramide* has been documented to improve gastric emptying and may therefore reduce vomition. Regurgitation should be countered by initial, and if necessary, periodic aspiration of oesophageal contents by oral or nasogastric intubation. This should lessen the risk of aspiration occurring. Total parenteral nutrition was used successfully in the short term management of one severely affected cat that could not tolerate any other means of feeding (Canton & Sharp, 1988).

External provision of heat is important as thermoregulation is disturbed in dysautonomia. Steam inhalation is reported to aid the lack of oronasal and lacrimal secretions. Gentle glycerol and liquid paraffin enemas to counter constipation are helpful, and cleansing of the perineal area combined with general grooming improves the cat's general demeanour. Manual evacuation of an atonic bladder is vital, even though dysautonomic cats may be seen to squat and make frequent attempts to pass small amounts of urine. If there is any evidence of respiratory or urinary tract infection, antibiotics should be administered.

After initial stabilisation, feeding by nasogastric intubation or via a gastrostomy feeding tube is preferable to oral intake in cats with marked oesophageal dysfunction. In severe cases, the bulk of an orally administered meal is retained and can cause oesophageal distention severe enough to provoke dyspnoea. Food given by tube needs to be liquidised and a small amount of Isogel bulk laxative should be mixed in. If gastric contents are vomited, *metaclopramide* may again prove valuable.

The technique for percutaneous gastrostomy intubation works well, but does require an endoscope (Matthews & Binnington, 1986). The cat must be anaesthetised to perform this proceedure, but once the tube is in place it can be managed successfully for months. Nasogastric intubation, following local anaesthetic spraying of the nares, is also well tolerated (Rochlitz, 1984). Pharyngostomy intubation has been unsuccessful in most cases (Sharp *et al*, 1984). The general lack of success with this technique may be a result of it causing a reflux into the flaccid oesophagus, or it may be that the few cats evaluated had poor gastric emptying. In one cat where gastric emptying was documented to be good, pharyngostomy did prove to be successful.

Once the cat has been stabilised on one of these feeding regimes, oral intake of food can be attempted, starting with aromatic meals. This will be aided by postural management such as by nursing the cat after feeding in an upright position for as long as possible. Corticosteroids or progestagens can be tried as short term appetite stimulants, although long term they are catabolic. Anabolic steroids can be used longer term and *diazepam* 2 mg orally immediately prior to feeding can be a successful appetite stimulant. Regular attention to bladder evacuation, and management of defaecation and hydration status are vital and much of the longer term nursing must be performed by the owner.

Adequate counselling of the owner regarding the amount of effort they will need to provide, likely length of the recovery period and the failure and complication rates are vital at the time of initial diagnosis so that a rational decision may be reached.

Early attempts at therapy included the use of various autonomic stimulants. Some of these, such as *pilocarpine* 1% or *physostigmine* 0.5% eye drops, may aid oronasal and lacrimal secretion and the latter given 20 minutes before feeding is also said to stimulate oesophageal function. However, these drugs can induce both muscarinic and nicotinic side effects such as abdominal cramps and muscular fasciculations. *Bethanecol* (total daily dose 2.5 mg and up to 7.5 mg, divided b.i.d. or t.i.d.), may promote useful glandular, bowel and bladder function but these drugs should not be used together. As well as the effects of overdose, in certain cats the phenomenon of denervation hypersensitivity could cause problems. Evidence to support this was seen in one cat in which *bethanecol* induced a profound bradycardia with arrhythmia.

Danthron poses less of a problem when combined with other parasympathomimetics and is used at 1—5 ml of a 5mg/ml solution orally per day.

Metoclopramide is a dopamine antagonist which has been documented to show fluoroscopic improvement in gastric emptying in dysautonomia. The dose used was 0.1 mg/kg IV and there would seem to be grounds to continue use of this drug either by parenteral or oral route. This dose needs to be further refined because, in man and in the horse, CNS side effects (excitation) are seen as the drug can cross the blood brain barrier. However, its potential benefits to gastric feeding of a cat with ileus are obvious.

Histopathology

This feature has been well described elsewhere (Sharp *et al*, 1984; Griffiths *et al*, 1985). Both sympathetic and parasympathetic divisions of the autonomic nervous system are equally affected. Although most severe at the postganglionic level, preganglionic neurones are also affected. Several nonautonomic neurones also degenerate to a much lesser degree including those in the nucleus ambiguus, oculomotor, trigeminal, facial and hypoglossal nuclei, and also ventral horn cells and dorsal root ganglion cells at the spinal level. The severity of the dysautonomia would appear to be proportional to the degree of neuronal dropout. One month after onset of the disease, all affected neurones have disappeared. The ganglion is occupied by the surviving neurones which are normal in appearance, and by an increased number of satellite cells and fibrous tissue in the supporting stroma.

There is no known aetiology that has a similar, relatively selective effect on autonomia neurones. At present the light and electron microscopic appearance of affected neurones is pathognomic for feline, canine and equine dysotonomia.

Prognosis

The grading system in Table 12.3 can also be used to gain some prognostic information. In general cats with Grade 3 or 4 clinical signs have a worse prognosis than those with grades 1 or 2. This is borne out by the improvement in prognosis (50 per cent survival) for cats seen in the last few years (Baxter & Gruffydd Jones, 1987). In general these cats appear less severely affected compared to those seen in the first two years of the epidemic (20 or 30 per cent survival) (Sharp *et al* 1984).

However, several cats of grade 4 severity have survived long term. They often show residual signs such as dilated pupils, low body weight and occasional regurgitation. These animals are likely to be less tolerant of severe stress. One cat recovered well from a grade 4 presentation, but at 5 months went into a profound state of cardiovascular and physiological collapse following a routine radiological examination, and died within two hours (Canton and Sharp, 1988). Cats have occasionally developed more unusual neurological signs after apparent recovery. Some mildly affected cases of grade 1 or 2 have made good progress but then developed faecal incontinence necessitating their euthanasia as late as nine months after the initial onset of illness.

Canine dysautonomia

Five cases have been described to date from both the United Kingdom and from Norway (Pollen & Sullivan, 1984; Presthus & Bjerkas, 1987). Dysuria seems to be a common feature, occurring in each dog together with a loss of the anal reflex. Four of the dogs showed decreased tear production, and regurgitation associated with oesophageal dysfunction was noted in all five dogs. The clinical picture was very reminiscent of feline dysautonomia and the histopathology in each case showed identical changes to the feline disorder. This condition has also recently been reported in the United States.

REFERENCES

BARSANTI,J.A. and DOWNEY,R. (1984). Urinary incontinence in cats. *Journal of the American Animal Hospital Association,* **20,** 979.

BAXTER,A. and GRUFFYDD-JONES,T. (1987). Feline dysautonomia. *In Practice,* **9,**58.

CANTON,D.D. and SHARP,N.J.H. (1984). Feline dysautonomia: a case report and literature review. *Journal of the American Veterinary Medical Association,* **192,** 1293.

GRIFFITHS,I.R., SHARP,N.J.H. and McCULLOCH,M.C. (1985). Feline dysautonomia (the Key Gaskell syndrome): an ultrastructural study of autonomic ganglia and nerves. *Neuropathology and Applied Neurobiology,* **11,** 17.

HOLT,P.E. (1983). Urinary incontinence in the dog. *In Practice,* **5,** 162.

HULTGREN,B.D. (1982). Ileocolonic aganglionosis in white progeny of overo spotted horses. *Journal of the American Veterinary Medical Association,* **180,** 289.

KEY,T. and GASKELL,C.J. (1982). (Correspondence). *Veterinary Record,* **110,** 160.

LEES, G.E. and OSBORNE, C.A. (1983). Use and misuse of intermittant and indwelling urinary catheters. In *Current Veterinary Therapy VIII.* (Ed. R.W. Kirk) W.B. Saunders Co., Philadelphia.

MATTHEWS, K.A. and BINNINGTON,A.G. (1986). Percutaneous incision-less placement of a gastrotomy tube utilising a gastroscope: preliminary observations. *Journal of the American Animal Hospital Association,* **22,** 601.

MICHELL,A.R. (1984). Ins and outs of bladder function. *Journal of Small Animal Practice,* **25,** 237.

MOISE,N.S. and FLANDERS,J.A. (1983). Micturition disorders in cats with sacrocaudal vertebral lesions. In *Current Therapy VIII* (Ed. R. Kirk) W.B. Saunders Co., Philadelphia.

MOREAU,P.M. (1982). Neurogenic disorders of micturition in the dog and cat. *Compendium of Continuing Education,* **4,** 12.

OLIVER,J.E. (1987). Disorders of micturition. In *Veterinary Neurology.* (Eds. J.E. Oliver, B.F. Hoerlein, and I.G. Mayhew). W.B. Saunders Co., Philadelphia.

OLIVER,J.E. and LORENZ,M.D. (1983). *Handbook of Veterinary Neurologic Diagnosis.* W.B. Saunders Co., Philadelphia.

POLLEN,M. and SULLIVAN,M. (1986). A canine dysautonomia resembling the Key Gaskell syndrome. *Veterinary Record,* **118,** 402.

PRESTHUS,J. and BJERKAS,I. (1987). Canine dysautonomia in Norway. *Veterinary Record,* **120,** 463.

ROCHLITZ,I. (1984). Feline dysautonomia (the Key Gaskell or dilated pupil syndrome): a preliminary review. *Journal of Small Animal Practice,* **25,** 587.

SHARP,N.J.H., NASH,A.S. and GRIFFITHS,I.R. (1984). Feline dysautonomia (the Key Gaskell syndrome): a clinical and pathological study of 40 cases. *Journal of Small Animal Practice,* **25,** 599.

WALTHAM SYMPOSIUM (1987). Feline dysautonomia. *Journal of Small Animal Practice,* **28,** 333.

CHAPTER 13

EPISODIC WEAKNESS

Michael E. Herrtage M.A., B.V.Sc., D.V.R., D.V.D., M.R.C.V.S.
Rosemary E. McKerrell, M.A., Vet.M.B., M.R.C.V.S.

Many neurological disorders may be episodic in nature, for example, seizures in idiopathic epilepsy, and recurrent paraparesis in thoracolumbar disc disease. These are, in the main, well recognised entities and are covered elsewhere in this Manual. There are a number of conditions, however, less well defined, which may show episodic weakness, neurological deficits or behavioural disturbances. This chapter aims to assist the clinician in the differential diagnosis of this group of disorders.

Episodic weakness is a prominent clinical sign in a large variety of diseases. It can be defined as a waxing and waning weakness interspersed with periods of apparent normality. The degree of weakness may vary from mild hindlimb ataxia to total collapse or syncope. Syncope or fainting is defined as a sudden, brief loss of consciousness. It is caused by a temporary lapse in cerebral function, usually as a result of reduced cerebral blood flow, inadequate oxygen delivery or inadequate glucose availability. Syncopal episodes are most frequently seen with cardiovascular, respiratory, metabolic or endocrine abnormalities. The same pathophysiological mechanisms may cause episodic hindlimb weakness or ataxia, but other conditions, for example, neuromuscular disorders, can also produce these clinical signs.

Primary neurological disorders, for example seizures, may cause syncopal-like signs and these require careful investigation in order to differentiate them from true syncope. A seizure, which is a period of abnormal behaviour caused by sudden, abnormal and excessive electrical discharge from the brain, frequently occurs in three stages; the prodromal phase (aura), the actual seizure or ictal phase and the post-ictal phase. This latter phase can sometimes be particularly difficult to differentiate from other causes of episodic weakness or syncope. In general, however, there are no prodromal signs and few post-ictal repercussions with other causes of episodic weakness or syncope. A detailed discussion of seizures can be found in Chapter 7 and only the major differential points will be mentioned in this chapter.

The differential diagnosis of episodic weakness presents a major diagnostic challenge to the clinician. Most of the animals are normal when they are initially presented to the veterinarian, thus meticulous attention to the information contained in the signalment, history and physical examination is important. Access to routine and sometimes specialized diagnostic aids is usually necessary to confirm a diagnosis.

DIAGNOSTIC APPROACH

A list of some of the conditions that may be associated with episodic weakness is presented in Table 13.1. The differential diagnosis is extensive and thus a logical and thorough investigation is essential if a diagnosis is to be made. A sequential diagnostic approach is given in Figure 13.1.

SIGNALMENT

Certain breeds are associated with diseases which cause episodic weakness (Table 13.1, see also Appendix). However, some breeds are associated with more than one condition and the association is by no means exclusive. Age and sex may limit the diagnostic possibilities or increase the index of suspicion in certain conditions.

Table 13.1
Differential Diagnosis of Episodic Weakness

Cardiovascular disorders

Bradyarrhythmia
Tachyarrhythmia
Congenital heart disease eg. aortic or pulmonic stenosis, tetralogy of Fallot, reverse shunting PDA
Acquired heart disease eg. valvular, myocardial, pericardial
Heartworm disease (Dirofilariasis, Angiostrongylosis)
Vasovagal syncope
Vasodilation
(Aortic) thromboembolism

Respiratory disorders

Laryngeal paralysis
URT obstruction especially brachycephalic breeds
Tracheal collapse
Severe coughing
Filaroides osleri
Pulmonary disease
Pleural effusions
Thoracic masses

Haematological disorders

Anaemia — regenerative eg. ruptured splenic
              haemangiosarcoma
              non-regenerative
Myeloproliferative disorders
Polycythaemia
Haemoglobinopathies
Pyrexia of unknown origin

Orthopaedic disorders

Degenerative joint disease particularly hips or stifles
Polyarthritis — various types

Neurological disorders

Congenital or acquired spinal disorders including Wobbler syndrome
Epilepsy (various causes)
Vestibular disease
Cerebellar disorders
Thiamine deficiency
Congenital disorders eg. hydrocephalus
Acquired disorders eg. old dog encephalitis, CVA, tumours
Lysosomal storage diseases
Giant axonal neuropathy

Neurological disorders — continued

Progressive axonopathy — boxer
Tetanus
Botulism
Narcolepsy/cataplexy — Doberman pinscher, poodle, Labrador retriever
Generalised tremor
Jack Russell ataxia
Scottie cramp — also seen in the Norwich terrier, Dalamatian and Jack Russell terrier
Episodic falling in the Cavalier King Charles spaniel .

Neuromuscular disorders

Myasthenia gravis
Polymyositis
Hereditary myopathy of Laborador retrievers
Sex-linked myopathy in Irish terriers, golden retrievers
Myotonia in chow chows, Staffordshire terriers
Hypokalaemic polymyopathy
Ischaemic neuropathy due to thromboembolism
Malignant hyperthermia
Mitochondrial myopathies eg. pyruvate dehydrogenase deficiency
Azoturia (rhabdomyolysis)

Metabolic disorders

Hepatic encephalopathy — portosystemic shunts,
                                 cirrhosis
Uraemic encephalopathy
Hyperglycaemia
Hypoglycaemia
Hyponatraemia
Hyperkalaemia
Hypokalaemia
Hypercalcaemia
Hypocalcaemia
Acidosis
Hyperthermia (heatstroke)
Hypoxia
Shock

Endocrine disorders

Insulinoma
Hyperadrenocorticism (Cushing's disease) – myotonia
Hypoadrenocorticism (Addison's disease)
Hypoparathyroidism
Hypothyroidism
Phaeochromocytoma
Diabetic ketoacidosis

Figure 13.1   Sequential Diagnostic Approach

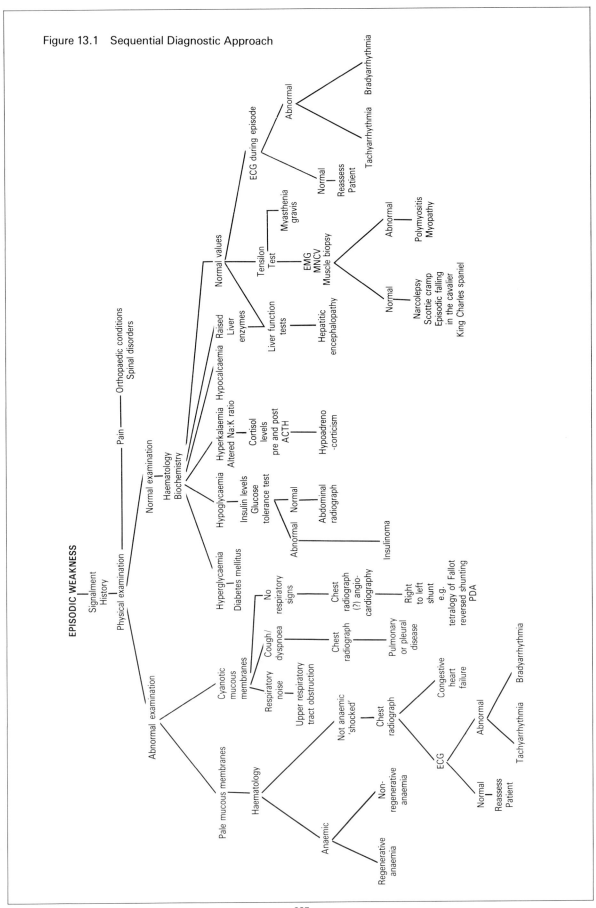

HISTORY

An accurate and detailed history is often critical to the eventual diagnostic success of a case. Questions concerning the episodes of weakness are of paramount importance, since the veterinarian may never actually witness an episode. Many observant owners can relate sufficient information to allow the clinician to reduce the number of possible differential diagnoses.

A detailed description of the episode should be gleaned from the information provided by asking the following questions:

How many episodes has the animal suffered?

Do the episodes follow a similar pattern?

Seizures and syncopal attacks tend to follow the same pattern on each occasion, whereas in most of the metabolic disorders, the clinical signs vary from episode to episode.

What time of the day do the episodes occur?

In idiopathic epilepsy, the seizures usually occur when the animal is at rest or on waking.

Are there any associations with the onset of an episode?

Weakness following excitement, exercise or stress is often associated with cardiovascular and neuromuscular disorders. The amount of exercise which causes weakness or collapse may be fairly constant and predictable as in myasthenia gravis or may be variable as in episodic falling in the Cavalier King Charles spaniel. Metabolic disorders are not usually associated with exertion.

There may be a relationship to feeding. In hypoglycemia, episodes occur either after fasting or just after eating. Feeding may also precipitate signs of hepatic encephalopathy, particularly if the food has a high protein content.

Seizures are often preceded by a prodromal phase (aura) which is characterized by a change in either behaviour (nervousness) or motor function (head turning or focal muscle twitching).

Does the animal lose consciousness?

With peripheral neuromuscular disorders, the animal will be totally aware of its surroundings and its eyes will tend to follow the owner. Animals with seizures, however, usually lose consciousness. Metabolic and endocrine disorders vary in severity but in cases severe enough to cause collapse, the animal will be depressed with occasional loss, or apparent loss, of consciousness. In cardiovascular disorders, the animal may be collapsed, dazed or unconscious.

What does the animal do during the actual episode?

The clinical expression of seizures varies depending on the area of the brain affected. Generalized motor seizures are usually characterised by symmetrical involvement of the entire body with tonic/clonic movements of the limbs and jaws, body tremor, loss of consciousness, salivation, tachypnoea, tachycardia, urination and defaecation. Syncope usually produces a flaccid collapse, although there may be vocalization, stiffening of the limbs and even urination, thus requiring careful differentiation from seizures. Syncope is not preceded by an aura nor followed by any unusual post-ictal behaviour.

Does the owner notice any change in the colour of the mucous membrane or in heart rate?

It may be necessary to ask the owner to check for these signs should the animal have another episode.

How long does an episode last?

Most episodes are brief. However, owners are understandably anxious and tend to overestimate the duration of an attack. Syncope usually lasts seconds to no more than a few minutes, whereas seizures often last one to five minutes. With metabolic or endocrine disorders, the animal may appear dazed, confused or weak for hours before slowly recovering. Patients with myasthenia gravis collapse on exercise, rest for a few minutes then appear to recover for a short time before collapsing again.

Is the animal normal afterwards?

The post-ictal phase of a seizure may vary from a few minutes to several days. Its length is not related to the severity or cause of the seizure. The animal may be depressed or overly excited, sleep or constantly pace and may be thirsty and/or hungry. The clinician may be misled if the owner misses the actual seizure and only observes the post-ictal phase when the animal is ataxic and weak. Enquire whether there was any sign of disturbance (eg. to bedding, furniture, etc.) or urination that might suggest a seizure.

From this information the clinician should be able to piece together a clear impression of the episode. Most animals appear normal between episodes but it is still important to ask about the general health of the patient. In hypoadrenocorticism, for example, the animal may show anorexia, weight loss, gastrointestinal upsets, polydipsia and polyuria even between bouts of weakness. In every case, information should be gained about appetite, thirst, urination, weight loss or in young animals failure to thrive, vomiting, diarrhoea and exercise tolerance.

PHYSICAL EXAMINATION

A complete physical examination including a full neurological assessment should be carried out in every case even if the clinician feels there are limited diagnostic possibilities. Animals with pain or discomfort due to orthopaedic or spinal conditions may be reluctant to move or incapable of walking normally and the owner may incorrectly assess this as weakness. Most of these animals will still be experiencing pain when they are presented for examination.

Clinical experience, history and physical examination may allow the clinician to differentiate or characterize the disorder so that only confirmation of the diagnosis is required. However, many cases of episodic weakness require careful and logical investigation to confirm the cause. This is particularly true when no abnormalities are found on physical examination. Further investigation will require some or all of the following examinations:

LABORATORY TESTS

Routine haematology and a biochemical profile including electrolytes, blood glucose, urea, liver enzymes (ALT, AP) and muscle enzymes (CPK, AST) should be considered the minimum data base. Interpretation of these results with respect to episodic weakness is given in Table 13.2. (Also, see Chapter 4).

In some cases the minimum data base will provide the diagnosis but in other selected cases further laboratory investigations are indicated.

Liver function tests — When hepatic encephalopathy is suspected, liver function tests should be performed. Bromsulphthalein (BSP) retention, bile acids and ammonia tolerance test have all proved useful in this regard.

Adrenocortical function tests — An ACTH stimulation test is necessary to confirm the diagnosis of hypoadrenocorticism. It is also a useful screening test for hyperadrenocorticism. The low-dose dexamethasone test has some advantages over ACTH stimulation in screening for hyperadrenocorticism, but it is not as useful in the detection of iatrogenic Cushing's disease and is affected by more variables. The high-dose dexamethasone test is used to differentiate adrenal-dependency from pituitary-dependency in hyperadrenocorticism if this has not already been determined.

Table 13.2
Interpretation of Laboratory Findings with
Respect to Episodic Weakness

HAEMATOLOGY

    Anaemia   —   regenerative
                      non-regenerative

    Polycythaemia

BIOCHEMISTRY

Blood urea	high	—	renal failure
			hypoadrenocorticism
	low	—	hepatic encephalopathy
			hyperadrenocorticism
Blood glucose	hyperglycaemia	—	diabetic ketoacidosis
			hyperadrenocorticism
	hypoglycaemia	—	insulinoma
			neonatal puppies
			toy and miniature breeds of dogs
			working/hunting dogs
			septicaemia
			nonpancreatic tumours (especially hepatocellular carcinomas)
			liver disease
			hypoadrenocorticism
			excess insulin therapy
Sodium	hyponatraemia	—	hypoadrenocorticism
Potassium	hyperkalaemia	—	hypoadrenocorticism
			acute renal failure
			diabetic ketoacidosis
			severe acidosis
	hypokalaemia	—	urinary loss (especially cats with hypokalaemic polymyopathy)
			severe vomiting and/or diarrhoea
			excessive fluid therapy
			insulin administration
Calcium	hypercalcaemia	—	hypoadrenocorticism
			primary renal failure
			certain malignancies
			lymphosarcoma
			anal gland adenocarcinoma
			bone metastases
			primary hyperparathyroidism
	hypocalcaemia	—	postparturient eclampsia
			hypoparathyroidism
			terminal renal failure
			protein-losing enteropathy
			severe alkalosis

Other hormone estimations — If hypothyroidism is suspected, a basal T4 level should be performed preferably followed by a TSH or TRH stimulation test. Insulin levels may be useful in cases of functional pancreatic islet cell tumour (insulinoma).

Immunological tests — In some of the immune-mediated disorders, immunological tests may provide useful information. For example, tests for antinuclear antibody (ANA) may be positive in cases of polymyositis and antibodies to acetylcholine receptors are diagnostic of acquired myasthenia gravis.

Blood gas and acid-base estimations — Blood gas analysis provides values for plasma pH, PCO_2 and PO_2 and these can be used to calculate bicarbonate and base excess levels. Arterial or venous blood samples can be used to evaluate PCO_2 and base excess levels, but oxygen levels are only meaningful on arterial samples. In cases of episodic weakness, pre- and post-exercise samples are usually required to aid the diagnosis. Blood gas analysis may be useful in obstructive pulmonary disease, upper respiratory tract obstruction, right to left cardiac shunts, diabetic ketoacidosis and mitochondrial myopathies.

Cerebrospinal fluid analysis — Examination of CSF is justified in most cases of seizures if an intracranial disorder is suspected.

RADIOLOGY

Thoracic radiographs are useful for ruling out significant cardiopulmonary disease. Particular attention should be paid to cardiac size and the clarity of the lung fields. If tracheal collapse is suspected, it will be seen on an inspiratory film in the cervical region but an expiratory film will be required if the tracheal collapse is intrathoracic.

Radiographs of the abdomen, spine, skull and limbs may be indicated from the findings of the physical examination.

Contrast studies may be required in selected cases, for example, angiocardiography, usually in combination with intracardiac pressures and blood gas estimations, is necessary for defining some congenital heart defects. Portal venography will identify the portosystemic shunts that cause hepatic encephalopathy and myelography may be required to rule out some spinal conditions.

Ultrasound and particularly echocardiography are useful for providing additional data in specific cases.

ELECTROCARDIOGRAPHY (ECG)

An ECG should be performed in all cases in which a cardiac cause is suspected. The rate and rhythm should be carefully assessed since conduction abnormalities and arrhythmias are a major cause of episodic weakness and syncope. When the arrhythmias are continuous, as in atrial fibrillation or third degree atrioventricular block, the diagnosis is relatively straightforward and may be made from one recording. However, certain types of arrhythmia, such as premature contractions, paroxysmal tachycardias or sinoatrial block, may be intermittent. In these cases a rhythm strip should be repeated after a vagal manoeuvre such as ocular pressure or carotid sinus massage and following exercise. Even so, the ECG is frequently normal in animals who have syncope associated with cardiac arrhythmias. In these cases 24-hour ECG monitoring is required using the Chiltern Box, Holter monitoring or in-hospital telemetry. Alternatively, adequate information regarding the arrhythmia may be obtained by simply teaching the owner how to monitor the heart rate during an episode, with a stethoscope if necessary.

ELECTROENCEPHALOGRAPHY (EEG)

An EEG may be indicated in some cases, though it is of greater value in the diagnosis of structural rather than functional diseases of the CNS (See Chapter 4).

ELECTROMYOGRAPHY (EMG) AND NERVE CONDUCTION VELOCITIES (NCV)

See Chapter 4. Measurement of motor nerve conduction velocity is of most value in those peripheral neuropathies where the primary lesion involves demyelination, resulting in a dramatic slowing in the conduction of the nerve impulse. In general, motor nerve conduction velocities are likely to be of little diagnostic use in cases of episodic weakness. However, repeated nerve stimulation may reveal a decremental response in the amplitude of the evoked response recorded from the muscle in cases of myasthenia gravis and this response can be shown to be abolished by the administration of anticholinesterase drugs.

Using the same equipment the electrical activity present within the muscle itself may be recorded. Normal relaxed muscle is electrically silent but in disease states spontaneous activity in the form of fibrillation potentials, positive sharp waves and bizarre high frequency discharges may be recorded. Although fibrillation potentials and positive sharp waves are most commonly seen in denervation, they may also be present in the muscles of animals with a variety of myopathic conditions including polymyositis. In other myopathic diseases such as Labrador retriever myopathy and golden retriever myopathy bizarre high frequency (pseudomyotonic) discharges are commonly recorded. Electromyography is of particular value in the diagnosis of myotonia in which high frequency discharges which wax and wane in frequency and amplitude (myotonic) are present.

MUSCLE AND NERVE BIOPSIES

See Chapter 4. Muscle biopsies may be obtained using an open surgical technique or by needle biopsy. Material obtained in this way may then be fixed in formalin and embedded in paraffin and examined for the presence of an inflammatory response (as in polymyositis) or parasites. If histochemistry and/or fibre typing is required pieces of fresh muscle must be snap frozen in liquid nitrogen and frozen sections cut in a cryostat. Alterations in the normal fibre type proportions are seen in some of the conditions described below, notably Labrador retriever myopathy.

Fascicular nerve biopsies of superficial peripheral nerves may be performed, but are generally only carried out in specialist and research laboratories.

'TENSILON' TEST

Tensilon is an ultra-short acting anticholinesterase (edrophonium chloride) and is used in the diagnosis of myasthenia gravis. A dose of between 0.1 mg and 1.0 mg, depending on the size of the animal, is given by slow intravenous injection. Oxygen should be available in case respiratory difficulty occurs. In cases of myasthenia gravis, administration of Tensilon produces a dramatic improvement in ability to exercise that is observed almost immediately and lasts for several minutes. Care should be taken over the interpretation of the test as occasionally there may be some non-specific improvement with Tensilon in other neuromuscular disorders. The Tensilon test is of particular value in the investigation of episodic weakness characterised by fatigue on exercise.

SPECIFIC CONDITIONS

CARDIOVASCULAR DISORDERS

Cardiac causes of episodic weakness and/or syncope are associated with either reduced cerebral blood flow or inadequate oxygen delivery to the brain (Beckett et al., 1978). These causes include:

Cardiac rhythm disturbances — severe supraventricular or ventricular tachyarrhythmias, or severe bradyarrhythmias including third degree AV block or sinus node disease. The episodes are most commonly associated with exercise or stress, but may occur at rest if the arrhythmia is severe. The diagnosis can only be confirmed by ECG.

Ventricular outflow obstruction — aortic stenosis, pulmonic stenosis, hypertrophic cardiomyopathy and heartworm disease. Outflow obstruction is usually associated with a systolic murmur and limits the overall ability of the ventricles to maintain cardiac output especially during exercise or excitement. Cardiac arrhythmias may complicate the situation. Diagnosis is dependent on physical examination, ECG, radiography and cardiac catheterization. Echocardiography is also helpful and may obviate the need for invasive procedures such as cardiac catheterization.

Heart failure — an inability to sustain forward flow is frequently observed in dilated cardiomyopathy and in severe mitral insufficiency. Pulmonary oedema may also lead to inadequate oxygen uptake. Under these circumstances exercise and excitement are most likely to cause episodic weakness and/or syncope. The diagnosis can be made on physical examination, radiography and ECG, but echocardiography can provide useful information about chamber size and contractility.

Cardiac tamponade due to pericardial effusion can cause weakness and syncope by restricting ventricular filling with consequent reduction in cardiac output. Weakness or syncope are rarely the sole presenting signs as ascites and dyspnoea are usually present as well.

Right-to-left shunts — weakness or syncope usually occur with exercise because lowered peripheral resistance increases the amount of deoxygenated blood shunted into the systemic circulation. Tetralogy of Fallot and reverse shunting patent ductus arteriosus are examples. In the latter case there is usually no murmur and the hindlimbs are more affected due to the anatomical position of the patent ductus arteriosus.

Vasodepressor or vasovagal syncope is poorly understood in animals, but probably explains some cases of syncope in brachycephalic breeds particularly the boxer. Syncope is caused by an increase in vagal tone which causes transient and usually profound bradycardia.

Cardiac drugs — overzealous use of diuretics that reduce plasma volume or of vasodilators (e.g. *hydralazine, prasozin* and *captopril)* that produce hypotension can cause weakness or syncope.

RESPIRATORY DISORDERS

Respiratory causes of episodic weakness and/or syncope are usually associated either with inadequate oxygen delivery to the brain or with reduced cerebral blood flow. Hypoxaemia can result from any form of respiratory tract obstruction or any disease process that reduces lung capacity or interferes with oxygen uptake. Episodic weakness and/or syncope from hypoxaemia is seen most commonly with laryngeal paralysis, upper respiratory tract obstruction in brachycephalic breeds and tracheal collapse. These conditions are associated with upper respiratory tract noise and/or coughing. Pleural effusions, intrathoracic masses and diffuse pulmonary disease can also lead to hypoxaemia. In all of these conditions, episodic weakness and collapse will usually follow a period of exercise, excitement or stress.

Severe coughing due to any cause may result in episodic weakness and syncope by reducing cerebral blood flow. During coughing, the intrathoracic pressure is markedly elevated causing a severe reduction in venous return to the heart. Cardiac output is reduced thus decreasing cerebral blood flow. Weakness or syncope occurs at the end of a bout of coughing.

History, physical and radiological examinations and blood gas analysis are useful in diagnosing respiratory causes of episodic weakness and collapse.

HAEMATOLOGICAL DISORDERS

Severe anaemia and sudden haemorrhage can give rise to hypoxaemia severe enough to cause weakness and collapse. In most cases, the weakness and collapse are associated with exercise, excitement or stress. In some, however, the clinical signs follow sudden and/or recurrent haemorrhage, for example, a ruptured splenic haemangiosarcoma (Brown *et al*, 1985).

Polycythaemia is a rare cause of episodic weakness and collapse, which is thought to occur because increased viscosity of the blood and increased vascular resistance result in reduced cerebral perfusion. These signs are precipitated by exercise and exertion.

Pyrexia of unknown origin may also cause episodic weakness and collapse. The differential diagnosis of pyrexia of unknown origin has been reviewed elsewhere (Dunn and Gorman, 1987).

PRIMARY CENTRAL NERVOUS SYSTEM DISORDERS

Most of the central nervous causes of episodic weakness and collapse listed in Table 13.1 are covered elsewhere in this Manual. Particular attention should be taken to differentiate seizures from other causes of episodic weakness and collapse. Narcolepsy/cataplexy complex, Scottie cramp and episodic falling in the Cavalier King Charles spaniel will be dealt with here in more detail. Lysosomal storage diseases should also be considered in the differential diagnosis. These diseases result from a genetic deficiency of a specific enzyme. Over fifty such diseases have been described in inbred domestic and wild animals. Affected animals present with a slowly progressive multifocal neurological problem usually in the first year of life. Clinical signs include ataxia, incoordination, weakness, blindness, nystagmus and tremor. Lysosomal storage diseases are dealt with in more detail elsewhere in this Manual.

NARCOLEPSY/CATAPLEXY COMPLEX

Narcolepsy is a disorder of sleep characterized by episodic sleepiness at inappropriate times. Cataplexy, the most common sign in animals, is characterised by sudden paroxysmal attacks of flaccid paralysis which may last from a few seconds to several minutes. The attacks are most commonly associated with excitement from eating or playing and may be reversed by petting or calling the animal's name. The respiratory and ocular muscles tend to be spared.

Narcolepsy/cataplexy has been reported in many breeds (Mitler *et al.*, 1976). It is believed to be an autosomal recessive condition in Doberman pinschers and is thought to be inherited in poodles and Labrador retrievers. Diagnosis is based on clinical signs which can be induced by exercise or feeding. Signs are usually present before six months of age, although adult dogs may develop the disease. During an attack, the animal is usually in sternal or lateral recumbency and appears unconscious and limp. There may be twitching of the eyelids, whiskers and paws but there is no salivation, urination or defaecation.

The disease is not life threatening and does not usually progress with time. Animals may respond favourably to *imipramine* (Tofranil) at a dose of 0.5 — 1.5 mg/kg orally two or three times daily.

SCOTTIE CRAMP

This is an inherited condition of Scottish terriers, which usually presents between six weeks and 18 months of age (Joshua, 1956; Meyers *et al.*, 1969). At rest the dog appears normal but after a variable amount of exercise the forelegs are abducted, the back becomes arched and the hindlegs appear to hyperflex. As the muscular tone increases the dog may fall over, curl into a ball and apparently stop breathing. There is no loss of consciousness and recovery usually begins after about 15 seconds. Attacks appear to be precipitated by anxiety and excitement and the frequency and severity varies between individuals.

Episodes may be induced by administration of serotonin antagonists, such as *methysergide* (Deseril). The drug is given orally at a dose of 0.3 mg/kg and the dog is then exercised two hours later. The underlying cause of the disease is not fully understood but it appears to be due to a disorder of neurotransmission in the CNS, probably a defect in the serotonergic neurons. *Chlorpromazine, acepromazine* and *diazepam* are effective in suppressing the clinical signs.

A similar condition has been described in the Dalmatian, in one Jack Russell terrier and recently a form of 'cramp' has been reported in Norwich terriers (Furber, 1984). In affected Norwich terriers spasms of the muscles of the hindquarters lasting approximately five minutes may occur during or after exercise. The condition has apparently been recognised for some years by breeders, who have suggested that dietary supplementation with seaweed or selenium may reduce the incidence.

EPISODIC FALLING IN THE CAVALIER KING CHARLES SPANIEL

This condition has been recognised by breeders for some years. The age of onset varies from three months to four years (usually three to four months) and episodes may be triggered by stress or excitement (Herrtage and Palmer, 1983). After a variable amount of exercise a bounding gait develops. The back is arched and the dog may 'bunny hop'. The hindlegs are abducted and appear stiff, although muscle tone is unaltered during attacks. The forelimbs may show excessive protraction to the extent that, when the animal collapses, the forelegs are held crossed over the back of the head. During the collapse there is no loss of consciousness and recovery is rapid. There is no response to *edrophonium chloride* (Tensilon) and the anticonvulsant drug, *carbamazepine* (Tegretol) may increase the frequency of the episodes. No abnormalities have been detected on either routine haematology, biochemistry or in either of the two affected animals on which post mortem examinations have been carried out. Episodic falling may be associated with 'fly-catching' and bears some resemblance to Scottie cramp in which there is thought to be a functional defect in serotonergic neurons.

Treatment with *diazepam* (Valium) may give some improvement but, usually, this is not permanent.

NEUROMUSCULAR DISORDERS

Neuromuscular disease is being recognised more frequently in veterinary practice as the conditions become more clearly defined. Neuromuscular causes of episodic weakness and collapse include peripheral neuropathies, disorders of neuromuscular transmission and myopathies. Peripheral neuropathies are dealt with in Chapter 14.

MYASTHENIA GRAVIS

Myasthenia gravis is a disorder of the neuromuscular junction which has been reported in both dogs and cats. In dogs, acquired and congenital forms of myasthenia are recognised (Palmer, 1980).

Acquired canine myasthenia gravis

Most cases occur in adult dogs of large breeds, especially German shepherd dogs. Signs are of severe muscular weakness, particularly of the forelimbs, and fatigue on exercise which improves with rest. The stride is short and, as the dog tires, the head is progressively lowered until eventually the dog refuses to continue or collapses. The condition is frequently associated with dysphagia and regurgitation due to megaoesophagus, which occurs because of the high proportion of striated muscle present in the oesophagus of the dog. Circulating antibodies to acetylcholine receptors of the neuromuscular junction are detectable; the condition is therefore considered to be immune-mediated and may be found in association with thymoma.

Diagnosis is based on clinical signs and on the response to Tensilon (see Tensilon test above). Affected dogs show a dramatic improvement on administration of Tensilon which lasts for several minutes. Repetitive nerve stimulation may demonstrate a decremental response in the amplitude of the evoked response recorded from the muscle, but this is seldom necessary for diagnosis. Most affected dogs have megaoesophagus which can be seen on thoracic radiographs. Treatment consists of the oral administration of longer acting anticholinesterase drugs, for example, *pyridostigmine bromide* (Mestinon). The dose of *pyridostigmine* required varies according to the size of the dog, the severity of the signs and the response to treatment. The dose may therefore range from 7.5 mg orally once a day in a Jack Russell terrier to 60 mg two or three times daily in a German shepherd dog. In some cases immunosuppressive levels of corticosteroids have been found to be beneficial, but they should not be given if the patient shows clinical signs of inhalation pneumonia. Some cases go into spontaneous remission and make a full recovery, but a proportion of cases develop complications such as inhalation pneumonia (due to megaoesophagus) and in others inadvertent overdose of anticholinesterase may prove fatal.

Congenital canine myasthenia gravis

Congenital myasthenia gravis is seen in the Jack Russell terrier, springer spaniel and the smooth-haired fox terrier, and is thought to be inherited as an autosomal recessive trait. Signs of weakness are first noticed at 6—8 weeks of age. Affected pups have difficulty standing or raising their heads and may be dysphagic. As in the acquired disease, diagnosis is based on the clinical picture and on the response to Tensilon. Prognosis is generally poor although it has proved possible to keep affected dogs alive for more than two years using small doses of oral anticholinesterase preparations.

There are no circulating antibodies to acetylcholine receptors in congenital myasthenia. The condition appears to be due to a reduced number of acetylcholine receptors present in the post synaptic membrane (Oda *et al.,* 1984).

Myasthenia gravis in the cat

Eight cases of myasthenia have been reported in cats (Joseph *et al.,* 1988). Of these, six were of adult onset and appeared to be acquired. In the other two cats, signs of Tensilon-responsive weakness first became apparent at four to five months of age. In these animals no antibodies to skeletal muscle could be detected in the serum and it was suggested that they may represent an example of congenital myasthenia. A ninth case of feline myasthenia examined by the authors was found to be associated with a thymoma.

POLYMYOSITIS

Polymyositis is a diffuse inflammatory disease of skeletal muscle. Adult dogs of either sex and of any breed may be affected although it is more common in large breeds of dogs. Presenting signs are variable, including weakness, which may appear to be episodic, fatigability, difficulty swallowing, lameness or stiffness and generalised muscle atrophy. About one third have pain on palpation of skeletal muscles and megaoesophagus may be present (Kornegay *et al.,* 1980).

On neurological examination no abnormalities are found but electromyography may reveal fibrillation potentials, positive sharp waves and increased insertional activity. Elevated serum enzymes may be present but since only some enzymes may be raised, CPK, AST (SGOT), aldolase and LDH should all be evaluated. Diagnosis is confirmed by examination of muscle biopsies in which necrosis of muscle fibres and infiltration of muscle by plasma cells and lymphocytes are seen. An immune-mediated aetiology is likely in most cases and treatment with steroids often produces rapid improvement. However, it is important that toxoplasmosis should be ruled out by serological testing and muscle biopsy before treatment with *prednisolone* (0.25 — 0.5 mg/kg every 8 hours) is started. Usually the response to treatment is dramatic, but if not, the dose should be doubled until improvement is seen and treatment continued for 5 — 10 days before reducing the dose gradually.

LABRADOR RETRIEVER MYOPATHY

This inherited disease has been reported in the United States (Kramer *et al.,* 1976) and in the United Kingdom (McKerrell *et al.,* 1984), and has been variously described as type II muscle fibre deficiency, myotonia, muscular dystrophy and heritable Labrador retriever myopathy (McKerrell and Braund, 1987). Onset of signs may occur between 8 and 12 weeks of age although a later onset at approximately six months has also been observed. At exercise, affected puppies move with a stiff, stilted gait and an arched back. The head carriage is often low and many of the puppies show abnormalities of joint posture such as overextended carpi or hyperflexed hocks. Exercise tolerance is reduced and in severe cases may be as little as 20 yards. As the animal tires, the stride shortens and the head is lowered until eventually the dog pitches forward onto its nose with no loss of consciousness. Considerable variation may be seen in the severity of the clinical signs both between individuals and within individuals from day to day, giving the impression that the weakness is episodic in nature. At approximately one year of age the clinical signs appear to stabilise although there is evidence that the pathological process continues to progress. However, exacerbations may occur if subjected to stress such as cold or infection, and recently three adult cases are known to have developed megaoesophagus. Despite reduced exercise tolerance and generalised muscle atrophy, these dogs can make acceptable house pets.

The condition affects males and females of both yellow and black coat colour and in the United Kingdom all the cases have occurred in dogs from working strains. The condition has been shown in America to be inherited as an autosomal recessive trait. Clinical examination usually reveals generalised muscle atrophy and hypotonia together with reduced or absent patellar and triceps reflexes. Administration of Tensilon has no effect, and CPK levels are within the normal range or only moderately elevated. Diagnosis is suspected from the clinical picture and confirmed by the results of electromyography and muscle biopsy. On electromyography, fibrillation potentials, positive sharp waves and bizarre high frequency discharges (pseudomyotonic) have been observed. The pathological change in the muscle is variable, ranging from changes indicative of mild denervation to those more suggestive of primary myopathic disease.

IRISH TERRIER: X-LINKED MYOPATHY

A degenerative myopathy has been described in a litter of Irish terriers (Wentink *et al.,* 1972, 1974). Affected puppies were all males and showed signs of dysphagia from eight weeks of age. By 13 weeks they had difficulty walking and at six months there was evidence of lumbar kyphosis, hypertrophy of the base of the tongue and marked stiffness of skeletal muscles. Examination of a six month old dog showed the stiffness to be most severe immediately after a period of rest. The gait then became normal until after walking approximately 500 metres the animal became tired, at which stage the stiffness returned. From seven months of age the signs appeared to stabilize until 14 months, at which time there was a rapid deterioration and the dog became unable to walk. At this stage the muscles were severely atrophied although still hypertonic and the dog was destroyed.

Affected dogs showed dramatically elevated serum CPK, with values recorded up to 14,000 iu/l. Although electromyography revealed the presence of persistent high frequency discharges similar to those seen in myotonia, there was no evidence of dimpling of muscle on percussion and no evidence of skeletal muscle hypertrophy. The condition has many features in common with golden retriever myopathy, and it has been suggested that the two conditions are analogous to Duchenne dystrophy of man. Histologically, the condition resembles vitamin E deficiency but serum levels of vitamin E were found to be normal and administration of vitamin E produced no improvement. Abnormalities of mitochondrial morphology were shown by electron microscopy and subsequent biochemical examination of the mitochondria revealed that, although they were capable of oxidative phosphorylation, they lacked respiratory control, so-called 'loosely coupled' mitochondria.

GOLDEN RETRIEVER MYOPATHY

A congenital sex-linked (males only) degenerative myopathy affecting golden retrievers has been described in the United States of America (Valentine et al., 1986; Kornegay 1988). Clinical signs become apparent in affected puppies by 6—8 weeks of age. The gait is abnormal, with a short stiff stride and they tire quickly. The condition progresses with atrophy occurring in most skeletal muscles over the next few weeks, although hypertrophy has also been observed in some muscle groups and in the tongue. One puppy was presented at 10 days of age with a history of inability to feed and respiratory difficulties due to gross hypertrophy of the tongue present from birth.

CPK is greatly elevated (values may be greater than 15,000 iu/l) and on electromyography, bizarre high frequency discharges (pseudomyotonic) are recorded. Histology of affected muscles shows necrosis and mineralization together with some evidence of regeneration. Many of the features of this condition are identical to those of the X-linked degenerative myopathy of Irish terriers described by Wentink et al in 1972. Breeding studies indicate that the mode of inheritance is the same as in the Irish terrier and the condition may be analogous to Duchenne muscular dystrophy of man.

MYOTONIA

Myotonia is characterised by the delayed relaxation of skeletal muscle following voluntary contraction or stimulation, and has been reported in man, goats, horses and dogs (Griffiths and Duncan, 1973; Farrow and Malik, 1981). A condition resembling myotonia congenita, an inherited condition of man, has been described in both chow chows (Great Britain, United States, Australia, New Zealand and Holland) and Staffordshire terriers (United States) (Shires et al., 1983). Signs first become apparent when puppies begin to walk. Affected animals have difficulty in rising, stiffness of all four limbs, respiratory stridor and a waddling 'bunny hopping' gait. The stiffness is worse when the dog first begins to move but improves with exercise. In some cases the generalised muscle spasm is so severe that the dog falls over and remains rigid in lateral recumbency for up to 30 seconds. Percussion of the tongue or skeletal muscles, which are usually greatly hypertrophied, results in the production of a myotonic dimple and on electromyography characteristic myotonic discharges are recorded. These high frequency discharges wax and wane in both frequency and amplitude, giving rise to the so-called 'dive bomber' sound when played over the amplifier. In both the chow chow and the Staffordshire terrier, an inherited aetiology is suspected, but so far the mode of inheritance has not been demonstrated.

Sporadic cases of myotonia-like conditions associated with myopathies have been reported in various other breeds, including a Cavalier King Charles spaniel, Rhodesian ridgeback and Great Dane.

Myotonia may also be seen in association with hyperadrenocorticism in the dog (Duncan et al., 1977). A few affected dogs develop signs of stiffness, and hypertrophic muscles which dimple on percussion. Both myotonic and pseudomyotonic discharges may be recorded from affected muscles. These dogs also show the more classic signs of hyperadrenocorticism (see below).

Diagnosis of myotonia depends on the clinical signs of stiffness, hypertrophy and dimpling on percussion and is confirmed by electromyography. Muscle biopsy may be of value in some cases.

HYPOKALAEMIC POLYMYOPATHY

Severe potassium depletion induces a characteristic syndrome of generalised muscle weakness, so-called hypokalaemic polymyopathy, in which muscle dysfunction results from the alteration in muscle cell membrane potential induced by the change in the intracellular-extracellular potassium gradient. Recent studies have shown that hypokalaemia and chronic potassium depletion is not uncommon in cats, especially older animals, and appears to be an intrinsic response of cats to deteriorating renal function (Dow *et al.*, 1987). In addition, periodic muscle weakness associated with hypokalaemia has been described in Burmese kittens and profound hypokalaemia has been reported in a cat with primary aldosteronism.

Affected cats develop generalised weakness with characteristic, persistent cervical ventroflexion, reluctance to move, poor exercise tolerance and apparent muscle pain. In most cases the onset of signs is acute. Occasionally, excessive salivation and vocalization may be observed. Sustained hypokalaemia has also been associated with impaired renal function, weight loss, gastrointestinal disorders, lethargy and poor hair growth.

The diagnosis should be suspected in a cat with typical clinical signs and concurrent hypokalaemia (<3.5 mmol/l and often <3.0 mmol/l) and elevated CPK levels (usually in the 5000 to 10,000 iu/l range). A positive response to dietary potassium supplementation is usually sufficient to confirm the diagnosis, although muscle biopsy to exclude inflammatory polymyositis may be prudent. Histological changes in hypokalaemic polymyopathy are minimal. EMG studies usually reveal evidence of generalised sarcolemmal hyperexcitability.

Severely hypokalaemic cats should receive 8 to 10 mmol potassium/day in divided doses. A response is usually noted in 1 to 2 days, although full strength may not return for several weeks.

ISCHAEMIC NEUROMYOPATHY DUE TO THROMBOEMBOLISM

This condition occurs most frequently in cats and is associated with cardiomyopathy (see Chapter 15). Emboli derived from the heart may be carried to any site within the arterial circulation. They most commonly occlude the distal aorta but may occasionally involve the brachial artery. Vasoactive substances released from the thromboemboli are important in the pathogenesis of the disease because they prevent the establishment of collateral circulation.

Clinical signs are of acute onset limb pain, paresis or paralysis. The femoral pulses may be weak or absent, the gastrocnemius muscles become firm and often painful, the limbs are cool and the nail beds often pale or cyanosed. The patellar reflex may be normal or absent. The pedal reflex is lost and pain sensation is absent in the distal limb. The clinical signs may not be symmetrical. CPK and AST levels are usually markedly elevated because of the muscle damage.

Auscultation of the chest may reveal a murmur or gallop rhythm. Thoracic radiographs usually show cardiac enlargement and echocardiography will differentiate dilated (congestive) cardiomyopathy from the hypertrophic form of the disease. Diagnosis of occlusive vascular disease can be confirmed by angiography.

If the cat survives, some improvement in motor function is common between 1 and 3 weeks. The prognosis, however, is guarded because of the potential for further thromboembolism. Medical therapy includes treatment of the underlying cardiac disorder and using *aspirin* at a dose of 25 mg/kg every third day for its anti-platelet aggregation properties. Low-dose *acepromazine* for alpha-adrenergic blockade or *cyproheptadine* (Periactin) for its anti-serotonin properties may help to prevent collateral blood vessel constriction. Analgesics should also be given for the first 24 to 48 hours (Robins *et al.*, 1982; Flanders, 1986).

MALIGNANT HYPERTHERMIA

Malignant hyperthermia is a hypermetabolic disorder of skeletal muscle. It is seen most frequently in man and in pigs, but also has been reported in the dog, cat, horse and in wild animals during capture.

In susceptible individuals the episodes of hyperthermia are usually initiated by administration of certain halogenated anaesthetic agents *(halothane* and *enflurane)* and depolarising skeletal muscle relaxants *(succinylcholine)*. The defect appears to lie in the sarcoplasmic reticulum; calcium is released but the membrane fails to take it up again leading to a sustained contraction. This results in the production of heat, acidosis, collapse, and death if untreated. In pigs the syndrome may be triggered by stress, and in a recent report in a greyhound the episode came on after an anaesthetic when the dog became excited on being reunited with its owner (Kirmayer *et al.,* 1984).

Malignant hyperthermia may also be induced by moderate amounts of exercise (Rand and O'Brien, 1987). The clinical and biochemical changes caused by exercise are conspicuously disproportionate to the intensity of the exercise. In normal dogs, exhaustive exercise (maximal heart rate for approximately one hour) is known to induce hyperlactacidaemia (lactate concentration increasing approximately threefold) hyperthermia (up to 41.8°C) haemoconcentration (PCV increasing 2% to 3%) and mild respiratory alkalosis. These changes, however, can occur after only a few minutes' exercise in susceptible dogs. Before diagnosing malignant hyperthermia, other possible causes should be excluded, for example heatstroke, pyrogens, thyrotoxic crisis, phaeochromocytoma, hypothalamic defect, drug or transfusion reaction, excessive coat or exhaustive exercise.

Treatment with *dantrolene* (Dantrium), a muscle relaxant acting specifically on skeletal muscle, at a dose rate of 5 mg/kg intravenously is currently recommended in cases of malignant hyperthermia.

MITOCHONDRIAL MYOPATHY

Mitochondrial myopathy in Clumber spaniels was first reported by Herrtage and Houlton in 1979. Affected puppies were eager to exercise but tired quickly, sinking into sternal recumbency after approximately one hundred yards. After ten to fifteen minutes they were able to rise but remained depressed for an hour after the collapse. During the period of collapse excessive panting and pronounced tachycardia were observed. Arterial blood samples revealed a severe acidosis after exercise, with lactate and pyruvate levels dramatically increased. In one animal the acidosis proved fatal. Resting levels of lactate and pyruvate were found to be higher than normal, and biochemical examination showed the defect to lie in the mitochondria, which were unable to oxidise pyruvate due to a deficiency in the pyruvate dehyrogenase complex. The condition has since been seen in the Sussex spaniel (Houlton and Herrtage, 1980) a breed known to be closely related to the Clumber.

A single case of myopathy in which bar-like inclusions were seen in the mitochrondria, was reported in a West Highland white terrier (Bradley *et al.,* 1988); and in 1972 Wentink *et al.,* described structural and biochemical abnormalities in mitochondria from the muscles of a litter of Irish terrier puppies with an X-linked recessive myopathy (q.v.).

METABOLIC DISORDERS

The differential diagnostic lists given in Tables 13.1 and 13.2 should help in the identification of specific problems. Hepatic encephalopathy will be dealt with in detail. Uraemic encephalopathy, however, is only seen in the terminal stages of renal failure when the diagnosis is usually straightforward.

HEPATIC ENCEPHALOPATHY

Hepatic encephalopathy is a syndrome of altered CNS function caused by hepatic insufficiency. It is seen most often in young dogs and cats with congenital portosystemic shunts, although occasionally animals with advanced liver disease and acquired portosystemic shunts will manifest clinical signs. While the exact mechanism by which these conditions induce hepatic encephalopathy remains obscure, the accumulation of toxins including ammonia, mercaptans and fatty acids is considered important. Ammonia is formed primarily in the colon by the action of urease-producing bacteria on protein and amino acids. Normally, the ammonia is absorbed into the portal vein and converted to urea in the liver. Portosystemic shunting of blood or severe hepatic disease results in excessive accumulation of ammonia in the blood, brain and CSF. Mercaptans are produced by bacterial action on methionine, which, ironically, is a constituent of some products used to treat liver disease. Short and medium chain fatty acids accumulate during hepatic failure and act synergistically with other toxins.

Neurological signs are variable and include depression, bizarre behavioural changes, ataxia, staggering, head pressing, circling, aimless wandering, blindness, seizures and coma. These signs usually fluctuate and are often precipitated by feeding, particularly if the food is high in protein. Other signs include stunted growth, weight loss, anorexia, vomiting, hypersalivation, diarrhoea and occasionally pica. Polydipsia, polyuria, ascites and jaundice may also be present in some cases. Anaesthetic and tranquillizer intolerance may be noted.

In most cases, a biochemical profile will identify changes suggestive of liver disease. Liver enzymes, however, are usually normal in young animals with portosystemic shunts, although increased when there is active hepatic damage. Blood urea is often low, since there is decreased conversion of ammonia to urea by the diseased liver. Albumin and cholesterol may also be reduced. Confirmation of reduced liver function can be obtained by bromsulphthalein (BSP) excretion, ammonia tolerance or bile acid analysis.

Congenital and acquired portosystemic shunts can be demonstrated by contrast radiography using operative portal venography. Liver biopsy is also useful to identify the cause of the liver disease.

Therapy should consist of a reduction in protein and fat intake, suppression or elimination of urease-containing intestinal bacteria and catharsis. Avoiding factors known to precipitate hepatic encephalopathy, for example increased dietary protein, gastrointestinal haemorrhage, excessive use of diuretics, sedatives or anaesthetic agents, uraemia, infection and constipation is considered important.

A diet high in carbohydrates and low in both fat and protein should be given. *Neomycin, metronidazole* or *ampicillin* with or without *lactulose* may be used to control ammonia production.

Congenital portosystemic shunts have been successfully ligated but care must be taken to check that patients have normal intrahepatic circulation after the shunt is ligated, or portal hypertension will develop with potentially catastrophic results.

HYPERGLYCAEMIA

Significant hyperglycaemia with glycosuria is seen mainly in diabetes mellitus, but it is not on its own responsible for episodic weakness and collapse except in the rare condition of non-ketotic hyperosmolar diabetic syndrome, where the blood glucose is so high that it dehydrates the cells especially in the brain. Diabetic ketoacidosis in uncontrolled or poorly controlled diabetic animals is seen more frequently. Polydipsia and polyuria may have been noted previously but anorexia, vomiting, diarrhoea, profound weakness and collapse are likely to be the presenting features. Weakness and collapse is caused by hypovolaemia and acidosis.

HYPOGLYCAEMIA

Hypoglycaemia is often caused by a functional islet cell tumour (insulinoma) in middle-aged to older dogs, but may also occur with liver disease, sepsis and excessive insulin administration. Transient hypoglycaemia may be seen in neonatal pups, toy and miniature dogs and working dogs.

HYPERKALAEMIA

Hyperkalaemia is found in association with hypoadrenocorticism, uncontrolled diabetes mellitus, acute renal failure and severe acidosis. High serum potassium is life-threatening and requires immediate correction.

HYPOKALAEMIA

Hypokalaemia is less common but may result from severe vomiting, diarrhoea, urinary loss, excessive fluid therapy or insulin administration.

HYPERCALCAEMIA

Hypercalcaemia may be associated with weakness and muscle wasting because increased calcium levels decrease cell membrane permeability in nervous tissue depressing the excitability of these tissues. Mild hypercalcaemia is often found in hypoadrenocorticism but more significant hypercalcaemia is seen with certain malignancies, particularly lymphosarcoma and anal gland adenocarcinoma, and in primary hyperparathyroidism. The differential diagnosis of hypercalcaemia is covered elsewhere (Weller *et al.,* 1985).

HYPOCALCAEMIA

Calcium is essential for muscle contraction and it stabilises the neuromuscular cell membrane by decreasing its permeability to sodium. In hypocalcaemia this stabilising effect is lost. Hypocalcaemic tetany can result from post-parturient eclampsia, terminal renal failure, primary hypoparathyroidism, protein-losing enteropathy and severe alkalosis.

ENDOCRINE DISORDERS

A number of endocrine disorders may be associated with episodic weakness and collapse. The most important in this respect are insulinoma, hypoadrenocorticism hypoparathyroidism and phaeo-chromocytoma. Hyperadrenocorticism (Cushing's disease), hypothyroidism and diabetic ketoacidosis or more rarely non-ketotic hyperosmolar diabetic syndrome may produce signs of weakness and/or collapse, but the history and other presenting signs are likely to suggest the diagnosis to the clinician.

INSULINOMA

Insulin-secreting pancreatic islet cell tumours (insulinomas) commonly present as episodic weakness or syncope due to hypoglycaemia. Most insulinomas in dogs are malignant and metastasis to regional lymph nodes and the liver is common. Secretion of the beta cells causes hyperinsulinism and hypoglycaemia. Glucose is the principal source of energy for neurons and since the brain cannot store significant amounts of glucose, a constant supply is required. Prolonged hypoglycaemia causes ischaemic neuronal cell damage identical to that caused by hypoxia.

Insulinomas usually occur in dogs over 5 years of age. There is no sex or breed predilection. Clinical signs are usually transient, lasting only a few minutes to an hour and occur days or even weeks apart. Episodes may include paraparesis, disorientation, blindness and abnormal behaviour and can progress to collapse and seizures.

Most animals will have a low blood glucose after fasting (<3.0 mmol/l). Some patients appear to adapt to the low glucose state by an unknown mechanism and may appear normal with a blood glucose of 1.5 mmol/l. Hypoglycaemia should suppress insulin secretion, so concomitant hyperinsulinism is suggestive of an islet cell tumour. An insulin : glucose ratio and an amended insulin : glucose ratio have been described, although some clinicians have questioned the value of these tests. An intravenous glucose tolerance test, oral glucose tolerance test or glucagon tolerance test can be performed. These tests transiently increase blood glucose, but the peak blood glucose level is lower and returns to normal much faster than in normal animals. When an insulinoma is strongly suspected and the laboratory results are equivocal, a laparotomy is indicated.

Surgical removal of the pancreatic mass and any involved lymph nodes can resolve the clinical signs for a year or more (Chrisman, 1980).

HYPOADRENOCORTICISM

Adrenocortical insufficiency has been associated with the following conditions: (a) primary idiopathic hypoadrenocorticism, (b) mitotane (o,p'DDD)-induced adrenocortical necrosis, (c) iatrogenic glucocortoid-induced adrenocortical atrophy, (d) haemorrhage or infarction of the adrenal glands, (e) mycotic or neoplastic involvement, (f) surgical adrenalectomy, and (g) secondary hypoadrenocorticism due to pituitary insufficiency (Herrtage, 1989). Primary idiopathic hypoadrenocorticism is due to atrophy of the adrenal cortex, probably as a result of autoimmunity, and results in mineralocorticoid and glucocorticoid deficiencies.

Aldosterone is the major mineralocorticoid and deficiency results in sodium and chloride loss and potassium and hydrogen retention. Hyponatraemia induces lethargy, depression, nausea, hypotension, impaired cardiac output, reduced renal perfusion, and hypovolaemic shock. Hyperkalaemia causes muscle weakness, hyporeflexia and impaired cardiac conduction. Glucocorticoid deficiency causes decreased tolerance of stress, loss of appetite and a normocytic, normochromic anaemia.

Other clinical signs include a chronic inability to gain weight, weight loss, periodic vomiting and/or diarrhoea, lethargy and weakness. Polydipsia and polyuria are also noted in some patients. These signs may vary over a period of weeks or months then suddenly culminate in acute hypotensive collapse. Addisonian crises occur acutely with or without any associated stress trigger.

Bradyarrhythmias are common and the ECG is useful for detecting the various changes associated with hyperkalaemia. The most common abnormalities include flattened P waves, increased T wave amplitude, broadened QRS complexes and atrial standstill. The latter is associated with profound bradycardia.

The biochemical findings include hyperkalaemia and hyponatraemia (Na:K ratio <25:1; normal >27:1). Additional abnormalities include mild to moderate hypochloraemia, uraemia, hyperphosphataemia and metabolic acidosis. Mild hypercalcaemia is often present, but hypoglycaemia is rarely seen. In rare cases, hypoadrenocorticism may be present with normal electrolytes. The definitive diagnosis is made by measuring serum cortisol levels before and after ACTH stimulation. Plasma cortisol levels are low and fail to respond to ACTH.

Treatment in an acute crisis includes correcting volume depletion with normal saline, correcting the electrolyte imbalance, replacing glucocorticoids and correcting life-threatening arrhythmias and acidosis. Maintenance therapy consists of mineralocorticoid replacement, salt supplementation and glucocorticoids given in times of stress.

HYPOPARATHYROIDISM

Primary hypoparathyroidism is an uncommon endocrine disorder characterized by decreased production and/or release of parathormone, which results in profound hypocalcaemia and mild to moderate hyperphosphataemia (Bruyette and Feldman, 1988). The clinical signs are caused by the physiological effects of hypocalcaemia on the neuromuscular system. Clinical signs include seizures, focal trembling, generalized muscle fasciculations, ataxia, weakness, panting and polydipsia and polyuria. Frequently, the neuromuscular signs are episodic and precipitated by exercise, excitement or stress.

The diagnosis is rarely difficult because resting hypocalcaemia (<2.2 mmol/l) is usually present even if the patient is asymptomatic. Laboratories usually measure total serum calcium, although only the ionized fraction is physiologically active. Hypoalbuminaemia may result in a reduction in total serum calcium, but does so at the expense of protein-bound calcium rather than the ionized fraction. Thus albumin levels should be determined at the same time as calcium.

PHAEOCHROMOCYTOMA

Tumours of the adrenal medulla (phaeochromocytomas) are rare in dogs and have not been reported in cats (Herrtage, 1989). Phaeochromocytomas are usually benign and may secrete excessive amounts of catecholamines.

Clinical signs may relate to an abdominal mass compressing adjacent structures or to the secretion of adrenaline and noradrenaline. Secretion of catecholamines may be intermittent or persistent and can cause hypotension or hypertension, tachycardia and tachyarrhythmias with associated weakness and trembling. Seizures, head pressing, epistaxis and retinal haemorrhages may also be noted. Intermittent secretion of catecholamines is very likely to give rise to episodic weakness and collapse.

Surgical removal of the tumour is the treatment of choice.

HYPERADRENOCORTICISM (CUSHING'S DISEASE)

Hyperadrenocorticism is associated with excessive production or administration of glucocorticoids and is one of the most commonly diagnosed endocrinopathies in the dog (Herrtage, 1989).

Affected dogs usually develop a classic combination of clinical signs. These signs include polydipsia/polyuria, polyphagia, abdominal distension, muscle wasting and weakness, skin and hair coat changes and anoestrus or testicular atrophy. Muscle wasting and weakness may be profound in some cases, leading to episodic weakness and/or collapse associated with exercise. Occasionally dogs with hyperadrenocorticism develop myotonia (see above).

Fairly consistent haematological and biochemical changes are found on routine laboratory tests. These include lymphopenia, eosinopenia, neutrophilia, increased alkaline phosphatase, ALT and cholesterol, high normal blood glucose and decreased blood urea. The diagnosis is confirmed by an ACTH stimulation test or a low-dose dexamethasone suppression test.

Treatment of hyperadrenocorticism is reviewed elsewhere (Herrtage, 1989).

HYPOTHYROIDISM

Hypothyroidism is the most common endocrinopathy seen in the dog and usually affects young to middle-aged dogs of the larger breeds. The clinical signs are very variable and often vague. Affected dogs may present with any one of a combination of the following clinical signs; lethargy, slow heart rate, poor exercise tolerance, obesity, intolerance to cold, alopecia, recurrent skin infections and abnormal oestrus cycles or a lack of libido. Occasional peripheral neuropathies and a myopathy are possibly thought to be associated with hypothyroidism. Episodic weakness and collapse may be seen in those patients in which lethargy, poor exercise tolerance, obesity and muscle wasting are most marked.

Confirmation of the diagnosis can be difficult. Reduced thyroid hormone levels and a subnormal response to TSH are considered the most sensitive tests. Thyroid supplementation should resolve the clinical signs.

SUMMARY

Despite intensive investigation, a few cases of episodic weakness and collapse will defy diagnosis. It is more likely that a diagnosis will be made in these cases if the episode can be precipitated and reproduced. Repeating the physical examination, rectal temperature, routine haematology and biochemistry, blood gas analysis and ECG during or immediately after an episode, is likely to be helpful in these difficult cases and may suggest further avenues to be considered.

REFERENCES

BECKETT, S.D., BRANCH, C.E. and ROBERTSON, B.T. (1978). Syncopal attacks and sudden death in dogs: mechanisms and etiologies. *Journal of the American Animal Hospital Association* **14**, 378.

BRADLEY, R., McKERRELL, R.E. and BARNARD, E.A. (1988). Neuromuscular disease in animals. In: *Disorders of Voluntary Muscle.* (Ed. Sir John Walton). 5th edn. Churchill-Livingstone, Edinburgh.

BROWN, N.P., PATNAIK, A.K. and MacEWAN G. (1985). Canine haemangiosarcoma: Retrospective analysis of 104 cases. *Journal of the American Veterinary Medical Association* **186**, 56.

BRUYETTE, D.S. and FELDMAN, E.C. (1988). Primary hypoparathyroidism in the dog. *Journal of Veterinary Internal Medicine* **2**, 7.

CHRISMAN., C.L. (1980). Postoperative results and complications of insulinomas in dogs. *Journal of the American Animal Hospital Association* **16**, 677.

DOW, S.W., LeCOUTEUR, R.A., FETTMAN, M.J. and SPURGEON, T.L. (1987). Potassium depletion in cats; hypokalemic polymyopathy. *Journal of the American Veterinary Medical Association* **191**, 1563.

DUNCAN, I.D., GRIFFITHS, I.R. and NASH, A.S. (1977). Myotonia in canine Cushing's disease. *Veterinary Record* **100**, 30.

DUNN, J.K. and GORMAN, N.T. (1987). Fever of unknown origin in dogs and cats. *Journal of Small Animal Practice* **28**, 167.

FARROW, B.R.H. and MALIK, R. (1981). Hereditary myotonia in the chow chow. *Journal of Small Animal Practice* **22**, 451.

FLANDERS, J.A. (1986). Feline Aortic Thromboembolism. *Compendium on Continuing Education for the Practising Veterinarian* **8**, 473.

FURBER, R.M. (1984) Cramp in Norwich terriers. *Veterinary Record* **115**, 46.

GRIFFITHS, I.R. and DUNCAN, I.D. (1973). Myotonia in the dog: A report of four cases. *Veterinary Record* **93**, 184.

HERRTAGE, M.E. (1989). The adrenal gland. In: *A Manual of Endocrinology* (ed. M.F. Hutchinson), British Small Animal Veterinary Association, Cheltenham.

HERRTAGE, M.E. and HOULTON. J.E.F. (1979). Collapsing Clumber spaniels. *Veterinary Record* **105**, 334.

HERRTAGE, M.E. and PALMER, A.C. (1983). Episodic falling in the cavalier King Charles spaniel. *Veterinary Record* **112**, 458.

HOULTON, J.E.F. and HERRTAGE, M.E. (1980). Mitochondrial myopathy in the Sussex spaniel. *Veterinary Record* **106**, 206.

JOSEPH, R.J., CORRILLO, J.M. and LENNON, V.A. (1988). Myasthenia gravis in the cat. *Journal of Veterinary Internal Medicine* **2**, 75.

JOSHUA, J.O. (1956). Scottie Cramp. *Veterinary Record* **68**, 411.

KIRMAYER, A.H., KLIDE, A.M. and PURVANCE, J.E. (1984). Malignant hyperthermia in a dog: Case report and review of the syndrome. *Journal of the American Veterinary Medical Association* **185**, 978.

KORNEGAY, J.N. (1988). Golden retriever muscular dystrophy. *Proceedings of the Sixth Annual Forum of the American College of Veterinary Internal Medicine,* Washington D.C.

KORNEGAY, J.N., GORGACZ, E.J., DAWE, D.L., BOWEN, J.M., WHITE, N.A. and DeBUYSSCHER, E.V. (1980). Polymyositis in dogs. *Journal of the American Veterinary Medical Association* **176**, 431.

KRAMER, J.W., HEGREBERG, G.A., BRYAN, G.M., MEYERS, K. and OTT, R.L. (1976). A muscle disorder of Labrador retrievers characterized by deficiency of type II muscle fibres. *Journal of the American Veterinary Medical Association,* **169**, 817.

MEYERS, K.A., LUND, J.E., PADGETT, G. and DICKSON, W.W. (1969). Hyperkinetic episodes in Scottish terrier dogs. *Journal of the American Veterinary Medical Association* **155**, 129.

McKERRELL, R.E. and BRAUND, K.G. (1987). Hereditary myopathy in Labrador retrievers: clinical variations. *Journal of Small Animal Practice* **28**, 479.

McKERRELL, R.E., ANDERSON, J.R., HERRTAGE, M.E., LITTLEWOOD, J.D. and PALMER, A.C. (1984). Generalised muscle weakness in the Labrador retriever. *Veterinary Record* **115**, 276.

MITLER, M.M., SOAVE, O. and DEMENT, W.C. (1976). Narcolepsy in seven dogs. *Journal of the American Veterinary Medical Association* **168**, 1036.

ODA, K., LAMBERT, E.H., LENNON, V.A. and PALMER, A.C. (1984). Congenital canine myasthenia gravis: I. Deficient junctional acetylcholine receptors. *Muscle and Nerve* **7**, 705.

PALMER, A.C. (1980). Myasthenia gravis. *Veterinary Clinics of North America: Small Animal Practice* **101**, 213.

RAND, J.S. and O'BRIEN P.J. (1987). Exercise-induced malignant hyperthermia in an English springer spaniel. *Journal of the American Veterinary Medical Association* **190**, 1013.

ROBINS, G.M., WILKINSON, G.T., MENRATH, V.H., ATWELL, R.B. and RIESZ, G. (1982). Long term survival following embolectomy in two cats with aortic embolism. *Journal of Small Animal Practice* **23**, 165.

SHIRES, P.K., NAFE, L.A. and HULSE, D.A. (1983). Myotonia in a Staffordshire terrier. *Journal of the American Veterinary Medical Association* **183**, 229.

VALENTINE, B.A., COOPER, B.J., CUMMINGS, J.F. and de LAHUNTA, A. (1986). Progressive muscular dystrophy in a golden retriever dog: light microscopic and ultrastructural features at 4 and 8 months. *Acta Neuropathologica (Berlin)* **71**, 301.

WELLER, R.E., CULLEN, J. and DAGLE, G.E. (1985). Hyperparathyroid disorders in the dog: primary, secondary and cancer-associated (pseudo). *Journal of Small Animal Practice* **26**, 329.

WENTINK, G.H., LINDE-SIPMAN, J.S. van der, MEIJER, A.E.F.H., KAMPHUISEN, H.A.C., VORSTENBOSCH, C.J.A.H.V. van, HARTMAN, W. and HENDRIKS, H.J. (1972). Myopathy with a possible recessive X-linked inheritance in a litter of Irish terriers. *Veterinary Pathology* 9, 328.

WENTINK, G.H., MEIJER, A.E.F.H., LINDE-SIPMAN, J.S. van der and HENDRIKS, H.T. (1974). Myopathy in an Irish terrier with a metabolic defect of the isolated mitochondria. *Zentralblatt für Veterinärmëdizin* **21A**, 62.

CHAPTER 14

CANINE AND FELINE PERIPHERAL POLYNEUROPATHIES

Ian D. Duncan B.V.M.S., Ph.D., M.R.C.V.S., M.R.C.Path.

The study of peripheral neuropathy in small animals has become an expanding field in veterinary neurology. While dogs with epilepsy and intervertebral disc disease are still likely to be the most common neurological diseases that the small animal practitioner encounters, dogs and cats with polyneuropathy will be more frequently recognised. This is more likely because of an increasing awareness of the symptomatology of animals with neuropathy, rather than an actual increase in the frequency of these disorders (Duncan & Griffiths, 1984) The symptoms of paresis and ataxia, so commonly associated with the myelopathy of intervertebral disc protrusion or other degenerative spinal cord diseases, are now also recognised as potentially being of peripheral nerve origin. In addition, peripheral nerves and the muscles they supply are much more accessible to both ancillary testing and biopsy than tissue in the central nervous system, thus increasing the likelihood of diagnosis. This chapter will succinctly review the current state of knowledge on polyneuropathy in small animals and provide the practitioner with a background to the range of these disorders and the means of diagnosing them.

THE PERIPHERAL NERVOUS SYSTEM (PNS)

The PNS is defined as consisting of those parts of motor neurones, primary sensory neurones and autonomic neurones that lie outside the boundaries of the central nervous system (CNS). Although motor neurones originate in the spinal cord or brain stem from ventral horn cells or cranial nerve nuclei, disorders of these structures are not classified as peripheral neuropathies. This may seem inconsistent as disorders of ventral horn cells will result in lower motor neurone signs. However, their exclusion from the overall 'neuropathy' classification is a useful separation from a nosological standpoint (Duncan, 1987).

CLINICAL EXAMINATION AND SYMPTOMS OF POLYNEUROPATHY

A standard approach to the examination should be carried out in any animal with neurological disease. After the history is taken, a complete physical examination is performed. A number of neuropathies are associated with a multisystemic disease, for example, diabetes mellitus and neoplasia, so the general examination should not be omitted even though the dog is clearly paretic and/or ataxic. This is then followed by the detailed neurological examination which is described elsewhere in this book. The first part is the evaluation of the animal's gait and muscle strength which should be done on a non-slippery surface. The animal's strength should be evaluated even if it is reported by the owner to be paraplegic or quadraplegic, as it may only be severely weak or the weakness may be asymmetric. If possible, the dog should be walked back and forth several times with the examiner viewing the animal from the back, front and side etc. It may be necessary to walk or run the dog up stairs to demonstrate weakness. With a cat, examination of the gait is performed in the examination room or on a carpeted area. After evaluation of the gait, the second part of the examination, evaluating the postural reactions, is performed. These tests will only be summarised as they have been described in detail elsewhere (Barker,1979; deLahunta 1983; Oliver and Lorenz, 1983 and in Chapter 3). Proprioception is assessed by testing paw position sense, sway response and reflex stepping. There may be some difficulty in distinguishing proprioceptive deficits from weakness, as the animal may be unable to replace the limb because of paresis and not as a result of proprioceptive deficits. However, paw position sense may be retained in animals which are paretic, almost up to the point of paralysis. Wheelbarrowing, hopping, hemi-stand/walk and postural thrust are tests used to demonstrate weakness in an individual limb or asymmetric weakness. Finally, visual and tactile placing reflexes are tested which require vision and intact tactile sensory receptors respectively, and the ability to flex the limb. The third part of the examination is the evaluation of spinal reflexes, muscle tone and muscle bulk. Reflexes are evaluated with the dog or cat relaxed in lateral recumbency. The patellar reflex is the most easily evaluated stretch reflex and should be graded (O-absent; + hyporeflexic; + + normal; + + + hyperreflexic; + + + + clonus). Front limb reflexes (biceps, triceps and extensor carpi radialis) should be tested but can be difficult to elicit and interpret. A pedal reflex should be elicited in each limb and the strength of flexion noted. At the same time, presence or absence of a pain response should be noted. Muscle tone is evaluated in all limbs and muscle bulk checked (already examined during postural testing). The final part of the neurological examination is the cranial nervous system. Both motor (V, V11 and X) and sensory deficits (V) to the head can be seen in neuropathies and so this should not be omitted.

SIGNS OF POLYNEUROPATHY

The most frequent presenting symptoms of animals with peripheral neuropathy are paresis, ataxia, muscle atrophy and hyporeflexia/hypotonia. In most instances, paresis is present from the onset of the exercise and thus is not exercise related, and frequently the history includes the report that the animal has difficulty in rising on the hind legs. There may be temporal progression of the weakness, with the development of tetraparesis and sometimes tetraplegia. In general, the hind legs are affected before the front legs, probably because of the greater length of the nerves of the hind legs. The length of the nerve is thought to explain why the recurrent laryngeal nerve is frequently clinically affected in neuropathy resulting in weakness of or loss of bark. On occasions, denervation of the skeletal muscle of the oesophagus can also result in local paresis, in these cases with resultant megaoesophagus.

Ataxia is a symptom often seen in neuropathy and results from involvement of large diameter proprioceptive fibres or their cell bodies in sensory ganglia. Hyporeflexia and hypotonia can also arise from lesions in sensory nerves or ganglia, and from disease of motor fibres. Finally, muscle atrophy is commonly seen in neuropathies and indicates degeneration of motor nerve fibres.

In most neuropathies, autonomic function and pain perception (nociception) remain intact and this may be useful in differentiating them from other neurological disorders. However, certain neuropathies almost exclusively affect either autonomic or nociceptive function, i.e. feline dysautonomia (see later and elsewhere in this book), and inherited sensory neuropathy (see later).

ANCILLARY AIDS

Routine serum chemistry profiles, special biochemical tests and complete blood counts are infrequently of assistance in the diagnosis of polyneuropathy. However, they are essential in the diagnosis of metabolic diseases in which neuropathy may occur secondarily e.g. diabetes mellitus-blood glucose; hypothyroidism-TSH response; hypoglycaemia (resulting from an insulinoma) - blood glucose, insulin/glucose ratio, etc. In cats, a rare inherited neuropathy associated with hyperlipaemia may be confirmed by measuring fasting lipoprotein levels (Jones, et al, 1986). Cerebrospinal fluid evaluation is also rarely helpful but it may demonstrate an albumino-cytological dissociation (raised total protein with a normal white cell count) in dogs (or cats) with polyradiculoneuritis. (Cummings,et al, 1982). In polyradiculoneuritis a lumbar collection of CSF is required as the lesions are predominantly in the lumbosacral area. (Cummings, et al, 1982).

Electrophysiological tests are often the mainstay of the diagnostic workup on a dog or cat with polyneuropathy. As these tests are detailed elsewhere in this book, they will only be summarised here. (See Chapter 4).

Electromyography — determines the level of innervation of a muscle (voluntary activity) or the electrical activity which arises after the muscle has become denervated (spontaneous activity eg. fibrillation potentials, positive sharp waves, high frequency discharges).

Nerve conduction studies — these tests measure the speed of conduction along the motor and sensory nerves and can be used to estimate the number of nerve fibres conducting and their normality. Because of the expense of the electromyographic equipment, these tests are usually only done at veterinary schools or in speciality small animal practices.

Finally, muscle and nerve biopsy are frequently useful in the investigation of peripheral neuropathy but often they indicate only the underlying pathology and not the cause. However, in certain neuropathies they may be diagnostic (e.g. canine giant axonal neuropathy and congenital protozoal infection — see later) and biopsy should always be considered, although it should only be done if the samples are submitted to a laboratory capable of processing the tissue properly. A muscle biopsy requires cryostat sectioning for routine histological stains and enzyme histochemistry, formalin fixation and sometimes fixation in aldehyde fixative for EM. Peripheral nerve should be fixed under slight tension in buffered glutaraldehyde before processing for embedding in epon (light and electron microscopy) and single nerve fibre teasing. (Dyck, *et al,* 1984).

DIAGNOSIS OF NEUROPATHY

It is rare that the diagnosis of a neuropathy can be made on clinical grounds alone, but in certain neuropathies a common antecedent event (e.g. in coonhound paralysis) or a familial trait (e.g. giant axonal neuropathy) can be diagnostic pointers. More often, the diagnosis is made from the combined information derived from the clinical examination, electrophysiology and muscle and nerve biopsy. Laboratory data may or may not implicate a metabolic cause and the electrophysiology will help determine the underlying pathology, i.e. whether it is a demyelinating or axonal disease. The muscle and nerve biopsy will confirm the latter and may permit a diagnosis to be made. The application of such an approach to diagnosis will undoubtedly increase the diagnostic rate but as in man, where more sophisticated testing is the norm (Dyck *et al,* 1984), many neuropathies will remain idiopathic in origin. Despite this cautionary note, such an approach has advanced the understanding and knowledge of small animal peripheral neuropathy greatly in the last decade and will continue to do so.

DIFFERENTIAL DIAGNOSIS

In most animals with paresis and ataxia, clinical examination will determine whether this is a result of disease of the CNS or neuromuscular system (PNS, neuromuscular junction and muscle). However, it is sometimes more difficult to differentiate a neuropathy from a myopathy, or a disturbance of neuromuscular transmission on clinical grounds alone. In most cases this differentiation is made, not on a single difference but on a combination of signs (Table 14.1). Differentiation of neuropathy from disorders of neuromuscular transmission is not usually difficult. Myasthenia gravis (MG), the most important of these, is usually associated with exercise intolerance and most cases have megaoesophagus (Duncan and Griffiths, 1986) which is much less common in neuropathy. The response to anti — cholinergic drugs in MG is the final clue.

Table 14.1. Differentiation between Neuropathy and Myopathy

	Neuropathy	Myopathy
Paresis	Yes	Yes
Ataxia	Yes (proprioceptive deficit)	No
Nociception	Can be lost in sensory neuropathy	Normal
Voice	Often changed or lost	Normal
Muscle bulk	Atrophy (not in demyelinating disease)	Frequent — sometimes hypertrophy
Muscle tone	Usually reduced	May be mildly reduced
Reflexes	Reduced to absent	May be reduced
Muscle pain	None (may be some tenderness on palpation in CHP)	Variable in polymyositis
Distribution of lesion	Frequently HL's first and worst, especially distal	Usually generalised but remember masticatory muscle myositis
Autonomic dysfunction	May be involved	None
Muscle dimple	None	Present in myotonic states
EMG/NCV	EMG — denervation potentials	EMG — spontaneous activity; myotonia
	NCV — reduced amplitude, slowed conduction	NCV — normal
Serum enzymes	Normal	CK — may be raised
Biopsy	Muscle — denervation, fibre type grouping	Muscle biopsy — often useful and diagnostic
	Nerve — **may** show abnormalities	Nerve biopsy — normal

HL's = Hind legs   CHP = Coonhound Paralysis   NCV = Nerve Conduction Velocity   CK = Creatinine Kinase

RESPONSE OF THE PERIPHERAL NERVE TO DISEASE

Peripheral nerves consist of large, medium and small myelinated nerve fibres and unmyelinated fibres, randomly mixed in groups known as fascicles which are surrounded by the perineurial connective tissue sheath. These structures have a very stereotyped response to injury. Transection of a nerve results in degeneration of all the fibres distal to the section (Wallerian degeneration) (Figure 14.1). Distal degeneration of nerve fibres can also occur in non traumatic situations; e.g. neurotoxic poisoning or certain familial neuropathies (Figure 14.1) Often this primarily affects long, large diameter myelinated nerve fibres and such a process is known as the dying back phenomenon, or distal axonopathy (Dyck *et al,* 1984). As this process initially affects long, large diameter nerve fibres, clinical evidence of neuropathy is first seen in the distal muscles of the hind legs e.g. gastrocnemius muscle, anterior tibialis muscle.

Demyelination is a random process in comparison and results in focal (paranodal or segmental) loss of the myelin sheath but leaves the axon intact (Figure 14.1). As a result, muscle fibres do not become denervated and no neurogenic atrophy is seen in the muscle biopsy, unlike in neuropathies where there is axonal degeneration with accompanying neurogenic muscle atrophy. Repair of the nerve following both axonal degeneration and demyelination is possible, although faster and more complete in the latter; this is reflected in the faster clinical recovery seen following demyelination. Successful re-innervation of muscle following the transection of a nerve will depend upon the distance between the muscle and the site of nerve trauma, the apposition of the cut ends of the nerve and the presence or absence of neuroma formation. The further from the muscle and the larger the gap between the cut ends the less the chances of recovery. Axonal regeneration in non – traumatic neuropathies also often occurs but may be abortive because of ongoing axonal disease.

Careful evaluation of the nerve biopsy (LM and EM, and single teased nerve fibres) will allow a pathological classification of the disease to be made, i.e., whether it is a predominantly axonal or demyelinating neuropathy or a mixture of both. Most often neuropathies are 'mixed' with pathological evidence of both degeneration and demyelination.

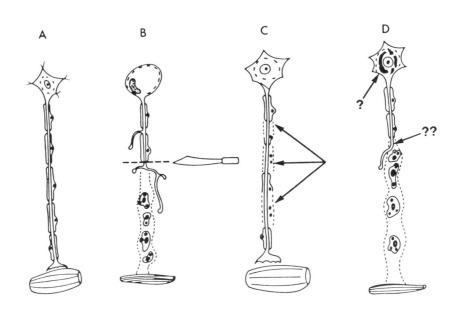

Figure 14.1
The basic disease processes affecting the peripheral nerves are detailed in this diagram.
A. Normal.   B. Wallerian degeneration causes central chromatolysis of the nerve cell body as well as distal degeneration of the axon.   C. Segmental demyelination of individual myelin sheaths or Schwann cells causes patchy damage.   D. In axonal neuropathy, the disease may affect either the cell body or the peripheral axon, causing axonal breakdown. In both forms of axonal degeneration, the muscle becomes atrophied.
(From Bradley, W. G.: *Disorders of Peripheral Nerves.* Oxford. Blackwell Scientific Publications, 1974, with permission.)

CLASSIFICATION OF NEUROPATHIES

There are a number of different ways of classifying neuropathies (Duncan, 1987) and these will be summarised.

Anatomical: Polyneuropathy is the term used for disease of multiple peripheral nerves. Many neuropathies symmetrically affect the distal parts of long, large diameter myelinated nerve fibres (distal axonopathy — see above), and so the distal limb muscles in the hind limbs are affected first and most severely. Occasionally the opposite can occur; i.e. proximal limb muscles first, but this is rare. Spontaneous neuropathies clinically affecting only one nerve are called 'mononeuropathy' (e.g. the left recurrent laryngeal nerve in the horse — roaring). If a number of nerves are affected randomly, the term 'mononeuropathy multiplex' is used. 'Polyradiculoneuropathy' is the term used if the site of the lesion is in the nerve roots.

Pathological: a) Axonal degeneration
               b) Demyelination
               c) Sensory Neuronopathies

Aetiological: the following list contains the known causes of peripheral neuropathy in animals, a) Genetic, b) Inflammatory, c) Traumatic, d) Immune mediated, e) Metabolic, f) Neoplastic, g) Infectious, h) Ischaemic, i) Toxic.

Clearly all causes of disease in general can affect the PNS. The final classification of a neuropathy usually includes all of the above types of classification e.g. the dog has a distal axonopathy with both axonal degeneration and demyelination caused by an autosomal recessive trait.

NEUROPATHIES

The following discussion briefly outlines the peripheral neuropathies seen in the dog and cat (Table 14.2). This discussion will emphasise those of most importance in the United Kingdom and will briefly describe those seen in North America. More details of these can be found elsewhere (Duncan and Griffiths, 1984; Griffiths and Duncan, 1986; Duncan and Griffiths, 1986).

Table 14.2.
Known Canine and Feline Polyneuropathies

Inherited		Acquired
CANINE		
Sensory neuropathy in Dachshunds	(autosomal recessive)*	Distal denervating disease
Sensory neuropathy in Pointers	(autosomal recessive)*	CHP/polyradiculoneuritis
Giant axonal neuropathy — GAN	(autosomal recessive)*	Sensory neuronopathy
Progressive axonopathy	(autosomal recessive)	Toxoplasma — polyradiculoneuritis
Hypertrophic neuropathy in Tibetan Mastiffs	(autosomal recessive)*	Brachial plexopathies
		Endocrine neuropathies
Globoid cell leucodystrophy	(autosomal recessive)	Trauma
		Paraneoplastic
		Neoplasia
		Individual case reports (usually idiopathic)
FELINE		
Neuropathy of inherited hyperchylomicroanaemia		Ischaemia
Niemann Pick disease*		Diabetes
		Feline dysautonomia
		Trauma
		Neoplasia
		Individual case reports
*Putative inherited trait.		

INHERITED CANINE NEUROPATHIES

SENSORY NEUROPATHY IN DACHSHUNDS

Aetiology and Pathogenesis: This disease appears likely to be inherited as an autosomal recessive trait. It has only been described to date in the United Kingdom (Duncan and Griffiths, 1982). Sensory nerve biopsy demonstrates a severe loss of myelinated fibres with diffuse unmyelinated fibre abnormalities (Duncan, Griffiths and Munz, 1982). A single case report in a Border collie described many similar clinical and pathological abnormalities to the dachshunds (Wheeler, 1987).

Clinical findings: Affected dogs are usually noted to have a hind leg ataxia from the time they start to walk. There is no paresis. Proprioception is slow to absent as are placing reflexes. Nociception is decreased or absent over the whole body and there may be rare evidence of self-mutilation. There may be autonomic involvement as the dogs may dribble urine and have a history of unexplained bouts of vomiting. Motor nerve conduction studies and EMG are normal but sensory nerve conduction is often abnormal. Confirmation of the diagnosis is made on biopsy of a sensory nerve.

Treatment: None, but affected dogs can usually survive quite normally without therapy.

SENSORY NEUROPATHY IN POINTERS

Aetiology and Pathogenesis: This neuropathy is inherited as an autosomal recessive disease. It is found in short-haired pointers in Europe and English pointers in the United States. The underlying lesion is a developmental disorder of primary sensory neurones with only minimal evidence of degeneration of these cells (Cummings, deLahunta and Winn, 1981a).

Clinical Findings: The first symptoms of neuropathy are usually seen under six months of age when mutilation of the extremities is found. In the hind limbs there is complete anaesthesia of the digits. This is reduced in thoracic limbs and trunk. By comparison, other sensory modalities, in particular proprioception, are intact, and the stretch reflexes are normal.

Treatment and Prognosis: There is no known treatment and self-mutilation will lead to considerable destruction of distal limb tissue.

GIANT AXONAL NEUROPATHY (GAN)

Aetiology and Pathogenesis: This is inherited as an autosomal recessive trait in German shepherds, although only one family of these dogs has been described in the United Kingdom (Duncan and Griffiths 1979; Duncan and Griffiths, 1981; Duncan et al, 1981). GAN is a classical distal axonopathy, with lesions being found first in distal nerves in the hind legs and at the end of long tracts in the CNS (Duncan and Griffiths, 1979). In both PNS and CNS, axons of both myelinated and unmyelinated fibres are focally distended with abnormally accumulated neurofilaments. These swellings finally result in degeneration of the distal axon.

Clinical Findings: The first symptoms are seen between 12-15 months of age when hind limb ataxia is noted. This progresses, with development of distal muscle weakness and atrophy, proprioceptive deficits, hypotonia and hyporeflexia. Pain sensation is reduced because of the involvement of small axons, and megaoesophagus always develops. By 18-24 months the dogs may be extremely weak in the rear with some foreleg weakness. EMG is useful in the initial demonstration of the distal nature of the denervation in the hind legs. Diagnosis is made on pathognomic nerve biopsy changes found in a motor or sensory nerve.

Treatment and Prognosis: None; poor outlook as megaoesophagus frequently leads to aspiration pneumonia.

PROGRESSIVE AXONOPATHY OF BOXER DOGS

Aetiology and Pathogenesis: This disease is inherited as an autosomal recessive trait. To date, it has only been described in certain breeding lines in the United Kingdom (Griffiths, 1980; Griffiths, 1986). Its early onset suggests that changes may be present at birth or begin in utero. Axonal swellings within the nerve roots of the lumbar cord, with resultant axonal atrophy in more distal portions of the nerves, are the hallmark of this neuropathy. The myelin sheath changes which occur are thought to be secondary to the underlying axonal pathology (Griffiths et al, 1987). Similar axonal changes are seen in the CNS.

Clinical Findings: The first symptoms are seen after 2—3 months of age but may be preceded by patellar areflexia at one month of age. The hind limbs show a marked ataxia with proprioceptive deficits, hypotonia and hyporeflexia, but no muscle atrophy. The forelegs may be involved late in the disease and there may be fine ocular tremor and head bobbing. The signs may not worsen after initial progression over the first two years of life. The diagnosis is made on a clinical and breed basis and is usually straightforward. Additional tests could include sensory nerve electrophysiology, which is abnormal, and a sensory nerve biopsy.

Treatment and Prognosis: There is no treatment, but affected animals may live comfortably for considerable periods of time.

CANINE HYPERTROPHIC NEUROPATHY

Aetiology and Pathogenesis: This neuropathy, which is found in the Tibetan mastiff in the USA, is inherited as an autosomal recessive trait (Cummings *et al,* 1981; Cooper *et al,* 1984). It is predominantly a demyelinating neuropathy unlike most other inherited canine neuropathies. Myelin sheath changes, associated with the accumulation of filaments in the cytoplasm of Schwann cells, occur early in life resulting in demyelination and remyelination. Subsequently, there is little further active demyelination and so, histologically, there is rare evidence of hypertrophic changes (i.e. onion bulbs).

Clinical Findings: The first signs are seen at about 6 weeks of age when paresis of the hind legs and then the forelegs (eight weeks) occurs. Hypotonia and hyporeflexia are seen but proprioception is intact. The weakness progresses with muscle atrophy developing and the adoption of a plantigrade stance. The voice may change as a result of involvement of the recurrent laryngeal nerve. These symptoms may not worsen and indeed, some strength may be regained if dogs are maintained on wood shavings and a smooth floor (Cooper *et al,* 1984).

Treatment and Prognosis: Apart from management changes during the early post-natal period there is no therapy but improvement, although not full recovery, can be seen.

ACQUIRED CANINE NEUROPATHIES

DISTAL DENERVATING DISEASE

Aetiology and Pathogenesis: This disease appears to be limited to the United Kingdom where it is one of the most common canine neuropathies (Griffiths and Duncan, 1979). The lesion is restricted to the intramuscular nerves or terminal motor branches of long motor nerves, where degeneration is found. Any age, breed or sex of dog can develop this disease and there are no known common epidemiological features such as a common antecedent event.

Clinical Findings: Affected dogs present with a history of progressive weakness involving all four limbs occurring over a few days to weeks, which often progresses to quadriplegia, with cervical weakness and loss of bark. Reflexes are absent and there is marked hypotonia. Proprioception is present up until the stage that the dog is too weak to stand, and pain perception is retained. With time, marked appendicular muscle atrophy develops. EMG examination reveals diffuse evidence of denervation in practically all skeletal muscles with abnormal motor nerve conduction studies. The diagnosis is made by the exclusion of other possible causes. Nerve biopsy is usually unhelpful as the lesion is distal to the point at which biopsies are taken.

Treatment and Prognosis: In practically all dogs with this disease, the outlook is excellent. As spontaneous recovery occurs, treatment consists of careful nursing care to prevent decubital ulcers, and hand feeding usually with soft food or gruel. Recovery should be seen within a 4—6 week period. Relapses have not been documented to date.

POLYRADICULONEURITIS/COONHOUND PARALYSIS (CHP)

Aetiology and Pathogenesis: The polyradiculoneuritis seen in dogs which have had a previous raccoon bite, is the most common peripheral neuropathy in North America (Cummings and Haas 1967; Cummings *et al,* 1982). Although raccoons are not present in Europe, occasional cases of polyradiculoneuritis have been reported. Similarly, cases of polyradiculoneuritis in some dogs in North America and in Europe which have not been bitten by a raccoon have also been documented (Northington and Brown, 1982; Griffiths *et al,* 1983). The actual relationship between the antecedent event in CHP, i.e. the raccoon bite and the development of the nerve root lesion, is not clear. The disease has been transferred by the injection of raccoon saliva into a dog that previously had bouts of CHP, but this has proved difficult to repeat (Holmes *et al*, 1979) There may be a delayed hypersensitivity reaction against myelin caused by a protein constituent of raccoon saliva. Although the antecedent events in the raccoon and non-raccoon associated polyradiculoneuritis may be different, the end stage is similar, with nerve root inflammation, demyelination and axonal degeneration.

Clinical Findings: In CHP, dogs that have been bitten by a raccoon 10—14 days previously develop a weakness in the hind legs, initially apparent by the development of a stilted gait . The weakness progresses to tetraparesis and often tetraplegia with a loss of bark. Likewise, the cervical muscles may also be weak with an inability to raise the head. Pedal reflexes are lost but the dog may be hyperaesthetic. An EMG examination shows diffuse evidence of denervation as in distal denervating disease. Nerve conduction studies may show some slowing of nerve conduction velocity and eventual failure of conduction (Cummings *et al,* 1982).

Treatment and Prognosis: As with distal denervating disease, the treatment consists of careful nursing but no specific medical therapy. These dogs can eat and drink if assisted and have never been reported to develop a megaoesophagus. Their outlook is excellent and recovery should take between 4—8 weeks depending on the initial severity of the neuropathy. Occasionally, the severe involvement of intercostal muscles can lead to respiratory difficulties and sometimes death. This should be watched and the dog placed on a respirator if necessary.

SENSORY NEURONOPATHY

Aetiology and Pathogenesis: There have been several recent reports of series and individual case reports of dogs with ataxia and sensory disturbance over the face and body that are of considerable interest (Carmichael and Griffiths, 1981; Cummings, deLahunta & Mitchell, 1983; Wouda *et al,* 1983; Steiss *et al,* 1987). In all of these dogs (except the first mentioned where only the sensory branches of cranial nerve V were involved), there was evidence of a loss of sensory neurones in the dorsal root ganglia with resultant loss of fibres in sensory nerves and in the sensory tracts of the spinal cord. This neuronal cell loss frequently was associated with collections of mononuclear cells with occasional degenerating neurones being noted. In all of these dogs the aetiology was unknown, but comparisons were made with similar human conditions and to neurotoxic poisons such as *adriamycin* which preferentially can cause sensory neuronal death.

Clinical Signs: In the majority of these dogs, the ataxia seen was associated with conscious proprioception deficits. There was evidence of hyporeflexia and hypotonia but no muscle atrophy, except of the masticatory muscles in some dogs (Cummings *et al,* 1983). Pain sensation was usually reduced or absent in the territory involved, i.e. over face or limbs. A megaoesophagus was seen in a few dogs. In the case of Carmichael and Griffiths (1981) there was a sensory loss only over the head (trigeminal nerve – maxillary and opthalmic branches) with no involvement of the mandibular nerve (motor branch) and absence of a sensory ataxia.

Treatment: There is no known therapy as the cause of these sensory neuronopathies is unknown. The course is likely to be progressive.

PROTOZOAL POLYRADICULONEURITIS

In utero infection of a pregnant bitch with a protozoan parasite, which recent work suggests to be due to *Neospora caninum* (Dubey *et al,* 1988) and not *Toxoplasma gondii* as previously thought, can cause a severe polyradiculoneuritis and polymyositis in pups. The first clinical signs are seen between 4—8 weeks of age when paresis and hind leg ataxia are noted. This progresses to paraplegia with extreme rigidity of the hind limbs and the development of muscle atrophy. Pain sensation is intact. The inflammatory nerve root lesion is extremely severe with a widespread loss of nerve fibres; (Jackson and Duncan, unpublished observations) as such, these lesions are not responsive to the standard medical therapy used in dogs with systemic protozoal infections which have myositis. The outlook therefore is hopeless.

BRACHIAL PLEXOPATHIES

Occasionally dogs will develop subacute/chronic fore-limb weakness and muscle atrophy (EMG shows denervation) without evidence of previous trauma (Duncan and Griffiths, 1986). These are usually idiopathic in nature although one report suggests an anaphylactic reaction associated with a horse meat diet as the cause. In this dog, microscopic studies of the brachial plexus showed a severe neuritis. In some dogs with brachial plexopathies, the hind legs may eventually become involved and so these cases should be regarded as generalised polyneuropathies. In those that remain restricted to the brachial plexus, this may indicate an inflammatory neuropathy and so steroids should be tried. A more distal nerve biopsy usually only shows evidence of axonal degeneration and so is not diagnostic.

ENDOCRINE NEUROPATHIES

Hypoglycaemia. A recent report suggests that dogs with insulinomas can have sub-clinical microscopic evidence of neuropathy (Braund *et al*, 1987a). This report followed anecdotal reports of clinical neuropathy in dogs with hypoglycaemia and insulinoma. We have seen one dog with insulinoma which had an acute onset of neuropathy with paresis, hypotonia, hyporeflexia and pathological evidence of an axonal neuropathy (Duncan, Panciera and Cuddon — unpublished data). However, most dogs with insulinomas do not have clinical evidence of neuropathy but the PNS should be carefully evaluated.

Diabetes mellitus. Neuropathy in diabetic dogs may occur but it appears to be less common than that seen in cats (see later).

Hypothyroidism. This association has been suggested but as yet is unproven.

TRAUMATIC NEUROPATHY

Avulsion of the nerve roots forming the brachial plexus, as a result of the road traffic accident, is the most common traumatic neuropathy in the dog and cat. This and sciatic nerve lesions caused by trauma, are discussed elsewhere in this book (see chapter 11).

PARANEOPLASTIC NEUROPATHY

There have been single case reports in the veterinary literature suggesting that there could be an association between a neoplasm and neuropathy. The connection between neoplasia (often a lung tumor) and neuropathy in man is well recognised and also with various non-neural neoplasms. A connection between various non-neural neoplasms and sub-clinical neuropathy in a large series of dogs (as seen on histological evaluation of the ulnar and peroneal nerves), has been proposed (Braund *et al*, 1987). The pathogenesis of the 'distant' effect of such a tumour is still unknown although there may be shared antigens between the tumour and nerve. A definitive association between clinical neuropathy and neoplasia in veterinary medicine has still to be made.

PERIPHERAL NERVE TUMOURS

These can occur and most often affect the brachial plexus and its roots. Affected dogs are often middle aged and present with insidious front leg lameness and pain on palpation of the limb (Carmichael and Griffiths,1980b). Deep palpation of the axilla may reveal a mass in the brachial plexus in only 50% of cases. With time, muscle atrophy occurs in the fore limb and if the tumour spreads up the nerves/nerve roots, compression of, or invasion into the spinal cord with upper motor neurone signs in the hind legs (e.g. hyper-reflexia) can be seen. These tumours can be neural (neurofibrosarcoma, Schwannoma, neurofibroma) or non-neural (e.g. osteosarcoma) in origin and they are uniformly difficult to treat. Early amputation of the limb may be successful but early diagnosis is uncommon (see chapter 11).

INDIVIDUAL CASE REPORTS

There are numerous single case reports of idiopathic neuropathy in small animals in the veterinary literature, predominantly in the dog. These have been reviewed elsewhere (Duncan and Griffiths,1984).

INHERITED FELINE NEUROPATHIES

NEUROPATHY OF INHERITED HYPERCHYLOMICRONAEMIA

Aetiology and Pathogenesis: This recently described neuropathy in cats in New Zealand appears likely to be inherited as an autosomal recessive trait (Jones *et al*, 1986). Affected cats were found to have resting hyperlipaemia, lipaemia retinalis and peripheral neuropathy (9 out of 20 with hyperlipaemia had neuropathy). The neuropathy was thought to result from compression of nerve trunks by the lipid granulomata (xanthomata) which develop. This compression affected peripheral nerves in a patchy fashion with notable axonal degeneration in either limb nerves, cranial nerves or the cervical sympathetic trunk.

Clinical Findings: The first signs seen were usually paralysis of an individual limb. The term mononeuropathy multiplex could be applied to this neuropathy as individual cats had involvement of the facial, tibial, peroneal, femoral,radial, trigeminal, or recurrent laryngeal nerves. In three cats, more than one nerve was involved. In addition, three cats developed a Horner's syndrome as a result of involvement of the cervical sympathetic trunk.

Treatment and Prognosis: Resolution of the neuropathy, associated with a lowering of the lipaemia, occurred in three cats which were placed on a low fat diet.

NEUROPATHY OF NIEMANN PICK DISEASE

Aetiology and Pathogenesis: The neuropathy was found in this lysosomal storage disease and has now been seen in three cats, two of whom were related (Cuddon *et al,* 1989). It may be inherited in an autosomal recessive fashion. There is deficiency in the enzyme sphingomyelinase which results in accumulation of sphingomyelin in neurones in the spinal cord and dorsal root ganglia, Schwann cells and in many cells (primarily associated with the mononuclear phagocyte system) in the viscera. In the PNS there is evidence of severe myelin breakdown and hypomyelination in the nerve roots.

Clinical Symptoms: In the three cats, there was some variation in the symptoms seen. In one cat, limb and trunk tremor with a 'stringhalt' like hind leg gait was noted from 4—6 weeks of age. This worsened over a 9-month period during which paraparesis, loss of tone and reflexes and muscle atrophy developed. The other two cats presented at 5—7 months of age with progressive tetraparesis, hyporeflexia and hypotonia.

Diagnosis during life can be made on enzyme quantitation of a liver biopsy or skin fibroblast cultures. A bone marrow biopsy can also be of use if foamy inclusions are seen in white blood cells.

Treatment and Prognosis: This is a progressive, debilitating disease and there is no treatment. Cats with tremor alone can live normally for a number of months.

ACQUIRED FELINE NEUROPATHIES

ISCHAEMIC NEUROMYOPATHY DUE TO THROMBOEMBOLISM

Aetiology and Pathogenisis: This is a fairly common sequelae of cardiomyopathy in which thrombus development results from the formation of emboli which occlude one or more branches of the aorta (Flanders, 1986). In particular, occlusion of the aortic trifurcation results in ischaemia to nerves and muscles in the hind limb and occlusion of the brachial artery can also occur with fore limb paralysis. It is not the loss of blood supply *per se* that results in muscle and nerve ischaemia, but the release of sertonin (5-HT) from platelets. In severe lesions there is ischaemia and degeneration of both muscle and nerve but demyelination proximal to the areas of degeneration in nerve is also seen (Griffiths and Duncan, 1979b). Regeneration of nerve can occur with re-establishment of blood supply. (Also see Chapter 15).

Clinical Findings: Following embolism of the aorta at its trifurcation, affected cats acutely develop paresis or paraplegia (depending on the degree of arterial block). Other symptoms include pain, loss of femoral pulses, cold limbs and pale foot pads and nails.

Treatment: This is aimed at treating the underlying cardiac disease, supply analgesics if required, and *aspirin* therapy to inhibit platelet function (low dose — 25 mg/kg, *per os*) every third day for the rest of the cat's life (Flanders, 1986). The prognosis depends on the initial severity of the ischaemia, the development of gangrene and the stage of the underlying cardiac disease. In all cases a guarded prognosis should be given as although recovery from the neuropathy can occur, further bouts are likely as the underlying heart disease is not curable.

DIABETIC NEUROPATHY.

Aetiology and Pathogenesis: Polyneuropathy has now been clearly demonstrated in a number of cats with diabetes mellitus (Kramek *et al,* 1984). Like human diabetic neuropathy, the exact causal relationship between the diabetes and the development of neuropathy is not known. In the cat the lesion appears to result in the distal degeneration of axons (distal axonopathy).

Clinical Findings: The neuropathy in these cats presents as hind limb paresis, affected cats often adopting a plantigrade stance. There can be noticeable distal muscle atrophy and hyporeflexia. EMG examination shows evidence of denervation and nerve conduction velocity may be slowed. A nerve biopsy of a distal hind leg nerve shows evidence of axonal loss and myelin sheath changes.

Treatment and Prognosis: Control of the diabetes, either in the newly diagnosed diabetic cat, or improved control in a cat already receiving insulin can reverse the signs of neuropathy. Severe, chronic neuropathy is less likely to respond to better diabetes control, however. Some cats will recover spontaneously from their diabetic state with subsequent partial to full clinical resolution of their accompanying polyneuropathy.

FELINE DYSAUTONOMIA

This is clearly the most important feline neuropathy in the United Kingdom at present. It is the only small animal neuropathy known so far that almost solely affected the autonomic nervous system. It is the subject of another chapter in this text (see Chapter 12).

REFERENCES

BARKER, J. (1979). Nervous system. In: *Canine Medicine and Therapeutics.* Eds. E. A. Chandler, J. W. Evans, W. B. Singleton, F. G. Startup, J. B. Sutton and W. D. Taverner. Blackwell Scientific, Oxford.

BRAUND, K. G., McGUIRE, J. A., AMLING, K. A. and HENDERSON, R. A. (1987). Peripheral neuropathy associated with malignant neoplasms in dogs. *Veterinary Pathology* **24**, 16.

BRAUND, K. G., STEISS, J. E., AMLING, K. A., TOIVIO-KINNUCAN, M., CASE, L. C., KEMPPAINEN, R. J. and COLEMAN, E. S. (1987a). Insulinoma and subclinical peripheral neuropathy in two dogs. *Journal of Veterinary Internal Medicine* **1**, 86.

CARMICHAEL, S. and GRIFFITHS, I. R. (1981). Case of isolated sensory trigeminal neuropathy in a dog. *Veterinary Record* **109**, 280.

CARMICHAEL, S. and GRIFFITHS, I. R. (1981a). Brachial plexus tumours in 7 dogs. *Veterinary Record* **108**, 435.

COOPER, B. J., deLAHUNTA, A. and CUMMINGS, J. F. *et al,* (1984). Canine inherited hypertrophic neuropathy: clinical and electrodiagnostic studies. *American Journal of Veterinary Research* **45**, 1172.

CUDDON, P. A., HIGGINS, R. J., DUNCAN, I. D., PARENT, J., MOSER, A. and MILLER, S. (1989). Feline Niemann-Pick disease associated polyneuropathy. Brain (In Press).

CUMMINGS, J. F., COOPER, B. J. and deLAHUNTA, A. *et al* (1981). Canine inherited hypertrophic neuropathy. *Acta Neuropathologica (Berlin)* **53**, 137.

CUMMINGS, J. F., deLAHUNTA, A. and WINN, S. S. (1981a). Acral mutilation and nociceptive loss in English Pointer Dogs. *Acta Neuropathologica (Berlin)* **53**, 119.

CUMMINGS, J. F., deLAHUNTA, A. and HOLMES, D. F. *et al* (1981) Coonhound Paralysis. Further clinical studies and electron microscopic observations. *Acta Neuropathologica (Berlin)* **56**, 167.

CUMMINGS, J. F., deLAHUNTA, A. and MITCHELL, W. J. Jr. (1983). Ganglioradiculitis in the dog: a clinical, light and electron-microscopic study. *Acta Neuropathologica (Berlin)* **60**, 29.

CUMMINGS, J. F. and HAAS, D. C. (1967). Coonhound Paralysis. An acute idiopathic polyradiculoneuritis in dogs resembling the Landry-Guillain Barré syndrome. *Journal of the Neurological Sciences* **4**, 51.

deLAHUNTA, A., (1982) *Veterinary Neuroanatomy and Clinical Neurology,* 2nd Edition. W. B. Saunders Co., Philadelphia.

DUBEY, J.P., HATTEL, A.L., LINDSAY, D.S. and TOPPER, M.J. (1988). Neonatal *Neospora caninum* infection in dogs: Isolation of the causative agent and experimental transmission. *Journal of the American Veterinary Medical Association* **193**, 1259.

DUNCAN, I. D. Etiology and Classification of Peripheral Neuropathies (1987). *ACVIM Proceedings* (San Diego), p 325.

DUNCAN, I. D. and GRIFFITHS, I. R. (1979). Peripheral nervous system in a case of canine giant axonal neuropathy. *Neuropathology and Applied Neurobiology* **5**, 25.

DUNCAN, I. D. and GRIFFITHS, I. R. (1981). Canine giant axonal neuropathy; some aspects of its clinical, pathological and comparative features. *Journal of Small Animal Practice* **22**, 491.

DUNCAN, I. D. and GRIFFITHS, I. R. (1982). A sensory neuropathy affecting long-haired Dachshund dogs. *Journal of Small Animal Practice* **23**, 381.

DUNCAN, I. D. and GRIFFITHS, I. R. (1984). Peripheral neuropathies of domestic animals. In: *Peripheral Neuropathy,* 2nd edn. (Eds.Dyck, P. J., Thomas, P. K., Lambert, E. H., Bunge, R. P.), W. B. Saunders Co., Philadelphia.

DUNCAN, I. D. and GRIFFITHS, I. R. (1986). Neuromuscular diseases. *In Neurologic Disorders.* (Ed. J. N. Kornegay). Churchill Livingstone, New York.

DUNCAN. I. D., GRIFFITHS, I. R. and CARMICHAEL, S. *et al.* (1981). Inherited canine giant axonal neuropathy. *Muscle and Nerve* **4**, 223.

DUNCAN, I. D., GRIFFITHS, I. R. and MUNZ, M. (1982). The pathology of a sensory neuropathy affecting Long-Haired Dachshund dogs. *Acta Neuropathologica (Berlin)* **58**, 141.

DYCK, P. J., THOMAS, P. K., LAMBERT, E. H. and BUNGE, R. (eds) (1984). *Peripheral Neuropathy.* 2nd Edn. W. B. Saunders Co., Philadelphia.

FLANDERS, A. (1986). Feline aortic thromboembolism. *Compendium of Continuing Eduction* **8**, 473.

GRIFFITHS, I. R. (1985). Progressive Axonopathy: an inherited neuropathy of Boxer dogs. 1. Further studies of the clinical and electrophysiological features. *Journal of Small Animal Practice* **26**, 381.

GRIFFITHS, I. R., CARMICHAEL, S., MAYER, S. J. and SHARP, N. J. H. (1983). Polyradiculoneuritis in two dogs presenting as neuritis of the cauda equina. *Veterinary Record* **112**, 360.

GRIFFITHS, I. R. and DUNCAN, I. D. (1979). Distal denervating disease. A degenerative neuropathy of the distal motor axon in dogs. *Journal of Small Animal Practice* **20**, 579.

GRIFFITHS, I. R. and DUNCAN, I. D. (1979a). Ischaemic neuromyopathy in cats. *Veterinary Record,* **104**, 518.

GRIFFITHS, I. R., DUNCAN, I. D. and BARKER, J (1980). A progressive axonopathy of Boxer dogs affecting central and peripheral nervous systems. *Journal of Small Animal Practice* **21**, 29.

GRIFFITHS, I. R. and DUNCAN, I. D. (1986). Neuropathies in domestic animals. In *Recent Advances in Neuropathology.* No. 3. (Ed. J. B. Cavanagh). Churchill Livingstone, Edinburgh.

GRIFFITHS, I. R., McCULLOCH, M. C. and ABRAHAMS, S. (1987). Progressive axonopathy: an inherited neuropathy of Boxer dogs. 4. Myelin Sheath and Schwann cell changes in the nerve roots. *Journal of Neurocytology* **16**, 145.

HOLMES, D. F., SCHULTZ, R. D., CUMMINGS, J. F. and deLAHUNTA, A (1979). Experimental Coonhound paralysis. Animal model of Guillain Barré syndrome. *Neurology* **29**, 1186.

JONES, B. R., JOHNSTONE, A. C., CAHILL, J. I. and HANCOCK, W. S. (1986). Peripheral neuropathy in cats with inherited primary hyperchylomicronaemia. *Veterinary Record* **119**, 268.

KRAMEK, B. A., MOISE, N. S., COOPER B. and RAFFE, R. (1984). Neuropathy associated with diabetes mellitus in the cat. *Journal of the American Veterinary Medical Association* **186**, 42.

NORTHINGTON, J. W. and BROWN, M. J. (1982). Acute canine idiopathic polyneuropathy. A Guillain-Barré-like syndrome in dogs. *Journal of the Neurological Sciences* **56**, 529.

OLIVER, J. E. and LORENZ, M (1983). *Handbook of Veterinary Neurologic Diagnosis.* W. B. Saunders Co., Philadelphia.

STEISS, J. E., POOK, H. A., CLARK and E. G. BRAUND, K. G. (1987). Sensory neuronopathy in a dog. *Journal of the American Veterinary Medical Association* **190**, 205.

WHEELER, S.J. (1987). Sensory neuronopathy in a Border Collie puppy. *Journal of Small Animal Practice* **28**, 281.

WOUDA, W., VANDEVELDE, M. and OETTLI, P. *et al* (1983). Sensory neuropathy in dogs: a study of four cases. *Journal of Comparative Pathology* **93**, 437.

CHAPTER 15

SPECIAL NEUROLOGY OF THE CAT

Richard J. Evans M.A., Ph.D., Vet.M.B., M.R.C.V.S.

INTRODUCTION

The principles of neurology are essentially the same in the cat as in the dog. There are, however, conditions which are unique to the cat which may produce neurological signs. Even amongst those conditions occurring in both species the pattern of diseases and the relative incidence of conditions vary. The objectives of this chapter are:-

1. To discuss the neurological conditions which occur in the cat but not in the dog.

2. To identify the differential diagnoses which must be considered when the most common neurological presenting signs are encountered in the cat.

3. To consider some important differences in the pattern of disease and/or therapy in the cat.

The conditions will generally be considered on the basis of presenting signs, with the sections organised in relation to the region of the brain affected. A number of important feline diseases may result in single or multifocal lesions which may affect any part of the nervous system. These conditions will be mentioned in relation to particular presenting signs. Detailed discussion of them will, however, be found in the section dealing with diseases producing multifocal signs.

SEIZURES

Seizures are an uncommon presenting sign in the cat. Although idiopathic epilepsy occurs, organic causes of seizures are relatively more common than in the dog (Kay, 1975). Convulsions need not necessarily be of cortical origin; effects at the spinal level (for example in strychnine poisoning) or the periphery (organophosphorous poisoning) may result in seizures which may be difficult to discriminate from those of central origin. Possible causes of seizures are given in Table 15.1.

Because of the relatively high prevalence of organic brain disease causing seizures in cats, it is essential to investigate thoroughly this possibility when collecting the history. Both when taking the history and when performing the neurological examination, it is pertinent to take note of the presence of neurological signs between seizure episodes since this strongly suggests the presence of organic pathological change. Clinical biochemical estimation, particularly plasma glucose, calcium, urea, total proteins, liver function tests, as well as routine haematology and urinalysis may all prove valuable in the investigation of the underlying pathology. In cases where either a space-occupying lesion or inflammatory disease is suspected CSF analysis may also prove helpful.

MANAGEMENT OF SEIZURES IN THE CAT

If the seizures are associated with organic disease treatment of the underlying cause should be instituted if appropriate.

In cases of functional epilepsy, or where therapy for organic underlying disease is not available or is ineffective, prophylactic anticonvulsant treatment will be needed if seizures are frequent. *Phenobarbitone* and *diazepam* are the only anticonvulsants which are suitable for prophylactic use in the management of fits in cats. *Phenytoin* is ineffective and *primidone* is toxic in the cat. *Phenobarbitone* is used most commonly, the dose generally lying within the range 7-30 mg b.i.d. or t.i.d.. For *diazepam* the dose is usually in the range of 1-5 mg b.i.d. or t.i.d.. It is important to titrate the dose and dosage interval so as to stabilise the patient on an effective treatment regimen, to maintain regular dosing and to avoid abrupt cessation of therapy.

In the event of status epilepticus, emergency treatment will be required. An airway should be established if necessary and oxygen given if there is marked hypoxia. The animal should be placed so as to minimise self-inflicted injury. *Diazepam* should be used as the first-line agent for the control of the seizures. 5-10 mg should be administered intravenously, preferably as the emulsion, or intramuscularly. If convulsions are not adequately controlled after 10 minutes, this may be followed by further doses up to a maximum total dose of 20mg. If this is still ineffective, *phenobarbitone* may be given intravenously or intramuscularly up to a maximum dose of 60mg or general anaesthesia may be induced using *pentobarbitone.* The patient should be monitored carefully.

PROGNOSIS

Cats with functional epilepsy can be kept seizure free for months or even for life if medication is carefully regulated. However, this requires careful attention to the detail of the dosage regimen. Where there is underlying organic disease this will generally determine the outcome.

Trauma

Cerebral inflammatory disease:

Feline infectious peritonitis (FIP)
Toxoplasmosis
Meningitis
Encephalitis
Meningo-encephalitis
Aujeszky's disease (pseudorabies)
Rabies
Cryptococcosis
Blastomycosis
Aberrant parasitic migration

Space-occupying lesions:
Neoplasms
Hydrocephalus
Coenurus cysts

Degenerations:
Cerebral ischaemia
Storage diseases and other heritable degenerations (see Progressive ataxia in young animals)
Thiamine deficiency

Intoxications:
Organochlorine pesticides
Organophosphorus pesticides
Lead
Ethylene glycol
Phenolics
Benzoic acid
Strychnine
Alphachloralose (high dose)

Metabolic abnormalities:
Uraemia
Hyperammonaemia (hepatic encephalopathy)
Hypoglycaemia
Hypocalcaemia

Table 15.1
Possible Causes of Siezures in Cats

SPECIFIC CONDITIONS ASSOCIATED WITH SEIZURES

Hydrocephalus.

Primary (congenital) hydrocephalus is relatively uncommon in the cat. When it is encountered the signs are variable but are noted within the first few days of life. Seizures are a common feature together with ataxia and visual deficits. Dullness, incessant circling and coma may also be encountered. The skull is domed and the fontanelle open. The prognosis is hopeless and affected kittens generally die early in life. Diagnosis may be made by pneumoventriculography.

Acquired (secondary) hydrocephalus is seen in the cat as a consequence of trauma, inflammation or space-occupying lesions which interfere with the drainage of CSF. Treatment is not practicable and death usually ensues rapidly.

Thiamine deficiency.

This presents with a variety of signs and severe seizures are common amongst these, particularly in advanced cases. The condition is uncommon and when seen it is generally in cats fed a diet rich in raw fish, due to high levels of thiaminase present (Jubb et al., 1956). Thiamine is heat-labile, so that the condition may also occasionally be seen in cats fed a diet of unsupplemented cooked meat.

Affected animals show progressive inappetance. The gait is characterised by ataxia and dysmetria, with high wandering steps. There may be head weaving and the head may be ventroflexed, often spasmodically. Mydriasis and slow light reflexes are common and there may be papilloedema and peripapillary neovascularisation (Barnett & Ricketts, 1985). Vestibular reflexes are absent. Spasticity may develop with the animals walking stiffly on extended toes and with the tail erect. Handling may increase the muscle tone. Seizures frequently develop. The most advanced cases become severely obtunded or semi-comatose and cry continuously. Persistent extensor tone with opisthotonus are seen in a proportion of advanced cases.

Early cases respond well to treatment with thiamine at 1—5 mg i.m. followed by oral supplementation although mild ataxia may persist for 2—3 weeks. The prognosis in advanced cases is very poor. The diet should be changed in cases which recur.

Hepatic encephalopathy.

The neurological signs commonly encountered in feline hepatic encephalopathy are behavioural changes, ataxia, fits, visual disturbances and mydriasis. The neural disturbances are associated with hyper-ammonaemia, although this may not be the major mechanism involved (see Chapter 13). Hepatic encephalopathy may be a consequence of chronic liver failure, but more frequently arises because of the presence of portosystemic shunts. These are congenital anomalies of the portal venous system connecting it directly to the systemic circulation. The liver is under-perfused by portal blood, with consequent hepatic insufficiency (Vulgamott et al, 1980).

The disease is seen in young cats, usually being detected before 6 months of age. Ptyalism is often the first clinical sign noted and precedes the development of encephalitic features. The neurological signs are episodic and are worsened following feeding. Only occasional affected individuals are stunted.

Increased basal ammonia levels are seen and there is reduced tolerance to an ammonium chloride challenge. Blood urea and plasma albumin concentrations may be in the reference range, as may the BSP clearance. Diagnosis therefore rests heavily on the demonstration of hyperammonaemia and on the use of contrast venography of the portal system to demonstrate shunting (see Chapter 5).

In many feline cases the shunts are outside the liver parenchyma and are accessible to surgical ligation, which has generally proved successful. In cases where ligation is not feasible medical management to reduce the degree of hyperammonaemia can be successful. A low protein diet, oral neomycin and lactulose may be helpful (Blaxter, 1987).

Intoxications.

Selected intoxicants which produce seizures are discussed in the following paragraphs. For further details of these and for discussion of the other intoxicants listed but not discussed elsewhere in this chapter the reader is referred to Burger and Flecknell (1985) and Evans (1988).

Organophosphorus and carbamate insecticides.

Cats are particularly susceptible to intoxicants (see Evans, 1988 for review). The widespread use of flea collars, insecticidal aerosols and vapourising strips for the control of parasites on the cat and insects in the environment results in a substantial risk of cumulative exposure to these agents via a variety of routes and cats are thus particularly at risk. The accumulation of acetylcholine, due to inhibition of cholinesterase by the organophosphorus compound or carbamate leads to peripheral nictonic, muscarinic and central effects. The signs include respiratory distress leading to apnoea, vomiting, diarrhoea, seizures, salivation and lacrymation. Coma and paralysis are also seen and death is due to respiratory paralysis. Treatment should be with atropine sulphate (0.2—0.25 mg/kg) by slow i.v. injection, repeated as necessary together with a similar dose intramuscularly.

In the case of organophosphorus compounds, but not carbamates, pralidoxime (20—40 mg/kg) may also be given if available but is of no value once four hours have elapsed beyond the time of exposure.

Intoxication with organochloride compounds —

Poisoning with organochlorine insecticides is relatively frequently encountered in the cat (Evans, 1988). The clinical signs produced by the organochloride insecticides are primarily due to increased neural excitability. Intermittent or continuous seizures are a frequent feature. Other clinical signs include muscle tremors, ataxia, depression, ptyalism, emaciation and alopecia.

Lead.

Lead poisoning is relatively uncommon in cats although this may represent underdiagnosis (Evans, 1988). The neurological signs are of lethargy or hyperexcitability and seizures. Anorexia, constipation and occasionally vomiting are also seen. Anaemia is rare. Treatment is with calcium ethylene diamine tetra-acetate (Ca-EDTA).

BEHAVIOURAL CHANGES

Behavioural changes in cats may reflect organic brain disease, disease of other systems or psychogenic abnormalities or normal behaviour patterns with which the owner is unfamiliar. For further discussion of psychogenic and behavioural problems the reader is referred to Mugford (1985). Some causes of behavioural changes are given in Table 15.2.

With the possible exceptions of psychomotor seizures and the early stages of rabies and pseudorabies, cats with behavioural changes of neurological origin will usually have other neurological signs.

Ischaemic encephalopathy.

Severe depression, acute in onset, sometimes with mild to moderate pyrexia characterises feline ischaemic encephalopathy. Partial or generalised seizures, mild ataxia, mydriasis, aggressive behaviour, unilateral postural deficits and circling to the contralateral side may also be seen. The majority of the signs regress within a few days but the unilateral postural defects and visual field defects may persist permanently. CSF analysis shows mild to substantial elevation of protein concentration with a normal cytological picture or a slight elevation in mononuclear cell numbers. The aetiology is unknown although commonly there is post-mortem evidence of cerebral infarction (Kornegay, 1981). There is no specific treatment; corticosteroids have been employed early in the course, but it is not known whether they have any beneficial effect.

Organic brain disease:

Tumour (particularly of the hypothalamus)
Other space-occupying lesions
FIP
Toxoplasmosis
Ischaemic encephalopathy
Hereditary degenerative disorders
  (Storage diseases and others)
Mercury poisoning
Lead poisoning
Rabies
Pseudorabies
Thiamine deficiency
Diabetes insipidus

Functional brain disorders:

Psychomotor seizures
Centrally-acting drugs
Hepatic encephalopathy
Uraemic encephalopathy

Psychogenic:

Spraying
Aberrant defaecation and/or urination
Exaggeration of any normal behaviour pattern
Feline psychogenic alopecia
Tail chasing

Normal behaviour:

Oestrus behaviour
Spraying
Territorial scratching

Disease of other systems:

Hyperthyroidism
Pain
Gastro-intestinal dysfunction
Genito-urinary dysfunction
Cardio-respiratory dysfunction

Table 15.2
Causes of Behavioural Changes in Cats

Space occupying lesions.

Neoplasms and other space-occupying lesions affecting the thalamic and hypothalamic areas may cause behavioural changes. The most commonly encountered neoplasms of the feline CNS are meningiomas (Zaki and Hurvitz, 1975). Astrocytomas and both extra — and intradural lymphomas also are relatively common. Lymphomas and meningiomas may be multiple. Pituicytomas and pituitary chromophobe adenomas may expand to compress or involve the hypothalamic region. Oligodendrogliomas, meningeal sarcomas and ependymomas also occur, but are rare. There may be depression and personality change, with a failure to respond to humans or there may be inappropriate rage and vicious behaviour or marked docility. Perturbation of normal habits is seen, with urination or defaecation around the house rather than in the garden or the litter tray. Appetite and thirst also may be disturbed. Seizures and circling (to the side of the lesion in 80 to 90% of cases) are also relatively common. There may be associated diabetes insipidus with polyuria and polydipsia. Feline pituitary tumours are non-functional and are not associated with hyperadrenocorticism.

Central nervous system causes:

Cranial trauma (notably road traffic accidents, and pellet/bullet injuries)

Encephalitides: (FIP, toxoplasmosis; rabies; pseudorabies (Aujeszky's disease) other viruses)

Hepatic encephalopathy

Uraemic encephalopathy

Other encephalopathies; thiamine deficiency

Meningitides: bacterial, blastomycosis, cryptoccosis

Space-occupying lesions; tumours, cysts

Hydrocephalus

Narcolepsy

Intoxications: alphachloralose, metaldehyde, ethylene glycol, phenolics, salicylates, barbiturates, narcotics

Hereditary degenerations (storage diseases and others)

Cerebrovascular accident

Generalised conditions and those affecting other systems:

Shock

Hypoglycaemia

Hyperglycaemia/hyperosmolarity/ketoacidosis

Anaemia/polycythaemia/hyperviscosity

Cardiopulmonary dysfunction/anoxia

Hypo- or hypercalcaemia

Hypoadrenocorticism

Weakness/muscle wasting/cachexia

Pyrexia/septicaemia/viraemia

Table 15.3
Diseases Causing Alteration in Consciousness in Cats

Rabies.

Rabies causes behavioural changes in the prodromal phase of the disease, which lasts 1-2 days, and in the furious stage (Gaskell, 1985). In the prodromal stage, shy cats may become more friendly, agitated or restless. Conversely, friendly cats may show unprovoked agression or may hide. The furious stage may be very dramatic in cats with the animal becoming very excitable and vicious, often making unprovoked attacks. Focal and cranial nerve signs and inco-ordination may be seen. Pharyngeal paralysis, masseter paralysis and drooling are less commonly seen than in the dog. The excitement phase then merges into the paralytic phase with ataxia, ascending paralysis and coma supervening. The furious stage is not invariably seen in dumb rabies; there may be direct progression to ataxia, followed by paralysis, coma and death. In the event of a suspected case in the United Kingdom the animal should be isolated and detained on the premises on which it has been examined. Immediate notification should be made to the Divisonal Veterinary Officer for the area of the Ministry of Agriculture, Fisheries and Food. Full details can be obtained in the Rabies Guidance Notes for Practising Veterinary Surgeons issued by the Ministry of Ariculture, Fisheries and Food.

Pseudorabies (Aujeszky's disease).

Aujeszky's disease is a rare condition in cats. After an initial period of anorexia and depression lasting 1-2 days, during which the cat may hide or cry piteously, frenzy develops as a result of severe pruritis (Dow and McFerran, 1963; Horvath and Papp, 1967). The cat rubs, claws and bites the offending areas causing severe self mutilation. The condition progresses rapidly to coma and death. Convulsions may be seen. The irritation and consequent mutilation are sometimes absent.

Psychogenic alopecia.

A much lesser form of self- mutilation, apparently of psychogenic origin, is seen in this condition, also called 'neurodermatitis' or 'feline hyperaesthesia'. This is a disease notably of Siamese cats but is also seen in animals of the Abyssinian and Burmese breeds. These cats excessively lick, groom and pluck hair, often from a localised area, for example one flank, the ventral abdominal wall, the medial aspect of the thighs, or the dorsum. Alopecia, with remarkably unblemished skin, or with moist, erythematous areas, and broken hair-shafts, results. Diagnosis rests on the elimination of physical and biological causes of the dermatological lesions and often on the elucidation of some underlying stress factor. Treatment is with *phenobarbitone* or *diazepam* coupled, where possible, with elimination of the underlying cause.

ALTERED/ABNORMAL CONSCIOUSNESS : DULLNESS : LETHARGY AND COMA

Altered states of consciousness may reflect disease of the central nervous system or of other systems. There is considerable overlap with conditions causing seizures or behavioural anomalies (see Table 15.3).

CRANIAL NERVE AND CERVICAL SYMPATHETIC TRUNK DEFICITS

Lesions of cranial nerve I are difficult to detect. Lesions of cranial nerves II, III, IV, and VI will be considered together, along with those of the cervical sympathetic trunk. Since all are involved in ocular function their deficits together constitute the subject matter of neuro-ophthalmology (see Chapter 9 for detailed discussion).

NEURO-OPHTHALMOLOGY

A detailed ophthalmological examination is an important part of the assessment of the neurological patient and this is particularly so in the cat because of the large number of multifocal diseases affecting the nervous system in this species. Uveitis is a particulary significant finding in cats with neurological signs. It is quite commonly present in cases of toxoplasmosis and of FIP affecting the central nervous system. Visual field defects are neither common nor easy to detect in the cat: when found they are, however, extremely illuminating. Perhaps the most common is bilateral loss of peripheral vision due to pituitary tumours compressing or ablating the optic chiasma. The orbit is not an uncommon site for lymphoma which may thus result in a proptosed globe together with deficits of some or all of the nerves innervating the eyeball. There may be strabismus or the globe may be totally fixed and Horner's syndrome may be present in such cases of retrobulbar lymphoma.

Horner's syndrome.

The clinical signs of Horner's Syndrome are described in Chapter 9 along with the neuroanatomical basis to these signs. Lesions at any level of the pathway may cause Horner's syndrome in cats. Damage to the sympathetic fibres in the cranial cervical spinal cord are accompanied by hemi- or quadriplegia. Injury in the cervicothoracic region results in a lower motor neurone deficit in the forelimbs and an upper motor neurone deficit in the hind limbs. Lymphomas and neurofibromas may affect the cervical sympathetic trunk alone in which case Horner's syndrome occurs in the absence of cranial nerve or motor neurone signs. Lymphoma, but more commonly otitis media, may involve the fibres as they cross the cavity of the middle ear. In this case there are associated vestibular signs and sometimes also a facial nerve paralysis.

Dilated pupils.

Dilated pupils may be due to excessive sympathetic or inadequate parasympathetic activity, or to damage to the retina or other sites on the optic pathway before the divergence of the fibres to the pretectal area. Pupillary dilatation is also seen late in the progression of tentorial herniation. Dilated pupils may be seen in fear, in atropine poisoning or in retinal degenerations. The most notable disease in which dilated pupils are seen is Feline Dysautonomia which is described in Chapter 12.

Strabismus or squint.

Strabismus or squint indicates either a deficit of one of cranial nerves III, IV or VI, abnormal projection of the visual pathways, vestibular dysfunction or a muscular or globe abnormality. Squints may be unilateral or bilateral. In true squints due to lesions of cranial nerves III, IV or VI, conjugate eye movements are preserved. In vestibular dysfunction, conjugate eye movements are normal in some head positions but not in others.

A congenital inwardly turning strabismus is encountered in Siamese cats. It is due to an abnormal projection of the retinal fibres in the lateral geniculate nucleus. It is of no clinical significance and cannot be corrected. This abnormality can also be encountered in 'crypto-Siamese' white cats in which the dominant white gene (see below) masks expression of the Siamese colouration pattern.

Blindness.

A hereditary progressive retinal atrophy occurs in Abyssinian cats (Narfstrom, 1985). The animals may present at any age from a few months onwards. The affected animals have dilated pupils and depressed pupillary light reflexes. Ophthalmoscopic examination reveals tapetal hyperreflectivity and atrophy of the retinal vasculature. Retinal degeneration is also a feature of many storage diseases. Familial photoreceptor degeneration has also been recorded in the cat (West-Hyde and Buyukmihci, 1982). FIP, toxoplasmosis and lymphosarcoma can all result in blindness of either retinal or central origin. Taurine deficient diets result in bilateral retinal degeneration which may eventually lead to blindness. Occasional cases of bilateral optic nerve aplasia are recorded (Barnett and Grimes, 1974). Blindness of central nervous system origin can otherwise occur due to a spectrum of causes closely resembling those encountered in the dog.

Nystagmus.

Nystagmus is a disturbance of ocular position in which there are eye movements which take the form of more or less regular oscillations of the eyes. Spontaneous nystagmus is associated with vestibular disease; fixating nystagmus is associated with cerebellar disease and is a form of intention tremor and positional nystagmus may be due to disease of either organ. In blindness there may be wide, irregular, wandering movements of the eyes.

In Siamese cats a congenital nystagmus is encountered. There are periodic bursts of fine, rapid horizontal eye movements. The condition is benign and apparently a physiological adaptation to abnormal central pathways.

OTHER CRANIAL NERVES (See Chapter 2).

Vth cranial nerve — damage by the impaction of objects across the fauces is much less common than in the dog. In the cat deficits are most commonly due to lesions in the cerebellopontine angle.

VIIth cranial nerve — is susceptible to damage in the same wide variety of sites and processes as in the dog.

VIIIth cranial nerve — Auditory division and the cochlea — Deafness has been difficult to assess in the cat until the advent recently of auditory evoked potentials. Congenital deafness in cats is associated with the dominant white gene. This should be distinguished from true albinism. In true albinism, in which the coat is white and the eyes are pink, the hearing is normal. Whether heterozygous or homozygous, the dominant white gene produces a white coat with 100% penetrance. The gene also has effects on the ear and on eye colour which are not fully penetrant. Up to 80% of cats carrying the dominant white gene are deaf in one or both ears. The eye involvement may also be unilateral or bilateral and affected cats may have blue eyes, yellow eyes or be odd-eyed. The deafness is due to degeneration of the organ of Corti and spiral ganglion (Elverland and Mair, 1980). There is no possibility of treatment. However, such cats can often lead a normal life.

Acquired deafness is rather rarely diagnosed in the cat though otitis media and interna are very common in the cat. Vestibular disturbances seem much more common, as a consequence of this, than is deafness. However, both unilateral and bilateral deafness can be encountered.

Cats are particularly susceptible to the ototoxic effects of the aminoglycoside antibiotics although administration of high dose levels for at least eight to ten days is required to produce the effects (Hawkins and Lurie, 1952, Hawkins et al, 1953). *Neomycin, streptomycin, dihydrostreptomycin* and *gentamycin* may all cause ototoxic effects but the distribution of lesions differs. *Neomycin* and *streptomycin* produce marked effects on the organ of Corti with loss of hair cells and to a lesser extent on the spiral ganglion.

ATAXIA

Ataxia or incoordination of the gait is probably the commonest neurological presenting sign in the cat. The examination of ataxic animals is discussed in Chapters 2 and 3, though it can be difficult to perform all tests in cats. Quiet observation of patients often reveals a significant degree of information in these cases.

ATAXIA OF VESTIBULAR ORIGIN

The signs of vestibular disease are described in Chapters 2 and 8.

Peripheral vestibular disease is common in the cat and is generally due to otitis media/interna. However, other causes must be considered, they include:-

> Congenital vestibular disease
> Ototoxicity (particularly methylmercury and aminoglycoside antibiotics)
> Idiopathic feline vestibular syndrome
> Tumours involving the petrous temporal bone (generally lymphoma)
> Tumours of the vestibular nerve (neurofibromatoma)
> Nasopharyngeal polyps
> Trauma

Congenital vestibular disease - has been recognised in a number of breeds including Burmese, Birman, British cream and Siamese cats. Signs may appear at any time between the first few weeks of life and three to four weeks of age. Severe rolling is seen in the kittens presenting very early in life. Later, a head-tilt and ataxia is seen in these kittens and also in those presenting once they are able to walk. Circling is only occasionally seen and deafness is not usually present. Many affected individuals recover, but in a proportion the signs are permanent.

ACQUIRED PERIPHERAL VESTIBULAR DISEASE

Idiopathic feline vestibular syndrome.

Idiopathic feline vestibular syndrome is a relatively common condition (Burke *et al,* 1985). The condition affects cats of all ages and both sexes and is more common in the summer and autumn than at other times. The condition is acute in onset with the development of severe head tilt, ataxia, and horizontal spontaneous nystagmus directed to the side opposite the head tilt. The patient often falls or rolls to the same side as the head tilt. The animals appear to be in pain and may cry out persistently. The signs gradually abate over one to two weeks without treatment. In many cases recovery is complete but slight ataxia or head tilt may remain permanently.

Ototoxicity.

The susceptibility of the cat to the ototoxic action of aminoglycoside antibiotics has already been noted. This sensitivity involves the vestibular as well as the auditory apparatus. Heavy metals, notably organic arsenical and mercurial compounds, can cause vestibular disease, as can salicylates. Lane (1985) has stressed the susceptibility of the cat's vestibular apparatus to iodine compounds, quaternary ammonium compounds and chlorhexidine, which can induce vestibular disease if used for irrigation of the ear.

Neoplasms.

Tumours of the vestibular nerve are rare and are generally neurofibromas. They are slow-growing and there is progressive development of unilateral vestibular signs and deafness. The lesion eventually results in compression of the brain stem and central signs then appear.

Rarely lymphomas may occur in the region of the tympanic bulla and petrous temporal bone and induce vestibular signs.

Motion sickness.

A small proportion of cats will vomit when transported by road vehicles or trains. A much higher proportion become extremely agitated and vocal but do not vomit. *Diazepam* at a dose of 0.5—2mg/kg given 45 minutes to one hour prior to the journey is usually a satisfactory prophylactic against both problems although, because of the variation between individuals, it may need some experience of a given cat to achieve the optimum dose for that individual.

ACQUIRED CENTRAL VESTIBULAR DISEASE

Acquired central vestibular disease has a wide variety of causes:-

> Trauma
> Space-occupying lesions — neoplasms, abscesses, hydrocephalus
> Inflammatory diseases — micro-abscessation of the brain stem, FIP, toxoplasmosis, cryptococcosis, nocardiosis, other meningitides/encephalitides
> Degenerations — thiamine deficiency, storage diseases
> Intoxications — lead, mercury

The neoplasms involving the central vestibular structures are gliomas, meningiomas, lymphosarcomas and extensions of neurofibromas from the VIIIth nerve.

ATAXIA OF CEREBRAL ORIGIN

The cerebral cortical causes of ataxia have been discussed above since they generally produce other more dramatic signs. They are:-

> Trauma
> Space occupying lesions — neoplasms, abscesses, hydrocephalus,
> Coenurus cysts
> Degenerations — (thiamine deficiency, ischaemic encephalopathy).

ATAXIA OF CEREBELLAR ORIGIN

In ataxia of cerebellar origin the characteristic findings are:- inco-ordination involving the head, trunk and all four limbs; a wide base stance; hypotonia; hyper-reflexia; dysmetria/hypermetria: intention tremor, head tremor and fixating nystagmus. In cerebellar hypoplasia the nystagmus frequently is absent.

The cerebellar causes of ataxia are:

    Congenital
        Cerebellar hypoplasia due to feline panleukopenia
        Non-inflammatory cerebellar hypoplasia
    Acquired
        Trauma
        Space occupying lesions —
                Neoplasms — astrocytomas, meningiomas, osteosarcomas
                involving the cranial vault or temporal bone
                Abscesses
                Coenurus cysts
        Inflammatory disease — (FIP, toxoplasmosis, cryptococcosis, other
                mengingitides/encephalitides)
        Degenerations
        Storage diseases, thiamine deficiency

Cerebellar hypoplasia.

Cerebellar hypoplasia due to feline panleucopenia virus was a common syndrome prior to the introduction of vaccination but has become decidedly rarer of late (Kilham *et al,* 1971). The signs are typical of cerebellar disease except that nystagmus is usually undetectable. The kittens show signs as soon as they are capable of walking. There is compensation with increasing age although the signs are present throughout life. Occasional cases of cerebellar hypoplasia are encountered which are non-inflammatory and therefore not due to feline panleucopenia. The aetiology of these is unknown.

ATAXIA DUE TO LESIONS OF THE SPINAL CORD
AND PERIPHERAL NERVOUS SYSTEM

These will commonly be associated with other signs of spinal cord or peripheral damage or dysfunction.

QUADRIPARESIS, AND ATAXIA OF ALL LIMBS

Lesions causing quadriparesis and ataxia affecting all limbs are described in Chapter 10. Some conditions are particularly prevalent in cats and thus are described here.

SPACE OCCUPYING LESIONS

At all levels of the brain stem and spinal cord space-occupying lesions are an important source of progressive ataxia and paresis. Most commonly these are tumours, but discospondylitis and inflammatory lesions are also relatively common. Intervertebral disc disease is a rare cause of these signs. Radiography and myelography are the most useful diagnostic aids (Wheeler *et al,* 1985).

Tumours.

Tumours in three locations may affect the spinal cord. They all produce slowly but progressively developing signs of spinal cord damage, often with pain present in the early stages. Occasionally, spinal seizures or hyperaesthesia may be seen. Extradural tumours are commonly lymphomas (Northington and Juliana, 1978) but meningiomas are also seen. Extradural tumours may arise from the nerve roots (neurofibromas and Schwannomas), or from the vertebrae (osteosarcomas and chondrosarcomas) or from extradural fat (lipomata). Very rarely metastases to the vertebrae may be encountered.

Meningiomas are the commonest intradural tumours but lymphomas and metastases are also rarely encountered.

Tumours within the cord are of neural origin and are usually gliomas or ependymomas.

Treatment with corticosteroids may temporarily suppress the signs but these will recur and progress and the prognosis is poor. Surgical treatment of spinal tumours is indicated in some cases, though medical management of spinal lymphoma may be possible (Gorman, 1986).

Vertebral osteomyelitis and discospondylitis.

Vertebral osteomyelitis and discospondylitis are (in the author's experience) more common in the cat than is generally supposed. The diagnosis is readily established by radiographic examination coupled with routine haematology which usually reveals a moderate to marked neutrophilia and left shift (Norsworthy, 1979). Long-term treatment (12 weeks or more) with *ampicillin* or *amoxycillin* is indicated. *Corticosteroids* may be helpful in reducing cord oedema and cage rest is required; sedation with *phenobarbitone* tablets (0.5−2 mg/kg) and analgesia with *codeine* tablets (0.25−1.0 mg/kg) may be helpful.

Intervertebral disc protrusion.

Intervertebral disc protrusion and collapse are relatively common radiographic and post mortem findings in cats and occur increasingly with age. The cervical and lumbar regions are particularly prone to be affected. However, neurological signs as a consequence of disc disease are extremely uncommon in the cat (Heavner, 1971). It is, therefore, essential to rule out the other causes of spinal ataxia and paresis before attributing them to disc disease. When neurological signs are encountered they should be managed as for the canine condition.

Multiple cartilaginous exostoses.

Multiple cartilaginous exostoses are characterised by the development of numerous partially calcified bony proliferations which arise from the cortex of the bone. The outgrowths may develop from the vertebral bodies and spinous processes of vertebrae, particularly in the cervical and lumbar regions. The ribs, sternum and scapulae may also be involved. The majority of cases have been in Siamese and domestic shorthairs. The animals usually present in early maturity. The vertebral lesions may lead to cord compression with tetraparesis if they are in the cervical region or paraparesis in the lumbar region. There is no treatment; euthanasia may be required but some patients live a relatively normal life.

ATAXIA AND PARESIS OF THE FORELIMBS

The majority of conditions leading to ataxia and paresis of the forelimbs may also affect the hindlimbs and are discussed in the next section. Hypervitaminosis A, however, far more commonly affects the forelimbs than the hindlimbs.

Hypervitaminosis A.

Hypervitaminosis A is due to excessive dietary intake of the vitamin and is generally a disease of the older cat. Liver and cod liver oil are the most likely foodstuffs to cause problems. The disease is commonly seen in cats that are addicted to a diet of liver. The condition is characterised by the development of exostoses which particularly involve the bones of the forelimb and the vertebrae. The vertebral exostoses may cause spinal cord compression or may compress spinal nerves or their roots. The neurological signs most commonly affect the forelimbs. There is paresis which varies greatly in severity, muscle wasting may be noted and localised areas of skin hyperaesthesia or anaesthesia may be present. The involvement may be uni- or bilateral.

In most cases withdrawal of liver from the diet leads to substantial improvement in the animal's condition but in the most severe cases significant deficits are likely to persist.

ATAXIA OF THE HIND LIMBS AND PARAPARESIS

Ataxia of the hind limbs and bilateral hindlimb weakness (paraparesis) or paralysis (paraplegia) can arise because of lesions at any level of the neuraxis. Evaluation of the level at which the lesion is present has been discussed in Chapter 3.

Conditions causing such signs are described in Chapter 10. Conditions which are particularly prevalent in cats are described in the above section and below.

Chronic organophosphorus intoxication.

Chronic organophosphorus intoxication with progressively developing posterior ataxia and paresis may follow 10-14 days after acute poisoning. Mercurial poisoning may also produce progressive posterior ataxia.

Mild paresis and spinal ataxia have been seen in some cases of intoxication with organochlorine compounds, occasionally these are the only signs found.

Progressively developing ataxia and ascending paralysis in young kittens are early signs of storage diseases (see below) and are a relatively marked feature in the neurolipidoses.

BLADDER AND VISCERAL DYSFUNCTION

Bladder dysfunction and faecal retention and/or incontinence is seen in a number of circumstances:

> Feline dysautonoma
> Sacral spinal cord lesions
> Avulsion or neuropraxia of the sacral spinal nerve
> Injury to the cauda equina
> Vertebral and spinal malformation

Avulsion of the sacral spinal nerves and neurapraxia of the pudendal nerve.

Avulsion of the sacral spinal nerves and neurapraxia of the pudendal nerve are quite common in the cat as a result of road traffic accidents, of attempts to catch or pull cats by their tail and of malicious attempts to swing them by their tail. There usually is urinary retention and overflow, constipation or faecal incontinence and tail flaccidity with complete sensation loss. There may also be weakness, ataxia, sensory loss or paralysis in the hindlimbs. Neurapraxia of the pudendal nerve is the more common of the two occurrences and most cases recover fully with conservative management. Cases of avulsion carry a poor prognosis but in occasional cases autonomous bladder contraction develops sufficiently although there is no control over when or where urination occurs. In either case, manual emptying of the bladder, or an indwelling catheter is required in the interim. *Bethanecol* (Myotonine) can be used to stimulate bladder contraction but manual expression or catheterisation are preferred.

Congenital abnormalities of the spinal cord and vertebral column.

A variety of spinal cord and vertebral column abnormalities are encountered commonly in Manx cats (Michael *et al*, 1969). The Manx condition is determined by a semi-lethal autosomal dominant gene and all Manx cats born alive are heterozygotes. Even amongst those considered normal, a proportion of these cats have megacolon, urinary retention or incontinence and mild paresis and ataxia of the hindlimbs. Many cats which are considered clinically abnormal have much more severe manifestations of the abnormality. They may have occult or open spina bifida, abnormalities of the pelvis, absence of the sacral vertebrae caudal to S_1 and of the coccygeal vertebrae. Exencephaly, kyphoscoliosis, vertebral fusion, and hemivertebrae may also be encountered. The caudal spinal cord may be histologically abnormal and there may be syringomyelia. The more severely affected individuals show faecal accumulation and incontinence; urinary retention and overflow with secondary cystitis; a hopping incoordinate hindlimb gait with plantigrade posture and dereased perineal sensation. Euthanasia is recommended in such cases.

Similar abnormalities are encountered from time to time in other breeds including domestic short and long hairs. Spina bifida has been recorded in the Siamese and Maltese breeds and in Siamese and Burmese crosses. The aetiology of these sporadic cases is unknown. Hemivertebrae, block and butterfly vertebrae are occasionally encountered in cats of all breeds but rarely give rise to any neurological problems.

DISORDERS OF PERIPHERAL NERVE

Disorders of the peripheral nervous system may be generalised or they may be localised and affect a single limb or cranial nerve. The localised conditions are commonly traumatic although very rarely they may be due to tumours or inflammatory lesions involving the nerve. The brachial plexus, sciatic nerve and radial nerve are most commonly involved in traumatic injury in the cat. The signs and treatment of these and other peripheral nerve injuries are essentially as in the dog, but in general the prognosis is less favourable in the cat. (See Chapter 11 and 14.)

Ischaemic neuromyopathy.

In aortic embolism ischaemic damage to the peripheral nerves of the hindlimb contributes to the signs. There is axonal degeneration and demyelination. Treatment depends upon re-establishing the circulation to the hind limbs and prevention of further embolic episodes. If this is successful, nerve regeneration can occur although there may be residual deficits (Griffiths and Duncan, 1979).

Polyneuropathies.

Inflammatory peripheral nerve lesions are extremely rare in the cat: there is one report (Flecknell and Lucke, 1984) of chronic progressive polyradiculoneuropathy in the cat. The signs waxed and waned over several months and consisted of a high stepping gait, ataxia, muscle twitching and loss of sensory perception. Polyneuropathy has been recorded in diabetes mellitus and cases of intoxication with lead, thallium and mercurials. The hereditary nervous system degenerations may involve the peripheral nerves.

WEAKNESS : DISEASES OF THE NEUROMUSCULAR JUNCTION

Botulism.

Occasional cases of botulism occur in cats. The disease is due to the ingestion of material containing the toxins of Clostridium botulinum. Generalised weakness or lower motor neurone type paralysis are seen. Diagnosis is by demonstration of the toxin. The prognosis is poor but supportive therapy is occasionally successful.

Myasthenia gravis.

Myasthenia gravis is a rare condition in cats, but both the acquired and the congenital forms have been recorded (Mason, 1976; Indrieri *et al*, 1983). The signs of the disease are generalised muscle weakness which is brought on by exercise, difficulty in respiration and in eating and altered voice. Megoesophagus occurs but is less frequent and less reliable as a diagnostic feature than in the dog. Diagnosis can be made by the demonstration of a decreasing end plate response to repetitive nerve stimulation. More commonly diagnosis must be made by performing a 'Tensilon' test (See Chapter 13). This should provide temporary relief of the signs leading to the animal being able to exercise for several minutes without tiring. Treatment is with *pyridostigmine bromide* (10-30 mg) orally once daily or *neostigmine methyl sulphate* (at a dose of around 0.25 mg) intramuscularly twice daily. It is essential that the dose is carefully adjusted for the individual animal. Overdosing leads to generalised cholinergic crisis, whilst underdosing leads to a recurrence of signs (see Chapter 13).

MUSCLE TREMOR AND SPASM, TETANY, TETANUS

Muscle tremor and spasm, tetany and tetanus may arise from the following causes:

Encephalitis
Tetanus *(Clostridium tetani* infection)
Hypocalcaemia (lactation tetany)
Hypoglycaemia
Uraemia

Intoxicants, notably:-	Strychnine	Lead
	Organophosphorous compounds	Ethylene glycol
	Organochlorine compounds	Metaldehyde

Unknown

Tetanus.

Tetanus is rare in the cat, but can follow accidental wounds or castration. The clinical signs may be very mild with only stiffness of a single limb. In more severe cases there may be stiffness of all limbs, inability to rise, tetanic spasms, protrusion of the nictitating membrane and curving of the tail up and over the back. (Killingsworth *et al*, 1977). Risus sardonicus, trismus and opisthotonus are rarely seen. Diagnosis is based on the history and signs. Treatment rests upon neutralising the toxin, eliminating the infection and minimising the clinical signs. The animal should receive 5,000 units of tetanus antitoxin, after a small test dose has been given and the absence of anaphylaxis confirmed. If the wound can be identified, although this is often not the case, it should be debrided and irrigated with hydrogen peroxide. *Procaine penicillin* G (60,000 units i.m. daily) should be given for a minimum course of five days and longer if signs persist. The animal should be kept in a quiet, dark place to minimise muscle spasms and *diazepam* (2.5 mg i.m. four times daily) or *phenobarbitone* (2.5 mg i.m. four times daily) given in order to minimise muscular activity. Fluid therapy, intravenous feeding and good supportive therapy are essential to success.

Strychnine poisoning.

Strychnine poisoning is the major differential diagnosis of tetanus. The signs are very similar but the spasms are more severe but with intervals of relaxation. Nictitating membrane protrusion is less frequently seen than in tetanus.

EPISODIC WEAKNESS OR COLLAPSE

Apart from myasthenia gravis which has already been discussed, episodic weakness and collapse is usually due to generalised disorders, metabolic disorders or to disease of other systems (see Chapter 13)

The causes in cats include:

Myasthenia gravis
Hypocalcaemia
Hypoglycaemia (including glycogenoses)
Hyperkalaemia
Hypokalaemia
Hypoxia
    Cardiopulmonary dysfunction
    Severe anaemia
Hyperviscosity of the blood
Toxoplasmosis

MULTIFOCAL SIGNS

Many feline diseases affecting the nervous system are generalised conditions that may affect any part of the nervous system. Frequently these conditions simultaneously involve the whole nervous system or more than one part, region or subsystem of it. Thus, clinical signs may be detected involving unrelated parts of the nervous system. In the cat, inflammatory processes generally of proven or presumed infective aetiology, storage diseases and other heritable degenerations feature prominently among the conditions producing multifocal nervous signs. The generalised metabolic diseases (other than the storage diseases), intoxications and neoplasms which affect the nervous system and may produce multifocal signs have already been discussed. The causes of multifocal signs are given in Table 15.4.

Storage diseases.

Storage diseases are a large group of genetically determined conditions in which the absence of a specific enzyme leads to the accumulation of its substrates. In many cases these substrates accumulate in lysosomes and eventually interfere with cellular function. In a few cases, notably the glycogenoses, the accumulations are cytoplasmic and the abnormality interferes with mobilisation of glycogen to maintain plasma glucose levels; weakness or collapse on exercise is therefore a clinical sign in these cases. Specific conditions occur in particular breeds and this is of help in identifying the abnormality under consideration. All of the conditions are progressive, are usually manifest in young animals and lead to death. The storage diseases are generally autosomal recessive in inheritance and only one or two animals which are homozygous for the condition will be affected in each litter. Since

Table 15.4
Diseases causing Multifocal Neurological Signs in Cats

Storage diseases*
Other heritable degenerations*
Other generalised metabolic disorders*
Disseminated neoplasms (notably metastatic disease or lymphomas)*
Intoxications (notably heavy metals)*
Infective/inflammatory processes
  Encephalitides
    Rabies
    Pseudorabies*
  Meningitides/generalised infections
    Feline infectious peritonitis (FIP)*
    Toxoplasmosis*
    Cryptococcosis*
    Aspergillosis*
    Nocardiosis*
    Actinomycosis*
    Histoplasmosis
    Blastomycosis
    Coccidiomyocosis
    Prototheccosis
  Aberrant parasitic migration
    Toxocariasis*
    Cutebriasis
    Dirofilariasis
    Angiostrongylosis

Only those conditions marked with an asterisk are likely to be encountered in cats raised and kept in the British Isles. The others occur in other areas of the world and may rarely be encountered in imported cats.

heterozygotes can usually be identified by suitable laboratory determinations they can be eliminated by selective breeding. The clinical signs vary somewhat with the condition involved but in general the affected animals show poor growth relative to their littermates. Progressively developing ataxia and paralysis which affects the hindlimbs first and then develops with an ascending pattern, are frequent findings. The storage diseases which have been recorded in the cat are shown in Table 15.5.

Diagnosis and the identification of heterozygotes require specialised laboratory facilities. There are a number of approaches to diagnosis and the most appropriate varies with the condition suspected. The activity of the lysosomal enzymes may be measured, usually in leukocytes. Stored product may be demonstrated by histochemistry, by electron microscopy or by biochemical isolation and characterisation, often in biopsy specimens. Since the appropriate organ(s) for investigation also vary according to the condition suspected, consultation at an early stage of a laboratory with experience of these conditions is recommended.

Other heritable degenerations.

Three other progressive degenerations with marked spinal cord and cerebellar signs have been recorded in the cat, two of which are clearly heritable. These are neuroaxonal dystrophy in domestic shorthairs (Woodward *et al*, 1974) and motor neurone disease characterised by neurofibrillar accumulation (Norby and Thuline, 1979) also in domestic shorthairs. The third condition is familial spongiform degeneration in the Egyptian Mau, the aetiology of which is uncertain (Kelly and Gaskell, 1976).

Feline infectious peritonitis.

The dry, pyrogranulomatous or non-effusive form of feline infectious peritonitis can involve the choroid plexus, meninges or brain parenchyma (Kornegay, 1978). Signs may be localised but they are more commonly multifocal. The eye is also commonly involved and uveitis should arouse suspicions of FIP. CSF analysis is helpful. The protein concentration is elevated to as much as 5g/l and is predominantly globulin and the nucleated cell count may reach 1×10^9/l. The nucleated cell population may be primarily mononuclear or there may be a large neutrophil polymorph component.

Other viral infections.

There are frequent reports of non-suppurative polio-encephalomyelitis and meningo-encephalomyelitis in cats. These are presumed to be viral but no causative organism has been identified (Borland and McDonald, 1965; Kronevi *et al*, 1974; Vandevelde and Braund, 1979; Hoff and Vandevelde, 1981).

Table 15.5
Storage Diseases Encountered in Cats

Disease	Breed	Absent enzyme
Glycogen storage disease Type I Pompe's disease	DSH	glucosidase
GM$_1$ gangliosidosis Type I	DSH	galactosidase
GM$_1$ gangliosidosis Type II	Siamese	galactosidase (partial)
GM$_2$ gangliosidosis Tay-Sach's disease	DSH	Hexosaminidase
Sphingomyelinosis Niemann-Pick disease	Siamese	Sphingomyelinase
Metachromic leukodystrophy	DSH	Arylsulphatase
Ceroid lipofuscinosis	Siamese	Uncertain
Globoid cell leukodystrophy Krabbe's disease	DSH	Galactocerebrosidase
Mucopolysaccharidosis I Hurler's syndrome	DSH	Alpha-L-iduronidase
Mucopolysaccharidosis IV Maroteaux-Lamy syndrome	Siamese	Arylsulphatase B
Mannosidosis	Persian	Mannosidase
?	Abyssinian	?

Toxoplasmosis.

Clinically apparent toxoplasmosis involving the central nervous system is much less common than FIP. Uveitis or retinitis may be seen. There may be an inflammatory polymyositis which may mimic neurological disease or may contribute to the signs if there is combined involvement. Liver, lung and gastro-intestinal involvement may also be prominent features (Hirth and Nielson, 1969). Pyrexia and lymphadenopathy are common. Oocyst shedding occurs for a very limited period of the sexual phase of infection, thus faecal examination is not of assistance in diagnosis. If there is lymphadenopathy the organism may be seen in aspiration biopsy smears of lymph node. The CSF has increased protein levels and a rather variable pleocytosis. Serology may be of some help in diagnosis. In many cases a definitive diagnosis is only made post mortem.

Fungal infections.

Both *Cryptococcus neoformans* and *Aspergillus fumigatus* are occasionally encountered as the causative organisms of central nervous infections, notably of meningitis. Either organism can enter from the nose or sinuses. On CSF examination the organisms are readily detected and can be cultured and identified. The CSF protein is raised and there is moderate pleocytosis.

Bacterial infections.

Bacterial infections are rare with meningitis being only slightly more common than encephalitis. In meningitis the CSF has markedly elevated protein concentrations, there is a florid neutrophil pleocytosis, organisms are usually visible on smears and can be cultured, and the glucose concentration is depressed. In encephalitis and brain abscessation the CSF changes may be much milder and may not be diagnostic.

REFERENCES

BARNETT, K. C. and GRIMES, T. D. (1974). Bilateral aplasia of the optic nerve in a cat. *British Journal of Ophthalmology* **58**,663.

BARNETT, K. C. and RICKETTS, J. D. (1985). The eye. In: *Feline Medicine and Therapeutics* (Eds: Chandler, E.A., Gaskell, C. J. and Hilbery, A. D. R.) Blackwell Scientific Publications, Oxford.

BLAKEMORE, W. F. (1975). Lysosomal storage diseases. *Veterinary Annual* **15**, 242.

BLAXTER, A. (1987). Feline hepatic disease. *Veterinary Annual* **27**, 329.

BORLAND, R. and McDONALD, N. (1965). Feline encephalomyelitis. *British Veterinary Journal* **121**, 479.

BURGER, I. H. and FLECKNELL, P. A. (1985). Poisoning. In: *Feline Medicine and Therapeutics* (Eds: Chadler, E. A., Gaskell, C. J. and Hilbery, A. D. R.). Blackwell Scientific Publications, Oxford.

BURKE, E. E., MOISE, S. and DeLAHUNTA, A. (1985). Review of idiopathic feline vestibular syndrome. *Journal of the American Veterinary Medical Association* **187**, 941.

DOW, C. and McFERRAN, J. B. (1986). Aujeszky's disease in the dog and cat. *Veterinary Record* **75**, 1099.

ELVERLAND, H. H. and MAIR, I. W. S. (1980). Hereditary deafness in the cat. An electron microscopic study of the spiral ganglion. *Acta otolaryngologica* **90**, 360.

EVANS, R. J. (1988). Toxic hazards for cats. *Veterinary Annual* **28**, 251.

FLECKNELL, P. A. and LUCKE, V. M. (1978). Chronic relapsing polyradiculoneuritis in a cat. *Acta Neuropathologica* **41**, 81.

GASKELL, R. M. (1985) Rabies. In: *Feline Medicine and Therapeutics* (Eds. Chandler, E. A., Gaskell, C. J. and Hilbery, A. D. R.). Blackwell Scientific Publications, Oxford.

GORMAN, N. (1986). Oncology. *Contemporary Issues in Small Animal Practice,* Vol 6. Churchill Livingstone, New York.

GRIFFITHS, I. R. and DUNCAN, I. D. (1979). Ischaemic neuromyopathy in cats. *Veterinary Record* **104**, 518.

HASKINS, M. E., JEZYK, P. F., DESNICK, R. J., McDONOUGH, S. K. PATTERSON, D. F., (1979). Mucopolysaccharidosis in a domestic short haired cat: a disease distinct from that seen in the Siamese cat. *Journal of the American Veterinary Medical Association* **175**, 384.

HASKINS, M. E., JEZYK, P. F., DESNICK, R. J. and PATTERSON, D. F. (1981). Animal model of human disease: Mucopolysaccharidosis VI Maroteaux-Lamy syndrome. Arylsulfatase B-deficient mucopolysaccharidosis in the Siamese cat. *American Journal of Pathology* **105**, 191.

HAWKINS, J. E. and LURIE, M. H. (1952). The otoxicity of streptomycin. *Annals of Otology, Rhinology and Laryngology* **61** 789.

HAWKINS, J. E., RAHWAY, N. J. and LURIE, M. H. (1953). The ototoxicity of dihydrostreptomycin and neomycin in the cat. *Annals of Otology, Rhinology and Laryngology* **62**, 1128.

HEAVNER, J. E., (1979). Intervertebral disc syndrome in the cat. *Journal of the American Veterinary Medical Association* **159**, 425.

HIRTH, R. S. and NIELSEN, S. W. (1969). Non-suppurative encephalomyelitis in cats suggestive of a viral origin. *Veterinary Pathology* **18**, 170.

HOFF, E.J. and VANDEVELDE, M. (1981). Non-suppurative encephalomyelitis in cats suggestive of a viral origin. *Veterinary Pathology* **18**, 170.

HORVATH, Z. and PAPP, L. (1967). Clinical manifestations of Aujeszky's disease in the cat. *Acta Veterinary Academy of Science Hungary* **17**, 49.

INDRIERI, R. J., CREIGHTON, S. R. and LAMBERT, E. H. (1983). Myasthenia gravis in two cats. *Journal of the American Veterinary Medical Association* **182**, 57.

JUBB, K. V. F., SAUNDERS, L. Z. and COATES, H. V. (1956). Thiamine deficiency encephalopathy in cats. *Journal of Comparative Pathology* **66**, 217.

KAY, W. J. Epilepsy in cats. *Journal of the American Animal Hospital Association* **11**, 77.

KELLY, D. F. and GASKELL, C. J. (1976). Spongy deterioration in the central nervous system in kittens. *Acta Neuropathologica* **35**, 151.

KILHAM, L., MARGOLIS, G. and COLBY, E. D. (1971). Cerebellar ataxia and its transmission in cats by feline panleukopenia virus. *Journal of the American Veterinary Medical Association* **158**, 888.

KILLINGSWORTH, C., CHIAPELLA, A., VERALLI, P. and DeLAHUNTA, A. (1977). Feline tetanus. *Journal of the American Animal Hospital Association* **13**, 209.

KORNEGAY, J. N. (1978). Feline infectious peritonitis: the central nervous system form. *Journal of the American Animal Hospital Association* **14**, 580.

KORNEGAY, J. N. (1981). Feline neurology. *Compendium for Continuing Education* **3**, 203.

KRONEVI, T., NORDSTROM, M., MORENO, W. and NILSSON, P. O. (1974). Feline ataxia due to a non-suppurative meningoencephalomyelitis of unknown aetiology. *Nordisk Veterinar Medecin* **26**, 720.

LANE, J. G. (1985). Ototoxicity in the dog and cat. *Veterinary Record* **117**, 94.

MASON, K. V. (1976). A case of myasthenia gravis in a cat. *Journal of Small Animal Practice* **17**, 467.

MICHAEL, C. C., LASSMAN, L. P. and TOMLINSON, B. E. (1969). Congenital anomalies of the lower spine and spinal cord in Manx cats. *Journal of Pathology* **97**, 269.

MUGFORD, R. A. (1975). Behavioural problems. In: *Feline medicine and therapeutics* (Eds: Chandler, E. A., GASKELL, C. J. and Hilbery, A. D. R.). Blackwell Scientific Publications, Oxford.

NARFSTROM, K. (1985). Progressive retinal atrophy in the Abyssinian cat: clinical characteristics. *Investigative Ophthalmology and Visual Science* **26**, 193.

NORBY, D. E. and THULINE, H. C. (1970). Neurofibrillar accumulations in neurons of cats with ataxia. *Nature* **227**, 1261.

NORTHINGTON, J. W. and JULIANA, M. M. (1978). Extradural lymphosarcoma in six cats. *Journal of Small Animal Practice* **19**, 409.

NORSWORTHY, G. D. (1979). Discospondylitis as a cause of posterior paresis. *Feline Practice* **9**, 39.

VAN DEN BERGH, BAKER, M. K. and LANGE, L. (1977). A suspected lysosomal storage disease in Abyssinian cats. Part I: genetic clinical and clinical pathological aspects. *Journal of the South African Veterinary Association* **48**, 195.

VANDEVELDE, M. and BRAUND, K. (1979). Polioencephalomyelitis in cats. *Veterinary Pathology* **16**, 420.

VANDEVELDE, M., FANKHAUSER, R., BICHSEL, P., WIESMANN, U. and HERSCHKOWITZ, N. (1982). Hereditary neurovisceral mannosidosis associated with alpha-mannosidase deficiency in a family of Persian cats. *Acta Neuropathologica* **58**,64.

VULGAMOTT, J. C., TURNWALD, J. C., KINGS, G. K., HERRING, D. S., HANSEN, J. F. and BOOTHE, H. W. (1980). Congenital portocaval anomalies of the cat: two case reports. *Journal of the American Animal Hospital Association* **16** , 915.

WEST-HYDE, L. and BUYUKMIHCI, (1982). Photoreceptor degeneration in a family of cats. *Journal of the American Veterinary Medical Association* **181**, 243.

WHEELER, S. J., CLAYTON JONES, D. G. and WRIGHT, J. A. (1985). Myelography in the cat. *Journal of Small Animal Practice* **26**, 143-152.

WILKINSON, G. T. (1979). Feline cryptococcosis: a review and seven case reports. *Journal of Small Animal Practice* **20**, 749.

WOODWARD, J. C., COLLINS, G. H. and HESSLER, J. R. (1974). Feline hereditary neuroaxonal dystrophy. *American Journal of Pathology* **74**, 551.

ZAKI, F. A. and HURVITZ, A. I. (1975). Spontaneous neoplasms of the central nervous system of the cat. *Journal of Small Animal Practice* **17**, 773.

ZAKI, F. A., PRATA, R. G. and WARNER, L. L. (1976). Necrotising myelopathy in a cat. *Journal of the American Veterinary Medical Association* **169**, 228.

FURTHER READING

AVERILL, D. R. (1973). Feline neurology. *Journal of the American Animal Hospital Association* **40**, 195.

BESTETI, G., BUHLMANN, V., NICOLET, J. and FANKHAUSER, R. (1977). Paraplegia due to Actinomyces viscosus infection in a cat. *Acta Neuropathologica* **39**, 231.

BLAKEMORE, W. F. (1975). Lysosomal storage diseases. *Veterinary Annual* **15**, 242.

CHRISMAN, C. (1982). *Problems in small animal neurology.* Lea and Febiger, Philadelphia.

DeLAHUNTA (1968). Feline vestibular disease. In: *Current veterinary therapy III* (Ed: Kirk, R. W.). W. B. Saunders Company, Philadelphia.

DeLAHUNTA, A. (1977). Feline neurology. *Veterinary Clinics of North America* **6**, 433.

DeLAHUNTA, A. (198?). *Veterinary neuroanatomy and clinical neurology.* W. B. Saunders Company, Philadelphia.

EVANS, R. J. (1985). The nervous system. In : *Feline medicine and therapeutics* (Eds: Chandler, E. A., Gaskell, C. J. and Hilbery, A. D. R.) Blackwell Scientific Publications, Oxford.

HOLIDAY, T. A. (1971). Clinical aspects of some encephalopathies of domestic cats. *Veterinary Clinics of North America* **1**, 367.

KAY, W. J. (1975). Epilepsy in cats. *Journal of the American Animal Hospital Association* **11**, 77.

KORNEGAY, J. N. (1981). Feline neurology. *Compendium for Continuing Education* **3**, 203.

LUGINBUHL, H. (1961). Studies of meningiomas in cats. *American Journal of Veterinary Research* **22**, 1030.

NAFE, L. A. (1979). Meningiomas in cats: a retrospective clinical study of 36 cases. *Journal of the American Veterinary Medical Association* **174**, 1224.

NAFE, L. A. (1984). Topics in feline neurology. *Veterinary Clinics of North America* **14**, 1289.

OLIVER, J. E. (1972). Neurologic emergencies in small animals. *Veterinary Clinics of North America* **2**, 341.

OLIVER, J. E. (1974). Neurogenic causes of abnormal micturition in the dog and cat. *Veterinary Clinics of North America* **4**, 517.

OLIVER, J. E. and LORENZ, M. D. (1983). *Handbook of veterinary neurologic diagnosis.* W. B. Saunders Co., Philadelphia.

PALMER, A. C. (1976). *Introduction to animal neurology.* Blackwell Scientific Publications, Oxford.

PARKER, A. J. (1973). Feline spinal cord damage. Part 1: degree and localisation. *Feline Practice* **5**, 36.

PARKER, A. J. (1973). Feline spinal cord damage. Part 2: differential diagnosis. *Feline Practice* **5**, 38.

PARKER, A. J., O'BRIEN, D. P. and SAWCHUK, S. A. (1983). The nervous system. In: *Feline medicine* (Ed. Pratt, P. W.) American Veterinary Publications, Santa Barbara.

ROCHLITZ, I. (1984). Scientific committee report. Feline dysautonomia (Key-Gaskell syndrome): preliminary review. *Journal of Small Animal Practice* **25**, 587.

SWAIM, S. F. and SHIELDS, R. P. (1971). Paraplegia in the cat: aetiology and differential diagnosis. *Veterinary Medicine small Animal Clinician* **66**, 787.

WILKINSON, G. T. (1984). *Diseases of the cat and their management.* Blackwell Scientific Publications, Oxford.

ZAKI, F. A. and LAFE, L. A. (1980). Ischaemic encephalopathy and focal granulomatous meningoencephalitis in the cat. *Journal of Small Animal Practice* **21**, 429.

NEUROLOGICAL PROBLEMS OF EXOTIC SPECIES

Martin P. C. Lawton B.Vet.Med., Cert.V.Ophthal, F.R.C.V.S.

An animal, being exotic, does not stop it from suffering neurological problems similar to those of the dog, cat and other domestic animals. Presentation of an exotic animal often causes a mental block in many veterinarians, but, by applying first principals, there is no reason why any such animal cannot be investigated as to the cause of its neurological deficit. In addition to general principles, an understanding of the dietary requirements of exotic animals is also beneficial.

Exotic animals may be divided into mammals, birds, and poikilotherms (the ectotherms). The poikilotherms include reptiles, fish and invertebrates. The distinction is not just academic but of practical importance. Mammals and birds are able to regulate their body temperature (endotherms) and respond in a standard way when examined. Those animals whose metabolism is affected by the external temperature (poikilotherms) may show different clinical signs at different temperatures. Similarly, reflexes also vary at different temperatures, due to metabolic affects on the speed of conduction of impulses through the nervous system.

Poikilotherms may also undergo hibernation if the external temperature falls too far below their preferred body temperature, causing their bodily responses to be diminished or to become virtually absent. However, even a tortoise that is in hibernation will move the forelimbs in response to gentle stroking of that leg, although this will be very slow. Problems may arise for the inexperienced in assessing whether or not a poikilotherm is alive or brain dead, a distinction most easily established by trying to return it back to its preferred body temperature by gradually increasing the temperature.

Neurological problems of exotics are divided into those resulting from diet, environment, toxic damage or trauma. Traumatic problems are often associated with too much 'furniture' and toys in the cage, resulting in crush injuries.

FERRETS

Ferrets may suffer neurological problems similar to those already described for the dog and cat in preceeding chapters, but are particularly prone to botulism and canine distemper.

Botulism

This may be seen in ferrets that are fed a raw meat diet which had been contaminated at some stage with butolin toxin. The ferret is moderately susceptible to toxin types A and B, but highly susceptible to type C (Andrews & Illman, 1987). Clinical signs, which start within twelve hours of ingestion of the contaminated food, initially are due to muscular stiffness and inco-ordination, but with time and progression of the disease, the ferret becomes ataxic and eventually paralysed. Death is the usual sequal due to paralysis of the respiratory muscles. Treatment may be attempted with antitoxin and supportive therapy, but the outcome depends on the amount of toxin ingested and how quickly the treatment is instigated.

Canine Distemper

Ferrets are extremely susceptible to canine distemper virus infection (Cooper, 1985a; Andrews & Illman, 1987). Mortality rate due to canine distemper virus is very high and the course of the disease is similar as that seen and described in the dog (Cornwell, 1984). If the ferret survives the initial systemic phase, then neurological symptoms may be seen, which are similar to that of myoclonus in the dog (Cooper, 1985a). There is no specific treatment, other than general nursing care and supportive therapy.

PRIMATES

It is difficult to assess all but the most severe neurological problems in primates, due to the problems in performing an adequate neurological examination safely and without the use of sedation.

Dietary problems

Primates, like birds and reptiles, are often fed an unsuitable and deficient diet, which results in problems due to calcium and phosphorous imbalance and lack of vitamin D. In addition to this they also have a dietary requirement for vitamin C.

Nutritional osteodystrophy in pet primates leads to inco-ordination, weakness, inability to grip and sometimes ataxia or true paralysis. Radiography will often show the obvious osteodystrophy, often with secondary pathological fractures. (Figure 16.1)

Treatment is aimed at the correction of the dietary imbalance and deficiencies, by changing to a more adequate diet and the use of vitamin and mineral supplementation, such as Vionate (Ciba Geigy) or ACE-High (Vetark).

Seizures

Seizures seen in primates may be associated with osteodystrophy or due to true epilepsy. Nelson (1979) reports the stress of handling as a cause of seizures. This is usually seen in juveniles and young adults, and is reproduceable upon repeated conditions and handling. Treatment with anticonvulsants may be attempted.

Paralysis

Paralysis seen in primates often is accompanied by atrophy and contraction of the affected muscles, preventing them from straightening their legs. This often is a result of inadequate cage size, and referred to as cage paralysis. It may also be associated with bad injection technique and resulting nerve damage (Nelson, 1979).

Paralysis associated with osteodystrophy may be due to pathological fracture or collapse of the vertebral column.

Other disorders

Other causes of neurological problems include rabies, poliomyelitis, or bacterial/viral encephalitis.

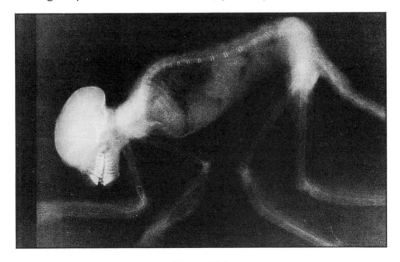

Figure 16.1
Squirrel monkey showing severe osteodystrophy and secondary pathological fractures

RABBITS

Neurological problems seen in rabbits are usually associated with infection or trauma.

Pasteurella multocida infection

Torticollis is a common presenting clinical sign (Figure 16.2), often associated with otitis media or interna, or encephalitis. The affected rabbit may have a slight head tilt or it may be so severe that balance is totally disrupted. Any attempt to handle or disturb the animal will result in it spinning and this is especially noticeable if it panics. Nystagmus also may be present.

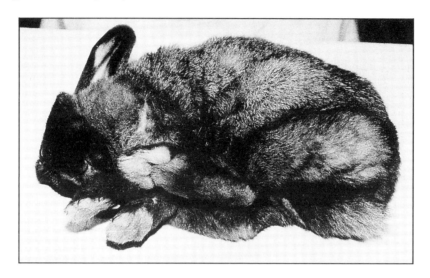

Figure 16.2
A rabbit affected with pasteurella infection showing torticollis

The usual cause of otitis media and interna is *Pasteurella multocida* (Harkness and Wagner, 1977, Flecknell, 1985a). As well as a cause of respiratory problems, *Pasteurella* is found frequently in the nares, conjunctiva, lung or pharynx but is usually asymptomatic (Harkness and Wagner, 1977). If the organism migrates via the eustachian tube it may result in otitis media, which eventually progress to otitis interna.

Treatment is generally ineffective (Flecknell, 1985a), but may be attempted with corticosteroids and a suitable antibiotic, such as *tylosin* or *oxytetracycline,* which may result in some remission.

Encephalitozoonosis

This is caused by the parasite *Encephalitozoon cuniculi,* which affects the central nervous system and kidneys. Occasionally it may be a cause of torticollis, paresis or convulsions, but most cases are chronic and sub clinical (Harkness and Wagner, 1977; Flecknell, 1985a).

Toxoplasma gondii

This may cause clinical disease in domestic rabbits (Flecknell, 1985a). Clinical signs include paralysis or convulsions and are usually followed by death in a few days. Diagnosis is at post mortem.

Spinal fractures

Fractures of the lumbar spine are common in rabbits (Baxter, 1975), usually due to the rabbit being dropped or struggling during restraint and handling (Harkness and Wagner, 1977; Flecknell, 1985a). The resulting degree of paresis, or paralysis, depends on the severity and location of the damage. Radiography is useful in making the diagnosis, but total recovery is unlikely. If there is contusion to the spinal cord in the absence of a true fracture, then steroid treatment together with cage rest and general nursing, may be helpful.

Arthritis

Severe arthritic change may also be seen clinically and may appear to be causing a neurological deficit. Usually there is total fusion of the joint associated with the arthritis, resulting in an inability to use the offending leg properly and is particularly noticed if it involves the hip joint (Figure 16.3).

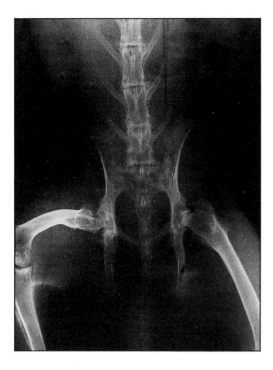

Figure 16.3
Radiograph of rabbit's hips with severe arthritis

RATS AND MICE

Pasteurellosis

As in rabbits, torticollis may be exhibited and may be due to pasteurella (Flecknell, 1985b), or a mycoplasma infection. Treatment may be successful after prolonged treatment with antibiotics.

Lymphocytic choriomeningitis

Lymphocytic choriomeningitis (LCM) can affect mice, guinea pigs, chinchillas, canines, primates, hamsters and humans. In humans it may cause a fatal meningitis or influenza-like signs. Fortunately, the fatal meningitis is rarely seen.

Although the natural host is the wild rodent population (Harkness and Wagner, 1977), LCM is usually asymptomatic in mice (Flecknell, 1985b), but may cause hind leg paralysis. Any rodent showing signs of a central nervous system disorder should be examined for serological evidence of LCM in view of the public health hazard.

Trauma

Traumatic injury in these small rodents is a common occurrence, due to being dropped by young owners, resulting in damage to the hind legs, spinal cord, concussion or intracranial damage. Radiology is required to diagnose or rule out these problems, and is best achieved using dental or non-screen film.

Other Disorders

Other viral causes of neurological problems include mouse encephalomyelitis virus, mouse hepatitis virus, and mouse poliomyelitis. Inheritable neurological disorders have also been described (Mullink, 1979).

GERBILS

Neurological problems discussed under rats and mice also occur in gerbils, although gerbils are more prone to spinal and hind limb injuries as they have no concept of height and easily leap (Toy, 1985a).

Gerbils have one peculiarity that requires special mention. They suffer epileptiform seizures which are provoked by handling. It is thought that these epileptiform seizures affect 20% of the population (Harkness and Wagner, 1977; Toy, 1985a), and are genetically influenced and thought to be a normal defensive mechanism against attack (Harkness and Wagner, 1977).

These seizures vary from a mild hypnotic state to a severe myoclonic convulsion followed by tonic extensor rigidity which may last from 30 seconds to 2 minutes. The seizures appear to have no adverse effects on the gerbil and they make a full recovery. These seizures can be very distressing to a young owner and control can be attempted by using anticonvulsant therapy (Harkness and Wagner, 1977; Toy, 1985a), although assessing a correct dose is difficult.

HAMSTERS

The neurological problems described for rabbits and rodents affect hamsters and include problems due to toxoplasmosis, nosematosis, (Sebesteny, 1979), bacterial otitis media interna or encephalitis (Harkness and Wagner, 1977; Sebesteny, 1979).

Lymphocytic choriomeningitis (LCM) has been reoprted in hamsters (Harkness and Wagner, 1977; Sebesteny, 1979; Toy, 1985b) and is of concern due to the popularity of these species as pets. LCM can result in incoordination or paralysis (Harkness and Wagner, 1977) but may be asymptomatic (Toy, 1985b). The virus is excreted in the urine and saliva and therefore general hygiene is an essential part of preventing the spread of this zoonosis.

Paralysis

Causes of paralysis include: —

Age (Toy, 1985b), due to the lack of exercise and a small cage. Moving the hamster to larger quarters and allowing it to exercise may bring about an improvement in this condition.

Muscular dystrophy (Caulfield, 1972; Toy, 1985b), is a genetic problem causing a hind limb paralysis, mainly of males, in the age group 6 — 10 months of age, although occasionally seen in females. (Figure 16.4).

Vitamin E deficiency (Granodos, 1968).

Miscellaneous problems such as falls, constipation, dystocia, or infected bite wounds have also been reported (Toy, 1985).

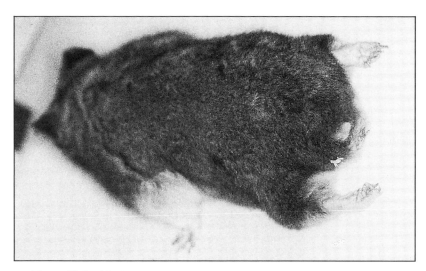

Figure 16.4   Hind leg paralysis of a hamster due to muscular dystrophy

Sleeper disease
This is a state of immobility which is found when the temperature exceeds 22°C (Toy, 1985b). The hamster, when faced with this high temperature, becomes lifeless, may tremble or shake and ataxia may be the final result. When the hamster is placed into a more suitable environment normal behaviour will return.

Hibernation
This occurs when the external temperature drops below 5°C and the hamster may be thought to be dead when in this state. The pulse and breathing are usually imperceptible and the hamster may also appear stiff and cold on handling. Any suspected 'dead' hamster should always be warmed to see if it awakens.

GUINEA PIGS

Guinea Pigs suffer with similar neurological problems as described above. Most common are otitis and fractured spines due to falls or incorrect handling (Harkness and Wagner, 1977; Wagner, 1979). Other problems include pododermatitis, enterotoxaemia and encephalopathies.

In addition there are three problems in guines pigs which warrant further mention.

Pregnancy toxaemia

Pregnancy toxaemia is seen in obese sows carrying twins or a single large baby and nearing parturition. The clinical signs may vary from anorexia with incoordination, to true convulsions. Treatment is by caesarian section accompanied by supportive treatment with fluids and corticosteroids.

Vitamin C deficiency

Guinea pigs are unable to manufacture their own vitamin C, therefore requiring a constant dietary source. Hypovitaminosis C may result in neurological signs associated with the inability to move or ataxia due to the swelling of the joints caused by this disease. Treatment is with vitamin C supplementation and a higher quality diet.

Back strain

Due to the size and weight of pet guinea pigs, which are often obese, back strain due to incorrect handling may be seen. Harkness and Wagner (1977) have reported this problem in laboratory guinea pigs, due to oedema and haemorrhage around the spinal cord. Clinical signs range from pain on movement to temporary paralysis.

Treatment is with strict rest, use of corticosteroids and diuretics. Training of owners in how to handle these creatures may prevent further distress.

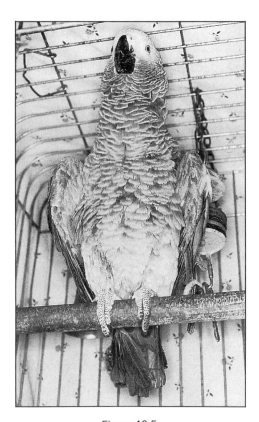

Figure 16.5
Wing fluttering in an African grey
associated with hypocalcaemic tetany

BIRDS

Neurological problems in birds may be due to dietary causes, toxins, trauma or infections.

Calcium: Phosphorus: Vitamin D_3 imbalance

Inadequate diets, particularly seeds such as sunflower, are very low in calcium but high in oils and phosphorus and metabolic bone disease is a common finding (Fowler, 1986a; Lawton, 1988a). Inadequate dietary calcium or vitamin D_3 may result in a fall in the blood calcium levels and result in hypocalcaemic tetany (Coles, 1988; Fowler, 1986a). Affected birds initially appear weak and drowsy or sway on their perch. There may be fluttering or uncontrollable flapping of the wings. (Figure 16.5).

Startling such a bird may cause a seizure as the hypocalcaemic bird is often hyperaesthesic. Seizures may last anything from fifteen seconds to several minutes, after which the bird will be weakened and unable to climb back onto its perch, laying exhausted at the bottom of the cage. A bird in this condition, if untreated, will die rapidly.

Treatment is with intravenous or intramuscular injection of *calcium borogluconate,* 0.6mg/kg giving a rapid response. Long term treatment is aimed at correcting the diet and calcium-vitamin D_3 supplementation.

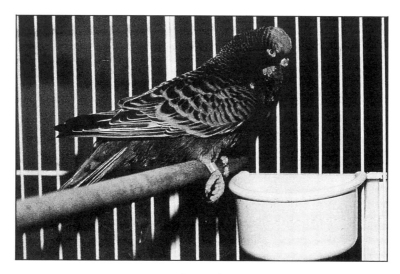

Figure 16.6
Paresis in a budgerigar due to abdominal mass

Vitamin E deficiencies

Birds so affected are seen with varying degrees of paralysis and respond to selenium and vitamin E supplementation (Harrison and Harrison, 1986).

In older birds, vitamin E deficiencies are characterised by central nervous signs (Coles, 1985; Lowenstine, 1986; Lawton, 1988a), in particular ataxia and torticollis. The underlying lesion is ischaemic necrosis with neuronal degeneration, demyelination and pronounced oedema (Lowenstein, 1986). Classical muscular dystrophy or white muscle disease also occurs in young birds.

Vitamin B deficiencies

Dietary problems in young birds result in inco-ordination, ataxia or so called 'star gazing' in chicks and are especially associated with the lack of thiamine. Fish eating water birds also may develop a thiamine deficiency and show central nervous signs similar to cerebrocortical necrosis in sheep (Humphreys, 1985).

Abdominal masses

Paresis/lameness in any bird may be associated with an abdominal mass, usually a gonadal or kidney tumour (Cooper and Lawton, 1988). The neurological signs may be directly due to the increased pressure on the sciatic nerve plexus causing an inability to perch (Blackmore and Cooper, 1982; Reece, 1987) or indirectly due to the altered centre of gravity resulting from the abdominal mass (Cooper and Lawton 1988). (Figure 16.6).

Toxicity

Birds, like reptiles, are very sensitive to certain drugs and chemicals. *Metronidazole* can cause convulsions which may be seen in pigeons treated for mouth canker or Trichomonasis.

Organophosphorus poisoning — can occur as a result of the use of the *dichlorvos* for treating external parasites. This is especially a problem in insectivorous birds, which eat insects already poisoned by the insecticide.

Botulism — water fowl are very prone to botulism toxicity. Developing maggots concentrate the toxin in their body tissues and are immune to its effects, but the level of toxin can prove lethal to the ducks that feed on such maggots (Barry, 1986).

The clinical signs include weakness and ataxia which may progress to total flaccid paralysis, but may be acute in onset, and death in ducklings may occur in fifteen minutes. Treatment with botulism anti-toxin may be effective (Barry, 1986).

Lead poisoning — has been reported in water birds (Humphreys, 1985) and psittacine birds (McDonald, 1986). In water birds it usually results from ingestion of lead weights cast aside by anglers or from lead gun shot. In psittacines, the lead poisoning may result from a wider range of sources, such as chewing the lead off stain glass windows, old cages or even discarded champagne tops.

Clinical signs appear several days after exposure to the source of the lead, but once the symptoms develop the course may be rapid and result in death. The severity of the disease is dependent upon the amount of lead ingested, the period of exposure and the size of the particles.

Lead encephalopathies result from diffuse perivascular oedema, increased cerebrospinal fluid and necrosis of neurons throughout the central nervous system (Smith *et al*, 1972). Lead may also act directly at the neuronal level by affecting metabolism. Muscular weakness, which commonly accompanies poisoning with lead, is thought to be due to the direct effect of demyelination (McDonald, 1986).

Clinical signs are vague and include lethargy, weakness, ataxia, torticollis, blindness, circling or convulsions. McDonald (1986) sites two key symptoms as haemoglobinuria and central nervous signs. Radiography may be helpful but is not diagnostic as there are other causes or radio-opaque foreign bodies in birds. Blood lead concentrations must be performed to give a definitive diagnosis, but often the presenting clinical signs and the dramatic response to treatment allows one to make a retrospective diagnosis.

Treatment is with *calcium EDTA*, 35—40mg/kg BID for five days, which binds with the lead to form a water soluble non-toxic complex capable of being excreted. Response to treatment is dramatic. The bird will become asymptomatic within 48—72 hours, providing the central nervous signs are relatively mild. The more severe the central nervous signs seen prior to treatment, the poorer is the prognosis. If seizures are present, control is attempted with *diazepam* at a dose rate of 0.5—1mg/kg intramuscularly 3 times daily.

Paramyxovirus infections

Infection by these viruses may lead to neurological signs, the best known being Newcastle disease. This virus affects most species of birds (Ashton, 1988; Clubb, 1983; 1986). It has been isolated from over 100 species of birds, 35 of which are parrots (Luthgen, 1981). There are 9 serologically distinct avian paramyxoviruses, and Newcastle disease is identified as paramyxovirus 1 (Ashton, 1988).

In most birds there are no pathognomonic lesions or clinical signs seen. However, with any neurological signs seen in pigeons, especially wing droop, a paramyxovirus infection should be suspected until it can be ruled out. The clinical signs may include inco-ordination, head shaking, tremors or nodding, torticollis and paralysis. Ataxia and neurological signs may persist in birds that recover from the infection. Diagnosis is by the isolation and culture of the virus, by demonstration of the haemaglutinating virus, or fluorescent antibody tests.

Trauma

Avulsion of the brachial plexus has been described in 5 birds as a cause of wing paralysis and muscle atrophy, and should be considered in any road traffic injured bird (Smiley *et al*, 1988). However, it should be noted that it may be difficult to assess the degree of damage because of the behaviour of these wild birds and the lack of responses to noxious stimulants even on the normal wing.

Behavioural Problems

These may be seen in birds (Lawton, 1988b). Neurosis, which in its early stages may not be very noticeable, is seen as agitation, such as hopping from perch to perch, or a continual shaking of the head in a figure eight pattern or a continuing dipping of the head from side to side (Dilger and Bell, 1982). It is possible that this may be mis-diagnosed as a neurological problem.

POIKILOTHERMS

SNAKES

Neurological signs seen in snakes are generally associated with a loss of righting reflex, convulsions, inability to constrict, inability to strike at their prey with resulting cachexia, or lack of muscle tone.

The righting reflex of the snake is easily assessed by turning the snake on to its back, in the same way of testing that of a mammal. Ataxia and inco-ordination of the snake is demonstrated by holding the snake by the mid body with the head down, and seeing whether or not it is able to raise up in a straight line without jerking or twisting to an unnatural position. Muscle tone is assessed by its ability to grip when draped around an arm, as it is the natural instinct for any snake, once looped around an object, to start constricting in order to hang on. Defects of the neurological system may well cause problems with any of these responses.

Convulsions

Convulsions, twitching or coma are commonly seen in snakes (Cooper and Jackson, 1981; Marcus, 1981; Lawrence, 1985a). The differential diagnosis includes dietary problems, septicaemia, colic, poisoning, dehydration, electrolyte imbalance, hypoglycaemia as well as spinal cord damage. Convulsions associated with terminal septicaemia are most commonly associated with respiratory disease.

Fractures

Fracture of the spine, usually traumatic (Frye 1981) can result in a flaccid paralysis distal to the fracture site, a distended cloaca and reduction, or lack of response to stimulae such as a needle prick, or pressure (Cooper and Jackson 1981). (Figure 16.7).

Diagnosis is by radiography. The prognosis is more favourable than the same injury seen in mammals. With conservative therapy, such as force feeding, diuretics and corticosteroids, there is a reasonable prognosis (Russo, 1985a). Usually, external casts are used; it is possible to use a plastic piping or tubing to stabilize the fracture site (Frye, 1981; Peavy, 1977).

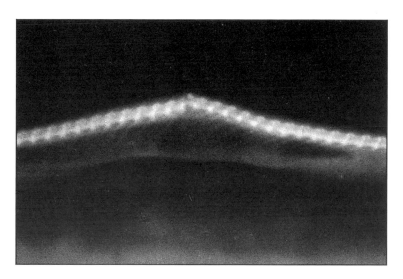

Figure 16.7
Fractured spine in a garter snake

Thiamine Deficiency

Snakes are fed on whole prey, therefore dietary problems are uncommon other than in fish eating snakes, such as garter and dice snakes. These snakes, in captivity, tend to be fed on a variety of frozen white fish. Freezing not only decreases the amount of vitamins readily available to the snake, but also, in certain types of fish, increases the amount of thiaminase activity which can result in a lack of available vitamin B_1 (Frye, 1979; Lawrence, 1985a).

The presenting clinical signs are convulsions, inco-ordination, torticollis, or inability to strike correctly at its prey.

Recovery in response to *thiamine* at 25 mg/kg is dramatic. Prevention of future problems is by providing a more suitable diet, reducing the thiaminase activity or by the addition of *thiamine* to the diet. Methods include heating the fish in boiling water for 60 seconds in order to deproteinize the thiaminase, and additional supplementation by placing *thiamine* directly into the fish. Garter snakes are easily encouraged to eat earthworms, pinkies (baby mice) or even cat food which do not result in problems. If at first they are not too keen, gently smearing the new food with white bait will attract the snake.

Toxicity

Convulsions in snakes may be associated with organophosphorus poisoning, for example, as a result of the use of *dichlorvos* for the treatment of external parasites. This is particularly prevalent if the snake is fed while in the presence of the dichlorvos strip. Treatment is supportive, partially cooling the snake will reduce the severity of the convulsions and lessen the risk of damage and injection with atropine is also recommended. Any remaining *dichlorvos* must be removed from the tank.

Certain other drugs, particularly antibiotics, can prove toxic towards reptiles, resulting in inco-ordination or even convulsions. These antibiotics include *metronidazol, gentamicin, canamycin, neomycin, streptomycin* and *polymyxin B* (Jackson, 1976; Holt, 1981; Marcus, 1981; Lawrence, 1985a). The amino-glycosides are particularly toxic when used in conjunction with anaesthetics, due to their action of neuromuscular blockade.

Other substances which may affect the snake include iodine tincture, iodoform, lime, sulphur, nicotine salts (including nicotine from smokers fingers), naphthalene, paraffin, ether, chloroform, alcohol, paint solvents, lactic base and wood preservatives (Lawrence, 1985a).

LIZARDS

Like most exotics, inadequate diets and supplementation are responsible for the majority of neurological problems.

Calcium: Phosphorus: Vitamin D$_3$ imbalance

A lizard fed an insectivorous, or vegetarian diet, which is low in calcium but high in phosphorus will develop nutritional osteodystrophy. The most common presenting sign in lizards is neurological deficits (Redisch, 1977; Fowler, 1986a; Russo, 1985b). Lack of calcium can result in hypocalcaemic tetany, seen as a bilateral or unilateral twitching of the muscles or paraplegia. True osteodystrophy can be presented as a lameness, either due to the presence of a pathological fracture, or mechanical interference to locomotion by the inflammatory changes of the surrounding tissues (Lawrence, 1985b). In the case of hypocalcaemic tetany, response to intravenous calcium is dramatic.

Nutritional osteodystrophy is treated by dietary supplementation, increasing calcium and vitamin D$_3$. The use of a baby food such as ''Millupa'' (fruit or vegetable types) force fed with the supplement to the lizard is the method of choice, as the lizards have a soft jaw which causes problems when they try to eat more solid food.

Fractures

Any lame lizard with a swelling in one of its limbs, should be radiographed to rule out pathological fractures, and if necessary a blood sample for calcium levels and a calcium: phosphorus ratio is also recommended (Figure 16.8). Treatment of secondary pathological fractures of the limbs only should be by external fixation, such as a light weight cast made from hexalite, plaster of paris, modified splints or dressings (Redisch, 1977; Frye, 1981).

Fractured spines, either simple or compression fractures, are usually traumatic and associated with osteodystrophy (Frye, 1981). The prognosis must always be guarded but, like snakes, nursing and confinement may well result in improvement. (Figure 16.9).

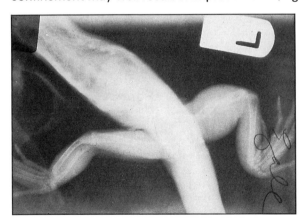

Figure 16.8   Pathological fracture of the femur of an iguana with nutritional osteodystrophy

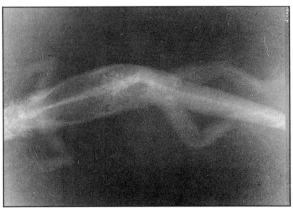

Figure 16.9   Iguana with fractured lumbar spine associated with nutritional osteodystrophy

Vitamin B Deficiencies

Other nutritional problems are associated with the B vitamin complex deficiencies. Biotin deficiency may be seen, particularly in monitor lizards fed raw eggs (Frye, 1979). The clinical signs are general muscle weakness, and diagnosis is based on the response to supplementation with vitamin B complexes, especially biotin. Lawrence (1985) advises the use of B vitamin complex routinely, when no other cause for paresis can be found.

TORTOISES

Neurological problems in tortoises include unilateral or bilateral paresis, circling, inability to hold the head up, or over extension of the head, together with inability to feed properly.

Egg Binding

Hind leg paralysis should always be investigated by radiography. Occasionally it may be due to trauma to the limb itself or to the carapace (dorsal part of the shell) and resulting damage to the spinal cord, as in injuries due to lawn mowers commonly seen affecting American Box tortoises.

However, hind leg paresis or paralysis is associated more usually with pressure in the abdomen due to egg binding and is diagnosed on a whole body radiograph. Such a tortoise may show excess wearing on the hind leg claws and sometimes on the plastron where they have been digging to lay their eggs. Others may show only an anorexia and an inability, or unwillingness to move.

Treatment is by injection with calcium 0.5 ml/kg on the first day, increasing the ambient temperature and bathing. The next day, *oxytocin* up to a maximum of 3 iu is given, continuing with the increased temperature and baths. If this is not successful in removing the number of eggs that have been counted on the radiograph, after a days rest, this procedure may be repeated. If this still is not successful, then laparotomy is indicated.

Freeze Damage

A tortoise walking around in circles may have neurological damage associated with a freezing episode suffered during hibernation. Such signs also may be due to toxaemia. Damage to the central nervous system often results in the head being held over to one side as shown in the Figure 16.10. Such a tortoise may keep its head to one side permanently, and walk in circles. This condition similarly is seen in tortoises suffering from hepatopathy due to gout or micro abscesses affecting the liver. Treatment is supportive, but the prognosis is guarded.

In the case of brain damage, diagnostic tests are of limited value, though there may be differences in the pupillary light reflex but they are not reliable (Cooper and Jackson, 1981). Reduced sensitivity to stimulae may be detectable, or conversely, there may be lower threshold, as a result of which the reptile exhibits excitability or hypersensitivity. Administration of *thiamine* to all cases may be useful.

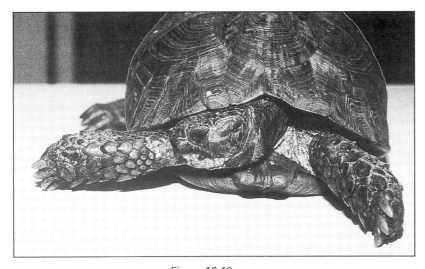

Figure 16.10
Mediterranean tortoise showing abnormal posture after
being exposed to over winter freezing

Blindness in the tortoise frequently is noted after freezing episodes and may be associated with hyphaema, unilateral or bilateral vitreal haze, unilateral or bilateral lenticular opacities, or true retinal damage. The retinal damage is noted on ophthalmoscopic examination as a general lack of reflectivity and normal structure of the retina, which instead of being the normal bright red, green and brown, tends to be a dull grey, with a lack of the cellular structure. Tortoises may show various signs associated with these freezing episodes partly dependent on the changes that have occurred to their eyes and all may be presented as neurological problems. A blind tortoise will not feed by itself and is reluctant to move about.

The retinal damage does respond well to supplementation with high doses of vitamin A but it may take anything up to 18 months for the sight to return. Even mild lenticular opacities may disappear with supportive therapy over a long period of time. In the meantime, it is essential that tortoises be hand fed until they are able to eat. Such tortoises, even without examining the eyes with an ophthalmoscope, should be suspected of being blind, by their lack of a menace response. On assessing the Jackson ratio they are found to be on or above the mean line, thus distinguishing from post hibernation anorexia.

Over extension of the head backwards, lack of movement or gasping is often associated with septicaemia or respiratory problems and, again, these may be diagnosed or ruled out by radiography.

Fractured legs occasionally are found in tortoises and are treated easily by replacing the leg into the shell and by use of epoxy resin to immobilize within the shell for a period of 3 months, which generally results in healing.

CROCODILES

Osteodystrophy and thiamine deficiencies may cause neurological signs similar to those already described.

Hypoglycaemia has been reported as a cause of neurological problems in crocodiles (Wallach, 1971; Frye, 1986). This is a stress-induced hypoglycaemia, which results in muscle tremors, loss of righting reflex, mydriasis and reduction of the metabolic rate. Treatment is with glucose, given orally, at 3 gm/kg and the removal of the stressful conditions (Frye, 1986).

FISH

Neurological problems in fish are associated generally with an inability of the fish to swim, or an abnormality of posture or buoyancy.

Buoyancy

Buoyancy is affected if the fish is floating upside down at the surface, or sinking to the bottom unable to support itself. Lack of buoyancy is often associated with failure of the swim bladder to function, which may be due to primary or secondary bacterial septicaemia (Collins, 1980). If due to secondary bacterial septicaemia, this is usually in the terminal phase. In goldfish, it is often a primary problem of unknown aetiology and with no signs of generalised disease (Collins, 1980). Affected fish may still live a normal life and feed, provided they are not unduly stressed.

Balance

The balance of fish is disturbed when the fish is seen tilting over to one side, usually due to an encephalitis (Collins, 1980).

Flashing

When the fish swims from side to side in an erratic or jerky motion, the result is that the shiny scales of the ventrum glint in the light, a phenomenon known as flashing. This type of swimming may be considered a neurological problem by the owner, but is probably due to external parasites, with the fish swimming and scraping against the bottom of the rocks in an attempt to rid itself of the external burden. Some fish may be seen to demonstrate erratic movements or spurts of activity and some may even jump out of the water. Treatment is by control of the causative parasite.

INVERTEBRATES

Invertebrates are very sensitive to chemical agents, especially insecticides, which may cause muscle spasms, inco-ordination and finally death. There are no specific treatments for toxicity other than to remove the invertebrates from the source of the insecticide and keep it in a well ventilated cage. Limbs may also be damaged or amputated due to incorrect handling or inappropriate furniture in their terrarium, but they will often regenerate (Cooper, 1985b).

REFERENCES

ANDREWS, P. L. R. and ILLMAN, O. (1987). The Ferret, in *The UFAW Handbook on the care and Management of Laboratory Animals* 6th edn. Ed. T. B. Poole, Longman Scientific and Technical, Avon. pp 436.

ASHTON, W. L. G. (1988). Newcastle Disease in *Manual of Parrots, Budgerigars and Other Psittacine Birds.* Ed. C. J. Price, BSAVA Publications, Cheltenham, pp 145.

BARRY, M. T. (1986). Botulism in an Outdoor Water Fowl Collection, *Avian and Exotic Practice 2 and 3,* 17.

BAXTER, J. S. (1975). Posterior Paralysis in the Rabbit. *The Journal of Small Animal Practice,* **16**, 267.

BLACKMORE, D. and COOPER, J. E. (1982). Diseases of the Reproductive System, in *Diseases of Cage and Aviary Birds,* 2nd edn. Ed. M. L. Petrak, Lea and Febiger, Philadelphia, pp 458.

CAULFIELD, J. B. (1972). Striated Muscle Lesions in Dystrophic Hamsters, in *Pathology of the Syrian Hamster.* Ed. F. Homburger, Progress in Experimental Tumour Research **16**, 274.

CLUBB, S. L. (1983). Viscerotropic Velogenic Newcastle Disease in Pet Birds, in *Current Veterinary Therapy VIII.* Ed. R. W. Kirk, W. B. Saunders Co., Philadelphia, pp. 628.

CLUBB, S. L. (1986). Velogenic Viscerotropic Newcastle Disease in *Zoo and Wild Animal Medicine,* 2nd edn. Ed. M. E. Fowler, W. B. Saunders Co., Philadelphia. pp 221.

COLES, B. H. (1985). *Avian Medicine and Surgery,* Blackwell Scientific, Oxford.

COLES, B. H. (1988). The Musculo-Skeletal System including the Feet, in *The Manual of Parrots, Budgerigars and Other Psittacine Birds.* Ed. C. J. Price. BSAVA Publications, Cheltenham, pp 127.

COLLINS, M. T. (1980). Medical Care of Tropical Fish, in *Current Veterinary Therapy VII.* Ed. R. W. Kirk, W. B. Saunders Co., Philadelphia, pp 606.

COOPER, J. E. (1985a). Ferrets, in *Manual of Exotic Pets.* Ed. J. E. Cooper and M. E. Hutchinson. BSAVA Publications, Cheltenham, pp 93.

COOPER, J. E. (1985b). Invertebrates, in *Manual of Exotic Pets.* J. E. Cooper and M. E. Hutchinson, BSAVA Publications, Cheltenham, pp 204.

COOPER, J. E. and JACKSON, O. F. (1981). Miscellaneous Diseases, in *Diseases of the Reptilia* Vol 2. Ed. J. E. Cooper and O. F. Jackson, Academic Press, London, pp 484.

COOPER, J. E. and LAWTON, M. P. C. (1988). The Urogenital System, in *Manual of Parrots, Budgerigars and Other Psittacine Birds.* Ed. C. J. Price, BSAVA Publications, Cheltenham, pp 91.

CORNWELL, H. J. C. (1984). Specific infections, in *Canine Medicine and Theraputics* 2nd edn. Eds. E. A. Chandler; J. B. Sutton and D. J. Thompson, Blackwell Scientific, Oxford, pp 340.

DILGER, W. C. and BELL, J. (1982). Behavioural Aspects, in *Diseases of Cage and Aviary Birds,* 2nd edn. Ed. M. L. Petrak, Lea and Febiger, Philadelphia, pp 18.

FLECKNELL, P. A. (1985a). Rabbits, in *Manual of Exotic Pets.* Eds. J. E. Cooper and M. E. Hutchinson, BSAVA Publications, Cheltenham, pp 59.

FLECKNELL, P. A. (1985b). Rats and Mice, in *Manual of Exotic Pets.* Eds. J. E. Cooper and M. E. Hutchinson, BSAVA Publications, Cheltenham, pp 70.

FOWLER, M. E. (1986). Metabolic Bone Diseases, in *Zoo and Wild Animal Medicine* 2nd edn. Ed. M. E. Fowler, W. B. Saunders Co., Philadelphia, pp 69.

FRYE, F. L. (1979). Reptile Medicine and Husbandry, in *The Veterinary Clinics of North America,* Symposium on Non-Domestic Pet Medicine. Eds. W. J. Bover, W. B. Saunders Co., Philadelphia, pp 415.

FRYE, F. L. (1981). Traumatic and Physical Diseases, in *Diseases of the Reptilia* Vol 2. Eds. J. E. Cooper and O. F. Jackson, Academic Press, London, pp 387.

FRYE, F. L. (1986). Feeding and Nutritional Diseases, in *Zoo and Wild Animal Medicine,* 2nd edn. Eds. M. E. Fowler, W. B. Saunders Co., Philadelphia, pp 139.

GRANDOS, H. (1968). Nutrition, in *Golden Hamster.* Eds. R. A. Hoffman; P. F. Robinson and H. Magalhaes. Iowa State University Press, Iowa.

HARKNESS, J. E. and WAGNER, J. E. (1977). *The Biology and Medicine of Rabbits and Rodents,* 2nd edn. Lea and Febiger, Philadelphia.

HARRISON, G. J. and HARRISON, L. R. (1986). Nutritional Diseases, in *Clinical Avian Medicine and Surgery.* Eds. G. J. Harrison and L. R. Harrison, W. B. Saunders Co., Philadelphia, pp 397.

HOLT, P. E. (1981). Drugs and Dosages, in *Diseases of the Reptilia,* Vol 2. Eds. J. E. Cooper and O. F. Jackson, Academic Press, London, pp 551.

HUMPHREYS, P. N. (1985). Waterbirds, in *Manual of Exotic Pets.* Eds. J. E. Cooper and M. E. Hutchinson. BSAVA Publications, Cheltenham, pp 136.

JACKSON, O. F. 1976, in *Manual of the Care and Treatment of Childrens and Exotic Pets.* Ed. A. F. Cowey, BSAVA Publications, London, pp19.

LAWRENCE, K. (1985a). Snakes, in *Manual of Exotic Pets.* Eds. J. E. Cooper and M. F. Hutchinson. BSAVA Publications, Cheltenham, pp 179.

LAWRENCE, K. (1985b). Lizards, in *Manual of Exotic Pets.* Eds. J. E. Cooper and M. E. Hutchinson, BSAVA Publications, Cheltenham, pp 165.

LAWTON, M. P. C. (1988a). Nutritional Diseases, in *The Manual of Parrots, Budgerigars and Other Psittacine Birds.* Ed. C. J. Price, BSAVA Publications, Cheltenham, pp 157.

LAWTON, M. P. C. (1988b). Behavioural Problems, in *The Manual of Parrots, Budgerigars and Other Psittacine Birds.* Ed. C. J. Price, BSAVA Publications, Cheltenham, pp 163.

LOWENSTINE, L. J. (1986). Nutritional Disorders of Birds, in *Zoo and Wild Animal Medicine.* 2nd edn. Ed. M. E. Fowler, W. B. Saunders Co., Philadelphia, pp 201.

LUTHGEN, W. (1981). *Fortschritte Der Veterinarmedizin.* 31 Verlag Paul Parey, Berlin and Hamburg.

MARCUS, L. C. (1981). *Veterinary Biology and Medicine of Captive Amphibians and Reptiles.* Lea and Febiger, Philadelphia.

McDONALD, S. E. (1986). Lead Poisoning in Psittacine Birds, in *Current Veterinary Therapy IX.* Ed. R. W. Kirk, W. B. Saunders Co., Philadelphia, pp 713.

MULLINK, J. W. M. A. (1979). Rats and Mice, in *Handbook of Diseases of Laboratory Animals.* Eds. J. M. Hime and P. N. O'Donoghue, Heineman Veterinary Books, London. pp 69.

NELSON, V. G. (1979). Monkeys and Apes, in *Handbook of Diseases of Laboratory Animals.* Eds. J. M. Hime and P. N. O'Donoghue. Heineman Veterinary Books, London pp 293.

PEAVY, G. M. (1977). A Non-Surgical Technique for Stabilisation of Multiple Spinal Fractures in Gopher Snake, in *Veterinary Medicine / Small Animal Clinician,* **72**, 1055.

REDISCH, R. I. (1977). Management of Leg Fractures in the Iguana, *Veterinary Medicine / Small Animal Clinician,* **72**, 1487.

REECE, R. L. (1987). Reproductive Diseases, in *Companion Bird Medicine.* Ed. E. W. Burr. Iowa State University Press, Ames pp 89.

RUSSO, E. A. (1985a). Anorexia and Spinal Fracture in a Boa Constrictor, *Avian and Exotic Practices,* **2**, 7.

RUSSO, E. A. (1985b). Nutritional osteodystrophy in an Iguana. *Avian and Exotic Practices,* **2**, 14.

SEBESTENY, A. (1979). Syrian Hamster, in *Handbook of Diseases of Laboratory Animals.* Eds. J. M. Hime and P. N. O'Donoghue. Heineman Veterinary Books, London, pp 111.

SMILEY, L. E., BONDA, M., GAYMOR, A., JUSTIN, R. B., VAN DER EEMS, K. L. and DE LAHUNTA, A. (1988). Avulsion of the roots of the Brachial Plexus in 5 birds. *Companion Animal Practice* **2**, 38.

SMITH, H. A., JONES, T. C. and HUNT, R. D. (1972). *Veterinary Pathology,* 4th edn. Lea and Febiger, Philadelphia.

TOY, J. (1985a). Gerbils, in *Manual of Exotic Pets.* Eds. J. E. Cooper and M. E. Hutchinson, BSAVA Publications, Cheltenham, pp 28.

TOY, J. (1985b). Hamsters, in *Manual of Exotic Pets.* Eds. J. E. Cooper and M. E. Hutchinson. BSAVA Publications, Cheltenham, pp 45.

WAGNER, J. E. (1979). Guinea Pigs, in *Handbook of Diseases of Laboratory Animals.* Eds. J. M. Hime and P. N. O'Donoghue. Heineman Veterinary Books, London, pp 137.

WALLACH, J. D. (1971). Environmental and Nutritional Diseases of Captive Reptiles. *Journal American Veterinary Medical Association,* **159**, 1632.

BREED RELATED NEUROLOGICAL DISORDERS

BREED	AGE	DISORDER
Afghan hound	Juvenile	Hereditary myelopathy
Australian shepherd	Juvenile	Deafness
Basset hound	Juvenile	Cervical vertebral malformation
	Adult	Intervertebral disc disease
Bernese mountain dog	Juvenile	Hypomyelinogenesis
	Juvenile	Necrotising vasculitis
Beagle	Juvenile	Narcolepsy
	Adult	Idiopathic epilepsy
	Adult	Intervertebral disc disease
Border collie	Juvenile	Cerebellar degeneration
	Juvenile	Deafness
Boston terrier	Juvenile	Hydrocephalus
	Juvenile	Deafness
	Juvenile	Vertebral abnormalities
	Adult	Primary brain tumours
Bouvier des Flandres	Juvenile	Laryngeal paralysis
Boxer	Juvenile	Progressive axonopathy
	Adult	Primary brain tumours
Brittany spaniel	Juvenile	Spinal muscular atrophy
Bull mastiff	Juvenile	Cerebellar degeneration
Bull terrier	Juvenile	Deafness
Burmese cat	Juvenile	Deafness
	Juvenile	Congenital vestibular disease
Cairn terrier	Juvenile	Globoid cell leukodystrophy
Cavalier King Charles spaniel	Juvenile	Collapsing syndrome
	Adult	Intervertebral disc disease
Chihuahua	Juvenile	Hydrocephalus
	Juvenile	Atlantoaxial subluxation
	Adult	Intervertebral disc disease
Chow chow	Juvenile	Myotonia
	Juvenile	Cerebellar hypoplasia
	Juvenile	Hypomyelinogenesis
Cocker spaniel	Juvenile	Deafness
	Adult	Idiopathic facial paralysis
	Adult	Intervertebral disc disease
Corgi	Adult	Intervertebral disc disease
Dalmatian	Juvenile	Cavitating leukodystrophy
	Juvenile	Deafness
Dachshund	Juvenile	Sensory neuropathy
	Juvenile	Narcolepsy
	Juvenile	Deafness
	Juvenile	Ceroid lipofuscinosis
	Adult	Intervertebral disc disease
Doberman	Juvenile	Deafness
	Juvenile	Congenital vestibular disease
	Juvenile	Narcolepsy
	Adult	Dancing Doberman disease
	Adult	Sensory neuronopathy
	Adult	Cervical spondylopathy

BREED	AGE	DISORDER
English bulldog	Juvenile	Spina bifida
	Juvenile	Hemivertebra
English pointer	Juvenile	Sensory (mutilating) neuropathy
English setter	Juvenile	Deafness
	Adult	Ceroid lipofuscinosis
Fox terrier	Juvenile	Deafness
	Juvenile	Congenital vestibular disease
	Juvenile	Congenital myasthenia gravis
	Juvenile	Hereditary ataxia
German shepherd	Juvenile	Congenital vestibular disease
	Juvenile	Deafness
	Juvenile	Glycogenosis
	Adult	Giant axonal neuropathy
	Adult	Idiopathic epilepsy
	Adult	Degenerative myelopathy
	Adult	Lumbosacral spondylopathy
Golden retriever	Juvenile	Muscular dystrophy
Great Dane	Juvenile	Cervical spondylopathy
Irish wolfhound	Juvenile	Cervical spondylopathy
Jack Russell terrier	Juvenile	Congenital myasthenia gravis
	Juvenile	Hereditary ataxia
Japanese akita	Juvenile	Deafness
Keeshond	Adult	Idiopathic epilepsy
Kerry blue terrier	Juvenile	Cerebellar degeneration
Labrador retriever	Juvenile	Narcolepsy
	Juvenile	Hereditary myopathy
Lhasa apso	Juvenile	Hydrocephalus
	Adult	Intervertebral disc disease
Manx cat	Juvenile	Sacro-coccygeal dysgenesis
Miniature poodle	Juvenile	Atlanto-axial subluxation
	Juvenile	Narcolepsy
	Adult	Intervertebral disc disease
	Adult	Idiopathic epilepsy
Miniature schnauzer	Adult	Idiopathic epilepsy
Old English sheepdog	Juvenile	Deafness
Pekingese	Juvenile	Intervertebral disc disease
Persian cat	Juvenile	Mannosidosis
Pomeranian	Juvenile	Hydrocephalus
Pug	Juvenile	Hemivertebra
	Adult	Encephalitis
Rhodesian ridgeback	Juvenile	Meningocoele
Rough collie	Juvenile	Deafness
	Adult	Degenerative myelopathy
Rottweiler	Juvenile	Neuraxonal dystrophy
	Adult	Leukoencephalomyelopathy
St Bernard	Juvenile	Narcolepsy
	Adult	Idiopathic epilepsy
Scottish terrier	Juvenile	Scotty cramp
Shih Tzu	Adult	Intervertebral disc disease
Siamese cat	Juvenile	Gangliosidosis
	Juvenile	Mucopolysaccharidosis
	Juvenile	Idiopathic vestibular disease
	Juvenile	Deafness
Siberian husky	Juvenile	Laryngeal paralysis
	Adult	Degenerative myelopathy
Springer spaniel	Juvenile	Congenital myasthenia gravis
	Adult	Intervertebral disc disease
	Adult	Fucosidosis
Staffordshire terrier	Juvenile	Myotonia
Tibetan mastiff	Juvenile	Hypertrophic neuropathy
Wiemaraner	Juvenile	Syringomyelia
	Juvenile	Hypomyelination
West Highland white terrier	Juvenile	Globoid cell leukodystrophy
Yorkshire terrier	Juvenile	Atlanto-axial subluxation
	Juvenile	Hydrocephalus
	Adult	Intervertebral disc disease

INDEX

LIST OF B.S.A.V.A. PUBLICATIONS

THE JOURNAL OF SMALL ANIMAL PRACTICE

An International Journal Published Monthly   Editor W. D. Tavernor, B.V.Sc., Ph.D., F.R.C.V.S.
Fifteen Year Cumulative Index published 1976
Available by post from: B.S.A.V.A. Administration Office, Kingsley House, Church Lane,
Shurdington, Cheltenham, Gloucestershire GL51 5TQ

Manual of Parrots, Budgerigars and other Psittacine Birds
Edited by C. J. Price, M.A., Vet.M.B., M.R.C.V.S.
B.S.A.V.A. Publications Committee 1988

Manual of Laboratory Techniques
New Edition
Edited by D. L. Doxey, B.V.M.&S., Ph.D.,M.R.C.V.S.
and M. B. F. Nathan, M.A., B.V.Sc., M.R.C.V.S.
B.S.A.V.A. Publications Committee 1989

Manual of Anaesthesia for Small Animal Practice
Third Revised Edition
Edited by A. D. R. Hilbery, B.Vet.Med., M.R.C.V.S.
B.S.A.V.A. Publications Committee 1992

Manual of Radiography and Radiology in Small Animal Practice
Edited by R. Lee, B.V.Sc., D.V.R., Ph.D., M.R.C.V.S.
B.S.A.V.A. Publications Committee 1989

Manual of Small Animal Neurology
Edited by S. J. Wheeler, B.V.Sc., Cert.V.R., Ph.D., M.R.C.V.S.
B.S.A.V.A. Publications Committee 1989

Manual of Small Animal Dentistry
Edited by C. E. Harvey, B.V.Sc., F.R.C.V.S., Dip.A.C.V.S., Dip.A.V.D.C.
and H. S. Orr, B.V.Sc., M.R.C.V.S., D.V.R.
B.S.A.V.A. Publications Committee 1990

Manual of Small Animal Endocrinology
Edited by M. F. Hutchison, B.Sc., B.V.M.S., M.R.C.V.S.
B.S.A.V.A. Publications Committee 1990

Manual of Exotic Pets
New Edition
Edited by P. H. Beynon, B.V.Sc., M.R.C.V.S.
and J. E. Cooper, B.V.Sc., Cert.L.A.S., D.T.V.M., F.R.C.V.S., M.C.R.Path., F.I.Biol.
B.S.A.V.A Publications Committee 1991

Manual of Small Animal Oncology
Edited by
R. A. S. White B.Vet.Med., PhD., D.V.R., F.R.C.V.S., Diplomate, American College of Veterinary Surgeons
B.S.A.V.A Publications Committee 1991

Manual of Canine Behaviour
Second Edition
Valerie O'Farrell, Ph.D., Chartered Psychologist
B.S.A.V.A. Publications Committee 1992

Manual of Ornamental Fish
Edited by R. L. Butcher, M.A., Vet.M.B., M.R.C.V.S.
B.S.A.V.A. Publications Committee 1992

Manual of Reptiles
Edited by P. H. Beynon, B.V.Sc., M.R.C.V.S.,
J. E. Cooper, B.V,Sc., Cert.L.A.S., D.T.V.M., F.R.C.V.S., M.C.R.Path., F.I.Biol.
and M. P. C. Lawton, B.Vet.Med., Cert.V.Ophthol., F.R.C.V.S.
B.S.A.V.A Publications Committee 1992

B.S.A.V.A VIDEO 1 (VHS and BETA)
Radiography and Radiology of the Canine Chest
Presented by R. Lee, B.V.Sc., D.V.R., Ph.D., M.R.C.V.S.
Edited by M. McDonald, B.V.M.S., M.R.C.V.S.
B.S.A.V.A. Publications Committee 1983

An Introduction to Veterinary Anatomy and Physiology
By A. R. Michell, B.Vet.Med., Ph.D., M.R.C.V.S.
and P. E. Watkins, M.A., Vet.M.B., M.R.C.V.S., D.V.R.
B.S.A.V.A. Publications Committee, 1989

Proceedings of the B.S.A.V.A. Symposium "Improved Healthcare in Kennels and Catteries"
Edited by P. H. Beynon, B.V.Sc., M.R.C.V.S.
B.S.A.V.A. Publications Committee 1991

Practical Veterinary Nursing
Second Revised Edition
Edited by C. J. Price, M.A., Vet.M.B., M.R.C.V.S.
B.S.A.V.A. Publications Committee 1991

Practice Resource Manual
Edited by D. A. Thomas, B.Vet.Med., M.R.C.V.S.
B.S.A.V.A. Publications Committee 1992

AVAILABLE FROM BOOKSELLERS

Canine Medicine and Therapeutics
Third Edition
Edited by E. A. Chandler, B.Vet.Med., F.R.C.V.S.,
D. J. Thompson, B.A., M.V.B., M.R.C.V.S.,
J. B. Sutton, M.R.C.V.S.
and C. J. Price, M.A., Vet.M.B., M.R.C.V.S.
Blackwell Scientific Publications 1991

An Atlas of Canine Surgical Techniques
Edited by P. G. C. Bedford, Ph.D., B.Vet. Med., F.R.C.V.S., D.V.Ophthal.
Blackwell Scientific Publications 1984

Feline Medicine and Therapeutics
Edited by E. A. Chandler, B.Vet.Med., F.R.C.V.S.
C. J. Gaskell, B.V.Sc., Ph.D., D.V.R., M.R.C.V.S.
and A. D. R. Hilbery, B.Vet.Med., M.R.C.V.S.
Blackwell Scientific Publications 1985

Jones's Animal Nursing
Fifth Edition
Edited by D. R. Lane, B.Sc., F.R.C.V.S.
Pergamon Press 1989